Infertility around the

2. Inequality around the Globe

Infertility around the Globe

*New Thinking on Childlessness, Gender,
and Reproductive Technologies*

EDITED BY

Marcia C. Inhorn
Frank van Balen

UNIVERSITY OF CALIFORNIA PRESS
Berkeley   Los Angeles   London

University of California Press
Berkeley and Los Angeles, California

University of California Press, Ltd.
London, England

© 2002 by
The Regents of the University of California

Library of Congress Cataloging-in-Publication Data
Infertility around the globe : new thinking on childlessness, gender, and reproductive technologies / edited by Marcia C. Inhorn,
Frank van Balen.
   p.   cm.
  Includes bibliographical references and index.
  ISBN 0-520-23108-2 (cloth : alk. paper)—ISBN 0-520-23137-6
(paper : alk. paper)
  1. Infertility—Developing countries.   2. Infertility—Social
aspects.   3. Infertility—Psycholgical aspects.
  [DNLM: 1. Infertility—psychology 2. Cross-Cultural
Comparison.   3. Feminism.   4. Reproduction Techniques. WP
570 I4335 2001]   I. Inhorn, Marcia Claire, 1957–   II. Balen,
Frank van.
  RC889 .I5613 2001
  616.6'92—dc21   2001007069

Manufactured in the United States of America

10 09 08 07 06 05 04 03 02 01
10 9 8 7 6 5 4 3 2 1

In memory of Dr. Mohammed Mehanna
and his dreams of advancing assisted conception in Egypt

M.C.I.

In memory of my beloved wife, Pauline

F.V.B.

CONTENTS

PART I

Discourses and Debates

ONE

Introduction

Interpreting Infertility: A View from the Social Sciences

Frank van Balen and Marcia C. Inhorn

After decades of scholarly neglect, human reproduction, as a biological phenomenon that is socially constituted and culturally variable through space and time, has slowly gained the attention of social scientists from a variety of disciplines. Largely as a result of the feminist movement and the entrance of greater numbers of women into the academy, the past twenty-five years have witnessed a veritable explosion of research on the social construction and cultural elaboration of women's reproductive experiences (Greenhalgh, 1995a). From menarche to menopause, few aspects of the human reproductive life cycle, particularly as it pertains to women, have been left unexamined by social scientists working in a wide variety of cultural settings. This interest in reproduction is clearly evident in the numerous articles, monographs, and major recent anthologies devoted in part or in toto to subjects of fertility, family planning, childbirth, breastfeeding, menopause, abortion, and the various reproductive technologies, old and new, being applied to facilitate, curtail, or in some way shape human reproductive processes (e.g., Davis-Floyd & Dumit, 1998; Davis-Floyd & Sargent, 1997; Franklin & Ragone, 1998b; Ginsburg & Rapp, 1995a; Greenhalgh, 1995b; Handwerker, 1990; Lock & Kaufert, 1998; Morgan & Michaels, 1999; Stuart-Macadam & Dettwyler, 1995). Rapp and Ginsburg, in "Relocating Reproduction, Generating Culture" (1999), note the diverse and pioneering range of research on reproduction that has been generated during the past decade, typifying it as a "cresting wave" of scholarly and activist interest. In their paper, intended in part as an update of their earlier theoretical reviews of the politics of reproduction (Ginsburg & Rapp, 1991, 1995b), they identify a dozen "recent genealogies" of social science research on reproduction, particularly in the domain of anthropology, their central discipline. Among these genealogies, they highlight work underscoring the dilemmas of "disrupted reproduction" in which the standard linear narrative of conception, birth, and the progress of the next generation is interrupted by pregnancy loss, reproductive pathology, abortion, and childlessness.

REPRODUCTIVE DISRUPTION: A SCHOLARLY LACUNA

It is to the last domain of disrupted reproduction—infertility leading to involuntary childlessness—that this volume is dedicated. We argue that, despite the inspiring proliferation of recent studies on the relationship of reproduction to culture and politics, certain reproductive topics continue to be overprivileged at the expense of others. In particular, we now know much more about what might best be called normative human reproduction—particularly "high" fertility that is "controlled" through "modern" contraceptive technologies, as well as successful childbirth at the hands of physicians and midwives, resulting in maternal and child well-being—than we do about non-normative reproductive scenarios and experiences. Unfortunately, the taken-for-grantedness of reproduction can never be assumed. Rather, in many cases, reproduction goes badly and sadly awry (Inhorn, 1994a), marring individual lives and even wreaking havoc on entire populations. Moreover, the ways in which reproductive trajectories may be disrupted, generating suffering and even death, are manifold. Such reproductive disruptions include various sexually transmitted diseases (STDs), including AIDS, that negatively affect sexuality, fertility, and maternal and child health and survival; ectopic (tubal) pregnancy that if undiagnosed can lead to maternal death; pregnancy loss through miscarriage and stillbirth; premature births accompanied by neonatal morbidity and mortality; births of children with congenital health problems and disabilities; lactational difficulties leading to poor neonatal and maternal outcomes; maternal deaths from pre- and postpartum complications; chronic, debilitating complications of childbirth in multiparous (as well as "circumcised") women; unwanted pregnancies leading to safe and unsafe abortions; life-threatening reproductive diseases such as cervical and ovarian cancer; endocrinological disorders leading to menstrual problems and premature menopause; and infertility leading to involuntary childlessness.

This volume interprets infertility from multiple global sites and disciplinary perspectives. It is the first attempt to bring together the work of social scientists, including anthropologists, sociologists, psychologists, and behavioral health scientists in schools of nursing, medicine, and public health, who have focused their empirical research on infertility and new reproductive technologies (NRTs) over the past two decades. This small group of scholars—and a handful of others who, for various reasons, are not represented here—have been committed to rescuing infertility from the aforementioned list of neglected reproductive subjects, in part by proving its relationship to some of the most hotly contested political and bioethical (thus morally contentious) issues of our time. These include, but certainly are not limited to, debates over (1) the transformative possibilities for kinship and family relations inherent in new technology-enhanced forms of reproduction; (2) the disposition of various forms of biogenetic material, such as donor eggs and frozen embryos; (3) "entitlement" to children and who should foot the bill for high-tech infertility treatments among disadvantaged segments of the (global) population; (4) the power of the media to shape reproductive expectations and desires, particularly when reproductive "miracles" become the focus of media frenzy; and (5) the nature of stress in our lives and its potential somatic effects, including adverse reproductive outcomes. Given the utility of infertility as a lens through which so many other compelling issues may be brought into focus, the question becomes, Why the relative neglect of infertility as a legitimate subject of social science inquiry? We believe that there are a number of answers to this question.

First, in Western societies infertility resulting in involuntary childlessness is often cast as a medical condition rather than as a social problem worthy of social analysis. This "medicalization" of infertility has served to restrict the research agenda to the domains of medicine, epidemiology, and medical psychology, the latter devoted largely to the psychological aspects of medical interventions. With the persistent growth of new forms of high-tech reproductive medicine, infertility continues to be a hot area of medical research and is the primary focus of two major journals, *Fertility and Sterility* and *Human Reproduction.* Thus it is somewhat ironic that infertility has attracted comparatively little attention in the social sciences, although the medical monopolization of the subject makes this lacuna somewhat understandable.

Second, in most Western societies at least, infertility has long been a taboo subject, one that is not easily discussed with others, even in "neutral" research settings. Infertility uncomfortably connotes sexuality, as babies are made through sexual intercourse. Thus when couples remain childless, issues of sexual "failure" come to the fore; particularly for men, infertility raises the specter of impotency and other emasculating disruptions of male virility (Inhorn, 2002). Indeed, around the world infertility can—and often is—read as the physical instantiation through childlessness of sexuality, particularly male sexuality, gone awry (see chap. 6, this volume). Seen in this way, it may be a deeply painful subject to investigate.

Third, in Western societies the taboo against talking about infertility also relates to changing notions of parenthood, women's roles, and the importance of children in women's and men's lives. Since the feminist revolution of the 1960s and 1970s, motherhood has come into question as an essential, even fetishized component of women's lives (Ginsburg & Rapp, 1995b), and as a result many women (and their partners) have chosen to remain childless. Thus childlessness in the West at least can be chosen as a lifestyle option and, for some, as a feminist statement. In other words, it can be voluntary as opposed to involuntary, and, in either case, it is something perceived as deeply personal. Thus when a Western couple is without children, it is difficult for others to know whether this is voluntary or involuntary. And this blurring tends to obscure the visibility and importance of the latter. Therefore, if childlessness is a desired outcome for some, it may be deemed as not a problem for those who did not choose this state of affairs. Or at least the uncertainty about whether any given case is "voluntary" or "involuntary" makes it difficult to ask the right questions and show compassion. This ambiguity has perhaps troubled social science investigators, who fear raising a delicate subject in their research or who, as feminist scholars themselves, do not want to appear committed to the essentializing notion that motherhood, and quests to achieve it, should be a woman's sole purpose in life.

Fourth, during the past two decades but particularly during the 1980s, infertility has been raised in scholarly circles primarily in the form of critique of the so-called new reproductive technologies. Much of this Western critique, emerging primarily from the fields of bioethics, science and technology studies, cultural studies, and women's studies, has been more philosophical than empirical; thus much of it remains highly speculative, polemical, and even somewhat dismissive of an individual's legitimate reproductive desires and experiences. As a result, infertility as actually lived by women in the West has been relatively understudied; for example, of the scores of books emerging from the United States on infertility and NRTs in the past two decades, only four have been solidly based on empirical studies of infertile women and men undertaken by social scientists (Becker [1990, 2000], Greil [1991], and Sandelowski [1993], all of whom are represented in this volume). Furthermore, the burgeoning Western literature on this subject has focused almost exclusively on a handful of Western societies—primarily the United States, the United Kingdom, and Australia, which have been the major "producer" nations of reproductive technologies. Hence this literature is blatantly Euro-American, rarely acknowledging the reproductive desires and dilemmas of infertile women and men living outside the West.

Yet in many non-Western countries infertile people's suffering is often exacerbated by strong pronatalist social norms that do in fact mandate parenthood. The scholarly silence in the West on the plight of the infertile in non-Western places—including, in some cases, their desire for high-tech reproductive medicine—mirrors the monolithic, even neo-Malthusian discourse of Western population policy makers, who are often obsessed with curbing the "hyperfertility" of non-Western subjects and who certainly do not see Third World women as worthy of high-priced, high-tech Western infertility interventions. In other words, helping infertile subpopulations in high-fertility non-Western settings—where infertile individuals may suffer more because of their "barrenness amid plenty"—has never been treated as a high priority in international population discourse and may even be viewed as contrary to the Western interest in global population control (Greenhalgh, 1995b; Lane, 1994).

Yet, as is apparent in this volume, focusing on infertility in "overpopulated" areas of the world reveals much about the "fertility-infertility dialectic" (Inhorn, 1994b, p. 23), or the relationship of tension and contrast that exists between fertility and infertility on both the microsociological level of individual human experience and the macrosociological level of reproductive politics. Many of the chapters in this book examine the inextricable relationship between fertility and infertility, asking how infertility is viewed—top down and then bottom up—in nation-states where fertility regulation is part of national political discourse and policy making. The very existence of infertility in high-fertility regimes represents a challenge to monolithic assumptions about the nature of population control and the extent to which fertility-control orthodoxies are in fact resisted and reconfigured in practice, particularly in non-Western populations among whom infertility is demographically significant and greatly feared.

GLOBAL CONTRASTS

In short, this volume is dedicated to countering the predominant Western view of infertility as a yuppie complaint of little concern to the rest of the purportedly overpopulated developing world. As we demonstrate, infertility is a global phenomenon, with some portion of every human population—estimated at 10 percent on average—affected by the inability to conceive at some point during their reproductive lives (Reproductive Health Outlook, 1999). This volume is dedicated to situating infertility in *global* perspective, which allows for two very general conclusions to be reached. First, infertility is, for most human beings everywhere, a distressing experience, leading to decreased levels of personal well-being. Second, women's well-being appears to be more seriously affected than men's in most parts of the world.[1]

Indeed, women worldwide appear to bear the major burden of infertility, in terms of blame for the reproductive failing; personal anxiety, frustration, grief, and fear; marital duress, dissolution, and abandonment; social stigma and community ostracism; and, in some cases, life-threatening medical interventions. Furthermore, in general these social and psychological consequences of infertility appear to be greater for women in the so-called developing societies of the non-Western world than for women in the West (Inhorn, 1994a; Kielmann, 1998; Sundby, 1997)—although, to be sure, the effects of infertility may vary greatly from one society to the next and among individuals in the same society, who may differ by virtue of gender, race, class, religion, age, sexual orientation, rural-urban location, and so on (Mohanty, Russo, & Torres, 1991). While never losing sight of these axes of "difference," several chapters in this volume certainly make clear that women in so-called developing societies may be blamed, sometimes unjustly, for reproductive failure and may become true social outcasts if they are unable to find a solution for their childlessness. Infertility thus profoundly affects women's moral identities and the local moral worlds in which infertile women live (Kleinman, 1992, 1995), given that suspicion, blame, guilt, and accusation are among the common by-products of the experience of continuing childlessness.

Certainly, in Western societies involuntary childlessness may also have important social consequences, especially for women. One's expectations and sense of personal identity are overturned; the prospect of a life without children (and, in turn, grandchildren) may lead to depression and marital turmoil; and the quest for high-tech medical interventions may lead to financial ruin, bodily harm, and, ultimately, lack of reproductive success. However, as implied in the very word *involuntary*, a childless life in the West tends to be much more accepted, and the social, psychological, and economic repercussions of involuntary childlessness are generally distinctively less severe. As pointed out by "voluntarily" childless adults, not having children may in fact have social, psychological, and economic advantages in many Western societies.

Thus to fully understand the consequences of infertility, the notion of child desire—the perceived importance of having children—must be interrogated in a variety of global settings. As more of this kind of research becomes available, salient global differences will become increasingly clear. In most Western societies, having children or not having them is generally perceived as a matter of choice. Other life goals, such as pursuing a fulfilling professional career, are often given equal weight. Thus in many Western countries motivations for having children often lie in the realm of personal happiness and involve notions of the unique parent-child relationship and the possibility of giving and receiving love and affection. In Western research settings, motivations involving continuity and old-age security are much less frequently mentioned (van Balen & Trimbos-Kemper, 1995).

On the contrary, in other global locations social and economic reasons for having children are often prominent. Frequently cited reasons for having children generally fall into three categories (Inhorn, 1996; see also Browner & Sargent, 1996): (1) social security desires, or the conviction that children are necessary in a number of ways to secure parents' and families' survival, often through their labor contributions and later their support of aging parents (in the absence of pensions, health insurance, nursing homes, and other forms of support for the elderly); (2) social power desires, or the belief that children serve as a valuable power resource, particularly for women confronted with patriarchal social relations within marriage and the family; and (3) social perpetuity desires, or the perceived need to continue group structures, particularly kin-based extended family systems, as well as ancestral "memories" into the future. Increasingly as well, having children may be seen as an important political investment or statement, as various ethnic, nationalist, and religious-fundamentalist movements use children to promote their causes and engage in demographic wars of relative survival vis-à-vis other groups in the political landscape (Inhorn, 1996; chap. 15, this volume).

The existence in many non-Western settings of such powerful social, economic, and even political rationales for having children does not mean that personal happiness and the joy of having children are not also important motivating factors. Indeed, the notion that children might be less loved, valued, and treated with affection in developing societies is not only ethnocentric but also belies much evidence to the contrary.[2] Loving, committed, highly affectionate parenting styles can be found throughout the world and are often abundantly evident in non-Western settings.

Given the multifaceted nature of child desire in many non-Western societies, not having children is seldom viewed as a choice or a lifestyle option. Children are often desired soon after a couple becomes sexually active (usually through marriage but increasingly through nonmarital consensual unions). And the failure to produce a child—especially a son in some societies—is readily recognized by the couple themselves, as well as by all those around them, as a major problem with numerous implications. As noted by anthropologists, including some in this volume, childlessness in most non-Western societies may not be "politely hidden," as it is in the West, and is often the source of much painful and direct discussion and gossip (see chap. 11, this volume; see also Inhorn, 1994b, 1996).

This is not to deny that painful social scrutiny of infertile couples also occurs in the West. They may meet with their share of insensitivity and incomprehension, for example, in comments such as "There are already so many children in the world," or "You have to be glad that you have so much spare time," or "You can't have everything," or "You can always adopt." These kinds of responses may be especially difficult to accept when they are expressed by couples with children.

Furthermore, widely held and highly valued beliefs in individualism, free choice, and control over one's own life may cause frustration for infertile Western couples that is not felt by those in societies where these values are less emphasized. Contraceptives preclude unwanted pregnancies, and in the case of a contraceptive failure, abortions are available (although less so in some countries such as the United States). Many couples plan the date of birth of their first child precisely, as well as the spacing of the next one(s). Moreover, Western biomedicine can increasingly control for the "quality" of the growing fetus through a variety of prenatal diagnostic tests and procedures (Browner & Press, 1995; Rapp, 1999; Rothman, 1986). In the case of a "positive" result (i.e., evidence of fetal "defect"), a "therapeutic" abortion is offered as an option. As a result of this highly medicalized climate of reproductive control, involuntary childlessness may be as hard to accept, but for different reasons, for couples in the West as it is for those in non-Western countries where reproductive control is never assumed.

MEDICINE AND MEANING

Thus another global contrast revolves around the role of medicine in infertile people's lives. Western-generated medical interventions to help achieve reproductive control—including high-tech infertility treatments—are simply unavailable or inaccessible for the vast majority of individuals living in developing countries. Even low-tech interventions are often out of reach for large segments of the population; if they are available, they may be delivered to patients under abysmal conditions, leading to iatrogenic consequences in some cases (see chap. 13, this volume; see also Inhorn, 1994b). Indeed, in many societies around the world, attempts to discover the etiology of and cure for infertility never involve "modern" Western medicine—let alone new reproductive technologies—and rely instead on ancient medical traditions and healing practices. In some societies with literate traditions, such ethnogynecological beliefs and practices can be documented to have existed for thousands of years (Inhorn, 1994b). Today the continuing presence of various ethnogynecologies—even in the midst of increasing Western technomedical hegemony—attests to the viability of traditional forms of healing and the continuing role that such alternative forms of medicine play in the contemporary world. Even in the West, bio-gynecology (i.e., Western, biologically based gynecology) is not entirely hegemonic; among infertile couples in some Western research settings, more than 10 percent report having used alternative medicine—including New Age healers, magical stones and crystals, religious amulets, and pilgrimages to places of worship—to overcome their childlessness (van Balen, Verdurmen, & Ketting, 1995).

Thus it is important to recognize the ways in which help seeking for infertility does not always involve resorting to the latest Western technologies. In fact, on a global level NRTs and even "lesser" forms of Western-based medical treatment for infertility are still rare, and the majority of infertile "patients" seek help in the ethnogynecological realm. Although high-tech reproductive medicine is being rapidly exported around the globe, it is often available only to elite segments of the population in developing countries (Inhorn, 2001). The class-based medical exclusion of large segments of the infertile population only serves to create increasing frustration and resentment among those less fortunate individuals who desire but are prevented from accessing new technologies. Inevitably, this frustration and resentment is bound to increase as more sophisticated forms of therapy become available in Third World sites and are heralded as "miracle solutions" to childlessness by global multimedia forces (see chap. 17, this volume).

In contrast, in those Western countries with socialized health care systems, NRTs are used by the majority of infertile couples. However, politicians continue to debate whether such treatments should be considered a basic health "right" and should be subsidized by governments or health insurers. In countries such as the United States that have dominant "free-market" systems of medical care, coverage of infertility treatments is neither a government priority nor a priority of most health insurers; thus, as in the non-Western world, high-tech therapies remain out of reach for disadvantaged American populations, including poor women of color, who, as a subpopulation, may suffer from higher rates of infertility than affluent white populations, who are able to gain access to infertility treatments (Nsiah-Jefferson & Hall, 1989).

Furthermore, contemporary political debates in a number of northwestern European countries are questioning the very meaning of the terms "infertility" and "involuntary childlessness" and their implications for national health care systems. Although these twin terms are often used interchangeably, they may in fact have very different connotations. Whereas infertility may be defined as the *process* of not being able to have children, involuntary childlessness may be viewed as the final *state or condition* resulting from infertility. In Western countries infertility is often thought of as a medical condition involving defective bodily parts and processes (see chap. 5, this volume), whereas involuntary childlessness refers to the social and psychological consequences of not having children. Although such distinctions may seem nothing more than semantic hair-splitting, the differing uses of these terms are of growing political concern in contemporary Europe, where current discussions center on whether not having a child is a medical problem (i.e., infertility) or an unfulfilled personal desire (i.e., involuntary childlessness). If it is the former, then infertile couples may be recognized as having a health problem and, consequently, their treatment for infertility is accepted as a necessity. Most important, the *costs* of such treatment must be paid or reimbursed by the national health care system. However, if not having a child constitutes a *social* problem of involuntary childlessness, as growing numbers of European politicians, ethicists, and even social scientists have argued, then the absence of children is a personal issue for which society bears no responsibility. From this perspective, children may just be one of the things in life that an individual may want but cannot necessarily have—like a steady partner, a house, a car, or a full-time job. In other words, childlessness is a matter of fate that one must accept, and it is not something that a society's health care system can be expected to remedy.

As this debate is being played out in European political circles, gynecologists, patient groups, and counselors are lobbying to accentuate infertility as a medical condition, to create positive societal attitudes toward reimbursement under national health care systems (see chap. 4, this volume). Although choosing this strategy may help to secure the future of insurance coverage for infertile individuals, it may also serve to diminish understanding of the essential pain of infertility, which is located less in the body (the site of medical interventions) and more in the psychosocial consequences.

The importance of language and meaning in debates over infertility can be seen further in the close examination of the Western medical definition of "infertility." In Western medical discourse, "infertility" is usually defined as the inability to achieve pregnancy after a year (or two) of trying to conceive a child through regular sexual intercourse. A distinction is also usually made between "primary" infertility, when such infertility occurs in the absence of a previous history of pregnancy, versus "secondary" infertility, when the infertility occurs after a pregnancy. Indeed, even a woman who has had only one short pregnancy (as determined by a chemical pregnancy test) that ended in an early spontaneous abortion is, by medical definition, considered to be secondarily infertile. Although such standard definitions may have utility in Western clinical settings, they can be shown to be an arbitrary cultural construction with limited utility for the rest of the world. In other regions, the Western medical definition of infertility may diverge considerably from individuals' subjective definitions, which are often based on socially relevant indigenous categories and systems of identity formation. Yet, because standard Western definitions of infertility have been adopted and disseminated globally—for instance, by the World Health Organization (WHO) in the infertility diagnostic criteria it publishes for worldwide consumption (1987b, 1989, 1993)—they underestimate the true extent of suffering that women (and men) endure as a result of their fertility problems, even when they already have living children.

Several chapters in this volume (see esp. chap. 10) show how purportedly universal definitions of infertility have little relevance for individuals actually *experiencing* infertility at various sites around the globe. For example, infertility may be experienced subjectively when pregnancy is not achieved within the first month or two of marriage—with a full year of infertility being perceived as grounds for marital dissolution. Or in some societies bearing no sons may be the social equivalent of having no children at all, making the parents infertile under the terms of a classic patriarchal social system (see chaps. 7 and 16, this volume). Or having only one or a few children may constitute a form of social infertility when community standards dictate that a "normal" woman bear seven, eight, or even more children (see chaps. 11 and 15, this volume). In other words, subjective meanings and experiences of infertility are culturally variable, pointing to the pitfalls of applying a standard Western, culturally constructed definition to the rest of the world; yet this is what is routinely done in demographic surveys and in Western-based clinical settings.

THE CRITIQUE OF NEW REPRODUCTIVE TECHNOLOGIES

"Standards" of infertility care in the West are constantly changing, given that "new" new reproductive technologies or new applications of existing technologies are being introduced continually. Yet it is crucial to recognize that "standard" infertility care does not automatically result in success. Rather, even in the best clinics in the West, the success rate of in vitro fertilization (IVF)—or what is often termed "the take-home-baby rate"—is never more than 40 percent and usually averages about 20 to 25 percent per cycle (Sciarra, 1994). Thus as many as 80 percent of infertile couples do not achieve viable pregnancies through NRTs—casting doubt on whether following a Western "standard of care" is a worthy goal in other regions (Okonofua, 1996; Sheth & Malpani, 1997).

Today in the West the most commonly used NRTs are (1) the oldest and least invasive method of intrauterine insemination, using either husband's or donor sperm that is ejaculated into a container, subjected to laboratory preparation procedures, and then inserted through the vagina into a woman's uterus; (2) IVF and several variants,[3] in which both sperm and ova are retrieved from individuals' bodies (either a husband and wife or egg and sperm donors), placed together in petri dishes under laboratory conditions (not in true test tubes, as the term "test-tube baby" implies) to be fertilized, and then transferred in the early embryonic stage (i.e., so-called embryo transfer) to the woman's uterus, with the hope that implantation and pregnancy will occur; and (3) most recently, intracytoplasmic sperm injection (ICSI), a variant of IVF involving micromanipulation techniques, whereby one spermatozoon is injected directly into an oocyte under laboratory conditions, in the hope of improving fertilization outcomes, particularly in cases of serious male-factor infertility. Indeed, in the most "extreme" cases of male infertility, in which no sperm are present in the ejaculate, microsurgical epididymal sperm aspiration (MESA) and testicular sperm extraction (TESE) provide means of invasively removing sperm from the testicles for the purposes of the ICSI procedure.

Together, these NRTs—also known as "advanced reproductive technologies" for the purposes of "medically assisted conception"—have clearly achieved an important status in the treatment of infertility in the Western world, where they have helped many couples, including several of the authors in this volume, to achieve pregnancy and become parents. However, NRTs have *not* proven to be a true panacea for the treatment of infertility, even in the major scientific producer nations. Given the relatively low success rates of all these technologies, their promise of a "take-home baby" can become a cruel chimera. For this and a number of other reasons, they have come under heavy criticism—even outright attack—from Western bioethicists, science and technology studies scholars, and feminist theorists and activists.

For one thing, because of the basic biological facts of life, women are the ones who must "embody" the new reproductive technologies, in the form of potent hormonal drugs, continuous monitoring of ovarian follicles and blood levels, invasive egg retrievals and embryo transfers, and, in some cases, surrogate pregnancies. This bodily surveillance and invasion has led women (usually not men) to assume significant levels of medical risk, leading feminist scholars and activists to ask if we really need all this technology. Furthermore, it has been argued that physicians actively participate in women's medical risk taking by encouraging their repetitive and often extreme use of the latest technologies—what Sandelowski (1991, 1993) has called the "never-enough quality" of NRTs—rather than by developing low-tech solutions, giving "nature" more time, advocating adoption or fostering, suggesting that treatments be stopped altogether and childlessness accepted, or searching for ways to *prevent* infertility.

The excesses of women's medical risk taking seem particularly pronounced in cases in which an otherwise fertile wife is being treated for her husband's infertility. The very nature of reproductive biology makes treatment for infertility in men themselves very difficult. Well-controlled studies have shown that male-directed treatments, such as varicocele surgery (i.e., surgery of the blood vessels in the scrotum) and low-tech treatments, such as hormonal therapy, biochemical therapy, and intrauterine insemination using a husband's sperm, have relatively low success rates (Devroey, Vandervorst, Nagy, & Van Steirteghem, 1998; Gerris, 1997; Kamischke & Neischlag, 1998). Only since the advent of ICSI and its attendant techniques, MESA and TESE, has the treatment of male infertility become more successful. With ICSI, a "subfertile" man and his wife can have offspring that are genetically related to both parents. However, ICSI is a high-tech version of IVF, in which the "treatment" is basically carried out on the woman's body. Thus feminist critics in particular have pointed to this basic inequality—of women being treated for male infertility by means of a risky, expensive, and not highly successful therapy—as a potent example of male bias in the practices of modern Western biomedicine.

Indeed, early radical feminist critiques—such as those in the works of Corea (1985; Corea et al., 1987), Klein (1989), Ratcliff (1989), and Stanworth (1987)—tended to describe NRTs as a conspiracy of male "techno-patriarchs" and the pharmaceutical industry against women, aimed at taking control of the female body and especially the childbearing process. Although more recent feminist critiques have been less condemnatory and more nuanced (see chap. 3, this volume), they have continued to point out the myriad problematic features and consequences of NRTs. Among these are the potentially lethal prescription of high doses of hormonal and chemical agents to stimulate "superovulation"; the manipulation of women's hormones so as to regulate cycles of IVF and ICSI according to physicians' office hours; the reluctance of the medical community to discuss and study possible negative, late-onset side effects of these therapies; the tendency of clinics to raise success rates by selecting only "promising" (especially younger) patients and manipulating the data presented to them; the presentation of incomplete and biased information to prospective patients; and the persuasion of poor childless women to donate oocytes in order to receive treatment themselves (which they would not otherwise be able to afford).

In addition, early feminist critics associated the new reproductive technologies with the glorification of traditional motherhood. Thus women who chose to use these technologies so as to fulfill a motherhood wish were often depicted as having "false consciousness" or being "cultural dupes" (see chap. 2, this volume). In feminist thought of the 1980s, motherhood was often criticized for its barriers to personal development and freedom, certainly not worthy of a high-stakes medical quest. Yet this feminist discourse proved oppressive in its own right: feminist or otherwise "emancipated" women who were experiencing infertility problems found it difficult to reveal their child desire and were forced to hide their infertility-treatment seeking from others. Some feminist scholars who were undergoing high-tech infertility treatments found themselves in the hypocritical position of denouncing the new reproductive technologies in lectures and at conferences.

Furthermore, most critiques tend to focus either explicitly or implicitly on the Western, white, socioeconomically elite, heterosexual couples who are able to afford high-tech reproductive medicine and who thus, to use Sandelowski and de Lacey's terms (chap. 2, this volume), provide the material and data for "commercial and academic exchange." In such discussions, the massive global spread of NRTs to individuals in the developing world (as well as the use of NRTs among single and lesbian women, particularly in the West) is rarely mentioned—an unexamined scholarly erasure that seems related prejudicially to what Ginsburg and Rapp (1995, p. 3) have called (following Colen, 1986) "stratified reproduction," a term indexing the power relations by which some categories of people are empowered to reproduce and nurture while others are devalued and even despised.

However, given the widespread prevalence of and suffering associated with infertility around the globe, particularly in pronatalist settings, it should come as no surprise that NRTs are being marketed to and readily consumed by those in the non-Western world who are able to afford them. In addition to the examples from Egypt, Israel, China, and India in this volume, limited reports and studies indicate that these technologies have spread to other parts of Asia (Sheth & Malpani, 1997), to Africa (Okonofua, 1996), and to Latin America (Nicholson & Nicholson, 1994). As is shown in this volume, such technologies do not enter cultural vacuums but rather are shaped by local considerations, be they cultural, social, economic, or political.

In particular, many of the moral quandaries surrounding the use of these technologies in the West take new forms in other cultural settings with varying religious traditions. An excellent example of this is afforded by the earliest "new" reproductive technology, artificial insemination with donated semen (AID), also known as donor insemination (DI) (see chap. 6, this volume). When carried out by a trained physician, this physically less invasive technology has about the same success rate as IVF and ICSI. Therefore, some feminist scholars have suggested it as a more acceptable strategy for the treatment of male infertility (Kirejczyk, 1996; van der Ploeg, 1995). What is missing in this essentially Western view of things are the cultural constraints against using donated semen among some groups, especially in the Muslim world (Inhorn, 1994b; chap. 14, this volume). Furthermore, donated semen must be assessed for the presence of HIV. This involves deep-freeze storage of semen for the period of HIV incubation (at least three months), thawing, and testing for HIV before the semen can be used. In other words, the spread of AIDS has changed the essentially low-tech method of DI into a relatively high-tech treatment. The need for such quality controls in the midst of other possible cultural constraints does not make DI a viable option for large parts of the developing world.

Ironically, it is AIDS and the increasing incidence of other sterilizing STDs that have finally brought infertility to the attention of international health policy makers. Not only are sexually transmitted infections a major risk factor for infertility, particularly in women (Cates, Farley, & Rowe, 1985; Reproductive Health Outlook, 1999), but women who are infertile

and desire a pregnancy are much less likely to use safe sex, thereby exposing themselves to the risk of HIV infection. Indeed, in some parts of Africa
infertile women have been shown to be two and a half times more likely
than pregnant women to be HIV-positive (Favot et al., 1997).

At the 1994 International Conference on Population and Development
in Cairo, in which various nongovernmental organizations and Third
World feminist groups were prominent, the international population establishment was heavily criticized for its top-down approach to population
and family planning that neglected many other urgent population issues,
such as sterilizing and life-threatening STDs, including AIDS. Thus the
Programme of Action adopted at that conference signaled a clear shift
toward the notion of reproductive health, broadly defined (Lane, 1994;
United Nations, 1995). And for the first time neglected populations of
"nonfertile" women—in the broad sense of menopausal women, girls, and
the infertile—were included on the agenda. The new agenda is therefore
intended to be based on the interests of populations themselves, including
populations among whom subfertility and infertility are perceived as serious threats.

In other words, infertility at last has been officially acknowledged in
international population and development circles as an important global
phenomenon in its own right, forecasting greater research and political
interest in this once-forgotten issue, especially in developing countries. The
fruits of official recognition are already becoming apparent. For example,
at the end of 1999 an international conference on infertility and the social
sciences, organized by two Dutch contributors to this volume, Frank van
Balen and Trudie Gerrits, was held at the University of Amsterdam. The
conference brought together approximately thirty researchers, most of
them social scientists, to discuss the results of their studies on infertility
from nearly every continent on the globe. At least half of the participants
were from the non-Western world, and several were conducting large-scale
studies of infertility funded directly by international health and population
organizations (e.g., the Ford Foundation). The sense of promise and momentum created by the conference was palpable, and plans were discussed
to hold an international meeting on infertility and the social sciences every
two years, in sites both Western and non-Western.

Thus the voices of the millions of infertile women and men around the
globe may finally be heard, as the results of these and other studies are
published. Indeed, we hope that the chapters in this volume, the first of its
kind to examine infertility in global perspective, will contribute to this new
international research agenda and, ultimately, to public health policies and
programs that will eventually alleviate the suffering of infertility wherever
it occurs.

THE AIMS AND ORGANIZATION OF THIS VOLUME

Allying ourselves with a growing number of social scientists who hope to place reproduction at the center of social and political-economic analysis (Franklin & Ragone, 1998a; Ginsburg & Rapp, 1995b; Greenhalgh, 1995b; Strathern, 1993), we are dedicated in this volume to interpreting infertility from a variety of positions and positionalities. Our dedication to multiple positioning means that we have drawn purposely from a wide range of disciplinary perspectives, theoretical frameworks, methodological approaches, discursive styles, and international locations, in terms of authors' institutional affiliations and their research venues. As a result of this multiplicity of scholarly interests, authors in this volume have adopted varying positions—for example, on the best uses of biomedicine and high-tech interventions for infertility, particularly in non-Western sites—that may seem less than uniform, even contradictory. Yet in our view this range of approaches and perspectives, coupled with the provocatively critical tone of many chapters, contributes to the heterodox richness of this globally inclusive volume.

Similarly, the authors in this volume bring a multiplicity of personal perspectives to their work. Most, but not all, are women, reflecting ongoing gender asymmetries in the study of human reproduction. Not surprisingly, many of the authors, including the editors, bring a keen sense of personal engagement to their studies, given their own life stories of non-normative reproduction, involving infertility, pregnancy loss, medically "assisted" conception, adoption, and childlessness. (See the contributor list at the back of this volume for details.) Thus, the professional *is* the personal for many of us involved in infertility research, as with research on reproduction in general (Rapp & Ginsburg, 1999). The studies, we argue, are richer because of this: not only do they bring us as researchers closer to our subjects through a kind of empathic interconnection, but they are also driven by a collective commitment to giving voice to the infertile, in an attempt to promote greater public understanding and compassion.

Furthermore, as suggested by this volume's title, *Infertility Around the Globe: New Thinking on Childlessness, Gender, and Reproductive Technologies,* we have a number of explicit aims. First, as suggested earlier, there is a need to destabilize standard, Western-based definitions of infertility, as well as the relationship of infertility to childlessness of an involuntary nature. Many of the chapters in this volume interrogate these concepts, thereby exposing the cross-cultural variability of the meanings associated with the inability to conceive and to produce desired children.

Second, this volume clearly exposes the deeply gendered nature of reproduction generally and infertility specifically. While we recognize the centrality of both women and men as reproductive actors, the chapters in this volume reveal the ways in which infertility, the world over, remains largely a *woman's* problem—despite Western medical rhetoric about the necessity of treating the infertile *couple*. Indeed, with few exceptions, even in the West, it is women who bear the burden of blame and social scrutiny for infertility, no matter how "infertility" is socially defined; who embody both popular notions of causation and actual medical diagnosis and treatment; and who live the untoward repercussions and social backlash associated with this affliction. Given this reality, the female experience of infertility is clearly foregrounded in this volume, although male infertility is also explored in a number of chapters (chaps. 6, 9, 12, 14, 15). Nonetheless, we acknowledge with dismay the relative lack of male "voices" in this volume—not only of the authors, three out of seventeen who are male, but also of male informants, who "speak" only in chapter 6 on donor insemination. Indeed, male infertility per se, as well as male experiences of partners' infertility, represents the great uncharted territory in the social science of infertility. Clearly, exploring this terrain is a most pressing research need for the twenty-first century, given that more than half of all cases of infertility globally involve so-called male factors (Reproductive Health Outlook, 1999). Exploring male infertility cross-culturally will require overcoming the stigma that currently prevents male researchers from initiating research on infertility—which, according to one male infertility researcher, is perceived as a "girly subject" (Bharadwaj, pers. com.).

Third, the explicit focus of this volume is on the global dimensions of infertility. This has meant moving beyond typical Western sites of research, debate, and technology production, to expose not only the cross-cultural prevalence of infertility but also global connections between societies that "produce" and "consume" reproductive technologies, both those that curtail fertility and those that enhance it. A major goal of this volume is to expose global interconnections, particularly with regard to reproductive technology transfer, on two levels. First, some societies are under international pressure to reduce population through the acceptance of family planning regimes and Western-generated reproductive technologies to regulate fertility. Yet even in societies that have accepted the inevitability of population reduction through fertility control, infertility is never considered a viable option, and infertile couples are under pressure to produce at least one child, sometimes with the assistance of new reproductive technologies, as in the case of China (see chap. 16, this volume). Thus, the second theme of global interconnectedness revolves around the cultural contextualization of new reproductive technologies, particularly as they reach societies where health care resources are limited and other indigenous systems of knowledge and healing are available. A number of chapters in this volume adopt a critical stance on the wholesale exportation of Western-generated reproductive technologies into new cultural sites, asking what happens when globalizing technologies are received in various non-Western localities far from their original source. In other words, this volume attempts to shift the discussion of new reproductive technologies away from typical Western solipsism to a multisited, critical ethnography of globalization and its impacts—one in which First and Third World consumers of technology are viewed not as we/they but rather as participants in the same historical trajectory (Greenhalgh, 1995a).

Part I. Discourses and Debates

The chapters in this volume are grouped into four sections, reflecting some of the issues raised above and a number of others as well. Part I is devoted to discourses and debates in the scholarly, activist, and popular literature on infertility and new reproductive technologies. The chapters in this section critically examine some of the implicit and explicit assumptions underlying the master tropes and metanarratives in the infertility literature, particularly since 1978, when Louise Brown, the world's first test-tube baby was born. In fact, Margarete Sandelowski and Sheryl de Lacey argue in chapter 2 that "in-fertility" was "invented" in 1978 with Baby Louise's birth, because in 1978 infertility became "a product of technology" in which virtually any obstacle to procreation could, at least purportedly, be circumvented. A "by-product" of this invention, according to these authors, is a profusion of (mis)representations of the infertile themselves in Western professional and popular discourses. Inspired by Foucauldian approaches to discourse analysis (Foucault, 1972), Sandelowski and de Lacey lay bare six of the most common tropes about infertile persons and the extent to which these different Western representations do or do not provide "experience-near" accounts of infertile persons' gendered subjectivities.

The gendered dimensions of infertility are also the explicit focus of chapter 3, in which Charis M. Thompson critically reviews feminist theorizing on infertility and NRTs during two phases: circa 1984–1991, when radical feminist critiques of NRTs prevailed, and circa 1992–1999, when feminist discourses on infertility shifted toward more nuanced representations of the technologies and those who use them. Thompson argues that infertility in the age of new reproductive technologies has, in fact, been performed as the "perfect feminist text," in which many of the rhetorical, personal, and political issues, conflicts, and debates within Western feminism have been played out. Both chapters 2 and 3 speak to the need for an ongoing commitment to deep empiricism and critical ethnography—particularly on the use of new reproductive technologies as cultural practices (Franklin & Ragone, 1998a)—to ground some of the more speculative discussions surrounding reproductive futures and dystopias in the age of NRTs.

The final chapter of this part, chapter 4, by Frank van Balen, shifts our attention to Western psychological discourses and especially the enduring "psychologization" of infertility over the past fifty years. Van Balen argues that Western psychiatric and psychological literature has attributed the underlying etiology of infertility to psychological disturbances, particularly of women in childless partnerships. He traces the shifting history of four models of psychological influence, describing the historical junctures at which particular models came to fruition and then waned. But he concludes that despite the discovery of biologically based, somatic causes for most cases of infertility, psychological thinking endures—leading to a "blame the victim" mentality that patients' rights groups are currently attempting to overcome. Thus van Balen asks us to consider what happens to the psyche of persons who are infertile and challenges us to interrogate age-old questions about the relationship of mind and body, psyche and soma.

Part II. Gender and Body Politics

The relationship between mind and body is also a theme of part II, which explores the embodied experience of infertility in the lives of individual women and men around the world. The emphasis in this part, however, shifts from scholarly discourse to individual experience: infertility and infertile bodies are explored in the most experience-near terms, by focusing primarily on infertile women's and men's own accounts, illness narratives, and life stories. The five chapters in this section, from disparate regions of the globe, speak to the magnitude of social suffering that infertile women (and to a lesser extent men) must endure, particularly as they strive to make sense of why their reproductive bodies have failed them. But they are also surprisingly hopeful in suggesting that the infertile are strategic actors, whose lives, marital relationships, and gender identities are not always permanently disrupted by the inability to produce desired children. Thus these chapters help to deconstruct the discourse of "desperateness" so common to both popular and professional accounts of infertility in women's lives around the globe (Franklin, 1990). The chapters also make abundantly clear that the gender and marital politics surrounding infertility and its treatment involve both conflict and accommodation. Most important, several of the chapters show that infertile marriages, instead of being destined for dissolution, may be surprisingly successful and enduring, even through the emotional turmoil of infertility treatment (see also Inhorn, 1996).

In chapter 5, Arthur L. Greil examines the ways in which the "social drama" of infertility is played out in the bodies of American women. He argues that in the discourse of Western medicine infertile women's bodies are often viewed metaphorically in "mechanical" terms—primarily as flawed machines in need of medical intervention. Although women internalize these metaphors, leading at times to self-blame, they are also not entirely passive in the face of medicalization and metaphorization. Instead, they are problem solvers, who actively and strategically "work the system" to push medical treatment in the direction they want it to go.

Chapter 6, by Gay Becker, examines how a similar social drama is played out in the lives of American couples who have chosen to use the "oldest" new reproductive technology, donor insemination, to overcome male infertility. Becker shows us that even though DI has been in place as a treatment option in the United States for several decades, couples who choose it still confront weighty decisions about whether or not to disclose this form of assisted conception to their children. She argues that no matter what stance they take, many parents lack clear confidence in their decisions and fear for the future well-being of their DI children. The discomfort and moral uncertainty faced by couples in this position reflect the ongoing social stigmatization of male infertility in American society—with all of its implications for masculinity and paternity—as well as the ongoing privileging of "biological" procreation and kinship connection in American society, where social parenthood is seen as being somehow less "real."

The next two chapters in part 2 explore Asian women's roles in society and expectations regarding marriage and motherhood. In chapter 7, Melissa J. Pashigian examines northern Vietnamese population discourse, which valorizes the "happy family" of two children and the "heroic" role of women as both mothers and workers. In this cultural setting, women feel motherhood is mandatory, not only to achieve adult gender identity, but also to establish bonds of emotional "sentiment" with a husband and, by extension, his patrilineal family. Thus this chapter examines desires for children within marriage and family life, placing the discourse of family within larger Vietnamese political discourses, which are simultaneously antinatalist and pronatalist.

By way of contrast, in chapter 8 Catherine Kohler Riessman argues for the nonmandatory nature of motherhood in the "progressive" South Indian state of Kerala. She provides a fine-grained sociolinguistic analysis of infertility narratives told by three South Indian women—narratives that throw into question whether women's lives, even in pronatalist societies such as India, are permanently and tragically marred by involuntary childlessness. Reissman suggests that by focusing on older, gainfully employed infertile women past reproductive age, we may gain new insights into the ways in which women fashion meaningful lives, gender identities, and marriages, even in the absence of motherhood.

Such "optimism" is also found in chapter 9, by Gwynne L. Jenkins, in conjunction with an infertile Costa Rican couple, Silvia Vargas Obando and José Badilla Navas, who were Jenkins's hosts and informants in the field. This poignant account of a couple's attempts to make meaning of and come to terms with long-term infertility in a socially intolerant cultural setting is a true testament to the human spirit, to the strength of marital love and commitment, and to the power of religious faith. The chapter explores the plight of the infertile in relation to the plight of unmarried teenaged mothers in Costa Rica, focusing on the "illegitimate" babies that are sometimes passed between them. And the chapter is also self-consciously reflexive, interweaving the experiences of the author, a young American woman anthropologist, with those of her hosts, who had kept their suffering over infertility hidden from her for many years. Their interwoven story, once finally told, is both heartrending and triumphant.

Part III. The Infertility Belt

Unlike part II, which highlights women's and men's experiences in disparate global locations, part III focuses on Central Africa, where reproductive morbidities and mortalities are related to each other in various complex ways. Specifically, the African continent is considered to have an infection-related "infertility belt" wrapped around its now AIDS-ridden center (Collet et al., 1988; Ericksen & Brunette, 1996; Larsen, 1994). With pockets of infertility reaching rates of 30 percent in some Central and southern African populations, infertility and AIDS represent twin threats for depopulation in this purportedly overpopulated region of the world (Feldman-Savelsberg, 1999).

But what is it like to be an infertile African woman living in the world's infertility belt? What are the social consequences of infertility, in terms of a woman's quotidian existence, her gender identity, her conjugal relations, her family support, her community acceptance, her future security? How are men implicated when conception fails to occur? And do men and women suffer, psychically, somatically, and socially, in the same ways? Is such suffering ameliorated by various forms of healing or social assistance? Are effective treatment options, including new reproductive technologies, available for the infertile? And do such forms of infertility treatment receive institutional support in countries committed, at least rhetorically, to population reduction? Indeed, can infertility be considered part of national and international efforts to promote family planning and women's reproductive health? Or is it a "luxury disease," a waste of valuable health resources, given that the inability to have children is not (apparently at least) life-threatening and may be perceived as mitigating population pressures?

These are questions that are taken up in the four chapters of this part, which explore Central and southern African infertility from a variety of disciplinary and local perspectives. In chapter 10, Lori Leonard takes us to Chad, where she contrasts local Sara women's accounts of their fertility "problems" with Western "scientific" accounts, both epidemiological and demographic in nature. She argues that despite the demonstrated existence of an infertility belt stretching across Central Africa and including Chad, standard demographic studies of infertility in Africa regularly miss many instances of indigenously defined problematic fertility in the lives of African women. This is because standard Western definitions of infertility, as well as demographic approaches to enumerating cases, are cultural constructions that may not be applicable in non-Western settings, where women's self-defined "fertility problems" are of much greater scope than standard definitions of infertility would suggest.

Similarly, in chapter 11, Pamela Feldman-Savelsberg challenges us to consider local emic, or indigenous, public health perspectives on infertility in the Grassfields of Cameroon. She examines the long-standing colonial and postcolonial interest in controlling fertility in this region, an area with uncontrolled "hyperfertility," according to international population policy makers. However, among the Grassfields Bamiléké, women view their fertility as deeply threatened and as tied to the troubled political positions of their chiefs, whose waning powers in a new era of Cameroonian nation-statehood symbolically index the infertility of both Bamiléké fields and women's wombs. Thus Feldman-Savelsberg argues that on a local level at least it is *infertility*, not hyperfertility, that is of paramount concern and the "unrecognized public health problem" for Grassfielders themselves. Thus chapters 10 and 11 demonstrate that in the politics of reproduction even numbers are "political artifacts" (Greenhalgh, 1995a, p. 26) and may be used variously and strategically on the international, national, and local levels.

In chapter 12 Trudie Gerrits takes us from the political to the ethnomedical as she explores the perceived causes of infertility in a matrilineal society in Mozambique. Gerrits argues that most of the studies of infertility on the African continent come from patrilineal societies, where women are typically blamed for infertility and expected to overcome it through a variety of ethnomedical treatment strategies. Therefore, the case of the Mozambican Macua, who are matrilineal, appears quite exceptional: not only are men typically diagnosed and deemed responsible for infertility problems in the Macua ethnomedical system, but women in infertile marriages are encouraged to "heal" their childlessness by procreating with other men, leading in some cases to female-initiated divorce. Gerrits concludes that although childless women are still stigmatized in some ways in Macua society (mainly through their exclusion from important fertility-related rituals), it is quite clear that matrilineality also protects them by preventing many of the profound social repercussions experienced by childless women in other patrilineal African societies.

The final chapter of part III explores the relationship between ethno-

medicine and biomedicine in sub-Saharan Africa, concluding with this cautionary and somewhat sobering note: as we enter the twenty-first century,
it is highly unlikely that Western-based infertility treatment and new reproductive technologies will supplant indigenous ethnogynecologies (Inhorn,
1994b) around the world, in part because of the poor distribution and
poor quality of gynecological care in biomedical settings around the world.
Indeed, the recourse to ethnogynecological medicine among infertile individuals the world over indexes in part the inability of Western-based biomedicine to "cure" all cases of infertility, even with the latest advances in
reproductive medicine. As shown in chapter 13, by Johanne Sundby, in the
developing world resources and competent medical personnel are often
scarce, and the great gulf between physicians and infertile patients (in
terms of their social status, education, and belief systems) makes patient
compliance with poorly explained and usually lengthy diagnostic workups
and treatment protocols unlikely. In such developing-country settings, it is
not surprising that infertile patients seek help in the realm of ethnomedicine, where rich indigenous traditions may exist to support infertile individuals, both medically and psychosocially (Inhorn, 1994b). Sundby examines this interplay between ethnomedicine and biomedicine in both The
Gambia and Zimbabwe, describing the undeveloped state of biomedicine
in these countries and suggesting what it would take to bring infertility
diagnostic and treatment facilities up to WHO standards. Thus Sundby
brings into critical focus issues of global inequality and contemporary international health debates about whether comprehensive "reproductive
health" services can ever really be achieved. In particular, she questions
whether Third World governments, plagued by limited health resources,
can be expected to broaden the scope of their reproductive health efforts
to include infertility and the various technologies required to diagnose and
overcome it, particularly in the midst of such other pressing crises as maternal mortality and AIDS.

Part IV. Globalizing Technologies

Despite the sobering conclusion to part III, part IV demonstrates that Western-based reproductive medicine, including new reproductive technologies, *is* spreading to the developing countries of the non-Western world.
Even in impoverished countries in Africa, Asia, and Latin America, NRTs
are being introduced and used by elite members of society. Thus, despite
the distributive injustice accompanying the globalization of NRTs, it is important to recognize that they are being rapidly exported and consumed
around the world, with far-reaching implications for societies on the receiving end of global technological transfer. The chapters in this final sec-

tion explore the globalization of NRTs in four non-Western societies, Egypt, Israel, China, and India, asking how these technologies are both accommodated and resisted in disparate settings.

In chapter 14 Marcia C. Inhorn explores the relationship of the global to the local, asking how NRTs, as purportedly universal, "culture-free," inherently beneficial medical technologies, are received locally in the "overpopulated," pronatalist Muslim nation of Egypt. Focusing on issues of embodiment, Inhorn shows how local cultural notions of reproductive bodies and physiology, as well as concerns about safety, efficacy, and the physical and emotional well-being of IVF children, deter many infertile Egyptians from pursuing NRT treatments and worry those who do use them. Furthermore, she demonstrates the profoundly gendered implications of the "newest" new reproductive technology—ICSI—when applied in the Egyptian context. In a Muslim society where all forms of egg, sperm, and embryo donation, as well as surrogacy, are strictly prohibited, the introduction of ICSI has led some infertile men to cast off their reproductively elderly wives in the hope of achieving biological parenthood with younger, more fecund women.

In chapter 15, based in neighboring Israel, Susan Martha Kahn provides a contrasting study of NRT use among Israel's ultraorthodox Jewish population. Although religion is equally if not more important in dictating the permissible uses of NRTs in this population, Kahn shows how the rulings of various ultraorthodox rabbis have led to very different conclusions about appropriate NRT use among ultraorthodox Israelis. Ironically perhaps, rabbinic interpretations of the permissibility of both sperm and ova donation are much more liberal than interpretations in Egypt, although restrictions still apply based on the perceived conferral of "Jewishness" through the recombination of procreative materials. Furthermore, unlike Egypt, where access to NRTs is restricted to the monied elite, they are widely available and significantly subsidized under the Israeli health care system; thus infertile ultraorthodox women, who are under pressure to produce numerous children, have essentially no choice but to undergo multiple trials of NRTs in the hope of achieving multiple births.

In contrast to the two pronatalist Middle Eastern societies described in chapters 14 and 15, Lisa Handwerker takes us in chapter 16 to the People's Republic of China, a nation with the largest population in the world and the most stringent one-child-only population policy. There, Handwerker examines the paradoxical growth of a major "high-tech baby-making industry." The new reproductive technologies have taken hold in China, she argues, because the one-child-only policy is indigenously interpreted as "you must have one child policy." That one child, furthermore, must be a "perfect" child to improve the fitness of the Chinese population as a whole. Thus Handwerker examines the use of NRTs as a method of "new eugenics," given widespread Chinese beliefs that IVF children are mentally and physically superior to children conceived without technological assistance. She concludes with a discussion of the potential bioethical implications of using new reproductive technologies for eugenic ends, particularly in societies with a culturally entrenched preference for sons and a resultant crisis of "missing females."

Finally, chapter 17 takes us to another "overpopulated" South Asian nation, India, where NRTs have also become available to urban elites. In this concluding chapter, Aditya Bharadwaj is less concerned with the uses of NRTs among advantaged Indians than with the fascinating controversy that is unfolding in India over "test-tube firsts." Bharadwaj describes the contemporary debate over which Indian doctor is truly responsible for introducing IVF to India and whether this is the same doctor who purportedly produced the second-ever test-tube baby in the world. Expanding on Latour and Woolgar's (1986) concepts of credit and credibility, Bharadwaj makes the case that in the age of NRTs multimedia forces are extremely important in ascribing "credit," as reward, to the scientists involved in the production of new scientific knowledge and, in this case, the production of human life itself. In other words, in India the media have played a major role in advancing the careers of particular IVF doctors and not others, which has led, among other things, to at least one suicide, an ongoing clash of medical egos, and a contemporary controversy over scientific "credibility" that Bharadwaj carefully lays out.

As with the other chapters in this section, the Indian case amply demonstrates how the availability of new reproductive technologies in disparate global sites may create new possibilities, new social imaginaries, and new arenas of cultural production, as well as new contradictions, new dilemmas of agency, and new regimes of control (Ginsburg & Rapp, 1995b). Yet an important point to bear in mind here is that despite all of the controversies described in the preceding chapters, NRTs are responsible for creating thousands of new lives around the world. Indeed, not all infertile persons remain infertile forever and at least some individuals move beyond the psychic suffering of infertility and childlessness to become parents, including of "test-tube" babies in places like India, China, and Egypt. But parenthood often brings with it new questions and quandaries, including concerns about the "fitness" of parents who have experienced the long-term trials and tribulations of infertility and IVF treatments, as well as the physical and social well-being of children conceived through such "extraordinary" means. Thus the optimistic conclusion of this volume—that childlessness can be overcome through perseverance and technological assistance—is also tempered by the reality that many societies, including those in the West, have yet to come to terms with infertility, new reproductive technologies, and the various strategies through which the infertile become parents, both inside and outside heterosexual unions. Globally, stigma endures and is a powerful force in the lives of the infertile and the children they love as their own.

Together, these chapters reveal much about the "lived experience" of infertility and childlessness the world over. Both collectively and individually, the infertile face a "medical and emotional road of trials" (Sandelowski, Harris, & Black, 1992, p. 282), one whose end is often not clearly in sight. Yet the chapters in this volume shed much light on the journeys of the infertile down that road—whether in Central Africa, western Europe, Latin America, South Asia, the Middle East, or Middle America. The local realities of infertility—with all the attendant suffering and hope for technological salvation—speak to the importance of infertility as a global phenomenon, one that deserves our attention and concern in the new millennium.

NOTES

1. For Western-based research on this subject, see Abbey et al. (1991); Greil (1997); Stanton et al. (1991); van Balen & Trimbos-Kemper (1993).

2. On a historical note, well-known pedagogical historians, such as Aries (1962) and Shorter (1977), argued that in preindustrial Europe parents were not affectionate to their children. The idea of loving and dutiful parents was supposedly a recent historical development. By implication, this was thought to be true as well in developing countries, where children are desired for their social and economic benefits. However, these ideas are being overturned by more recent scholarship.

3. Such variants include gamete intrafallopian transfer, zygote intrafallopian transfer, tubal embryo transfer, and, most recently, intracytoplasmic sperm injection using micromanipulation techniques. Additional spin-offs of the IVF procedure include cryopreservation of unused embryos, the use of donor eggs, and combining donor sperm and/or eggs in various types of surrogate gestational relationships (Turiel, 1998).

REFERENCES

Abbey, A., Andrews, F. M., & Halman, L. J. (1991). Gender's role in response to infertility. *Psychology of Women Quarterly, 15,* 295–316.

Ariès, Ph. (1962). *Centuries of childhood: A social history of family life.* New York: Knopf.

Becker, G. (1990). *Healing the infertile family: Strengthening your relationship in the search for parenthood.* Berkeley: University of California Press.

Becker, G. (2000). *The elusive embryo: How women and men approach new reproductive technologies.* Berkeley: University of California Press.

Browner, C. H., & Press, N. A. (1995). The normalization of prenatal diagnostic screening. In F. D. Ginsburg & R. Rapp (Eds.), *Conceiving the new world order: The global politics of reproduction* (pp. 207–322). Berkeley: University of California Press.

Browner, C. H., & Sargent, C. F. (1996). Anthropology and studies of human reproduction. In C. F. Sargent & T. M. Johnson (Eds.), *Medical anthropology: Contemporary theory and method* (pp. 219–234). Westport, CT: Praeger.

Cates, W., Farley, T. M. M., & Rowe, P. J. (1985). Worldwide patterns of infertility: Is Africa different? *The Lancet, September 14,* 596–598.

Colen, S. (1986). "With respect and feelings": Voices of West Indian childcare and domestic workers in New York City. In J. B. Cole (Ed.), *All American women: Lines that divide, ties that bind.* New York: Free Press.

Collet, M., Reniers, J., Frost, E., Yvert, F., Leclerc, A., Roth-Meyer, C., Ivanoff, B., & Meheus, A. (1988). Infertility in Central Africa: Infection is the cause. *International Journal of Gynecology & Obstetrics, 26,* 423–428.

Corea, G. (1985). *The mother machine: Reproductive technology from artificial insemination to artificial wombs.* New York: Harper & Row.

Corea, G., Klein, R. D., Hanmer, J., Holmes, H. B., Hoskings, B., Kishwar, M., Raymond, J., Rowland, R., & Steinbacher, R. (1987). *Man-made women: How new reproductive technologies affect women.* Bloomington: Indiana University Press.

Davis-Floyd, R., & Dumit, J. (Eds.). (1998). *Cyborg babies: From techno-sex to techno-tots.* New York: Routledge.

Davis-Floyd, R. E., & Sargent, C. F. (Eds.). (1997). *Childbirth and authoritative knowledge: Cross-cultural perspectives.* Berkeley: University of California Press.

Devroey, P., Vandervorst, M., Nagy, P., & Van Steirteghem, A. (1998). Do we treat the male or his gamete? *Human Reproduction, 13 (suppl. 1),* 178–185.

Ericksen, K., & Brunette, T. (1996). Patterns and predictors of infertility among African women: A cross-national survey of 27 nations. *Social Science & Medicine, 42,* 209–220.

Favot, I., Ngalula, J., Mgalla, Z., Klokke, A. H., Gumodoka, B., & Boerma, J. T. (1997). HIV infection and sexual behavior among women with infertility in Tanzania: A hospital-based study. *International Journal of Epidemiology, 26,* 414–419.

Feldman-Savelsberg, P. (1999). *Plundered kitchens, empty wombs: Threatened reproduction and identity in the Cameroon Grassfields.* Ann Arbor: University of Michigan Press.

Foucault, M. (1972). *The archaeology of knowledge and the discourse on language.* New York: Pantheon.

Franklin, S. (1990). Deconstructing "desperateness": The social construction of infertility in popular representations of new reproductive technologies. In M. McNeil, I. Varcoe, & S. Yearley (Eds.), *The new reproductive technologies.* London: Macmillan.

Franklin, S., & Ragone, H. (1998a). Introduction. In S. Franklin & H. Ragone (Eds.), *Reproducing reproduction: Kinship, power, and technological innovation* (pp. 1–14). Philadelphia: University of Pennsylvania Press.

Franklin, S., & Ragone, H. (Eds.). (1998b). *Reproducing reproduction: Kinship, power, and technological innovation.* Philadelphia: University of Pennsylvania Press.

Gerris, J. M. R. (1997). *A comparative investigation in the real efficacy of conventional therapies versus advanced reproductive technology in male reproductive disorders.* Antwerp: Universiteit van Antwerpen.

Ginsburg, F. D., & Rapp, R. (1991). The politics of reproduction. *Annual Review of Anthropology, 20,* 311–343.

Ginsburg, F. D., & Rapp, R. (Eds.). (1995a). *Conceiving the new world order: The global politics of reproduction.* Berkeley: University of California Press.

Ginsburg, F. D., & Rapp, R. (1995b). Introduction: Conceiving the new world order. In F. D. Ginsburg & R. Rapp (Eds.), *Conceiving the new world order: The global politics of reproduction* (pp. 1–17). Berkeley: University of California Press.

Greenhalgh, S. (1995a). Anthropology theorizes reproduction: Integrating practice, political economic, and feminist perspectives. In S. Greenhalgh (Ed.), *Situating fertility: Anthropology and demographic inquiry* (pp. 3–28). Cambridge: Cambridge University Press.

Greenhalgh, S. (Ed.). (1995b). *Situating fertility: Anthropology and demographic inquiry.* Cambridge: Cambridge University Press.

Greil, A. L. (1991). *Not yet pregnant: Infertile couples in contemporary America.* New Brunswick, NJ: Rutgers University Press.

Greil, A. L. (1997). Infertility and psychological distress: A critical review of the literature. *Social Science & Medicine, 45,* 1679–1704.

Handwerker, W. P. (Ed.) (1990). *Births and power: Social change and the politics of reproduction.* Boulder, CO: Westview Press.

Inhorn, M. C. (1994a). Interpreting infertility: Medical anthropological perspectives. *Social Science & Medicine, 39,* 459–461.

Inhorn, M. C. (1994b). *Quest for conception: Gender, infertility, and Egyptian medical traditions.* Philadelphia: University of Pennsylvania Press.

Inhorn, M. C. (1996). *Infertility and patriarchy: The cultural politics of gender and family life in Egypt.* Philadelphia: University of Pennsylvania Press.

Inhorn, M. C. (2001). Money, marriage, and morality: Constraints on IVF treatment seeking among infertile Egyptian couples. In C. M. Obermeyer (Ed.), *Cultural perspectives on reproductive health.* Oxford: Oxford University Press.

Inhorn, M. C. (2002). "The worms are weak": Male infertility and patriarchal paradoxes in Egypt. *Men & Masculinities,* in press.

Kamischke, A., & Neischlag, E. (1998). Conventional treatments of male infertility in the age of evidence-based andrology. *Human Reproduction, 13 (suppl. 1),* 62–75.

Kielmann, K. (1998). Barren ground: Contesting identities of infertile women in Pemba, Tanzania. In M. Lock & P. A. Kaufert (Eds.), *Pragmatic women and body politics* (pp. 127–163). Cambridge: Cambridge University Press.

Kirejczyk, M. (1996). *The blessings of technology? Gender and the debated introduction of in vitro fertilization in the Dutch health care system.* Utrecht: Van Arkel.

Klein, R. D. (1989). *Infertility: Women speak out about their experiences of reproductive medicine.* London: Pandora Press.

Kleinman, A. M. (1992). Local worlds of suffering: An interpersonal focus for ethnographies of illness experience. *Qualitative Health Research, 2,* 127–134.

Kleinman, A. M. (1995). *Writing at the margin: Discourse between anthropology and medicine.* Berkeley: University of California Press.

Lane, S. D. (1994). From population control to reproductive health: An emerging policy agenda. *Social Science & Medicine, 39,* 1303–1314.

Lane, S. D., & Cibula, D. A. (2000). Gender and health. In G. L. Albrecht, R. Fitz-patrick, & S. C. Scrimshaw (Eds.), *Handbook of social studies in health and medicine* (pp. 136–153). London: Sage.

Larsen, U. (1994). Sterility in sub-Saharan Africa. *Population Studies, 48,* 459–474.

Latour, B., & Woolgar, S. (1986). *Laboratory life: The social construction of scientific facts.* 2d ed. Princeton, NJ: Princeton University Press.

Lock, M., & Kaufert, P. A. (Eds.). (1998). *Pragmatic women and body politics.* Cam-bridge: Cambridge University Press.

Mohanty, C. T., Russo, A., & Torres, L. (1991). *Third World women and the politics of feminism.* Bloomington: Indiana University Press.

Morgan, L. M., & Michaels, M. W. (Eds.). (1999). *Fetal subjects, feminist positions.* Philadelphia: University of Pennsylvania Press.

Nicholson, R. F., & Nicholson, R. E. (1994). Assisted reproduction in Latin America. *Journal of Assisted Reproduction and Genetics, 11,* 438–444.

Nsiah-Jefferson, L., & Hall, E. J. (1989). Reproductive technology: Perspectives and implications for low-income women and women of color. In K. S. Ratcliff (Ed.), *Healing technology: Feminist perspectives* (pp. 93–117). Ann Arbor: University of Michigan Press.

Okonofua, F. E. (1996). The case against new reproductive technologies in devel-oping countries. *British Journal of Obstetrics and Gynecology, 103,* 957–962.

Rapp, R. (1999). *Testing women, testing the fetus: The social impact of amniocentesis in America.* New York: Routledge.

Rapp, R., & Ginsburg, F. (1999). Relocating reproduction, generating culture. Pa-per presented at the invited session, The Anthropology of Reproduction: Trends and Trajectories, American Anthropological Association, 98th Annual Meeting, Chicago, November 19.

Ratcliff, K. S. (Ed.). (1989). *Healing technology: Feminist perspectives.* Ann Arbor: Uni-versity of Michigan Press.

Reproductive Health Outlook. (1999). Infertility: Overview and lessons learned. Web site: http://www.rho.org.

Rothman, B. K. (1986). *The tentative pregnancy: Prenatal diagnosis and the future of motherhood.* New York: W. W. Norton.

Sandelowski, M. (1991). Compelled to try: The never-enough quality of conceptive technology. *Medical Anthropology Quarterly, (NS) 5,* 29–47.

Sandelowski, M. (1993). *With child in mind: Studies of the personal encounter with infer-tility.* Philadelphia: University of Pennsylvania Press.

Sandelowski, M., Harris, B. G., & Black, B. P. (1992). Relinquishing infertility: The work of pregnancy for infertile couples. *Qualitative Health Research, 2,* 282–301.

Sciarra, J. (1994). Infertility: An international health problem. *International Journal of Gynecology & Obstetrics, 46,* 155–163.

Sheth, S. S., & Malpani, A. N. (1997). Inappropriate use of new technology: Impact on women's health. *International Journal of Gynecology & Obstetrics, 58,* 159–165.

Shorter, E. (1977). *The making of the modern family.* New York: Basic Books.

Stanton, A. L., Tennen, J., Affleck, G., & Mendola, R. (1991). Cognitive appraisal and adjustment to infertility. *Women and Health, 17,* 1–15.

Stanworth, M. (Ed.). (1987). *Reproductive technologies: Gender, motherhood and medicine.* Cambridge: Polity Press.

Strathern, M. (1993). Introduction. In M. Strathern (Ed.), *Reproducing the future: Anthropology, kinship and the reproductive technologies* (pp. 1–12). Manchester: Manchester University Press.

Stuart-Macadam, P., & Dettwyler, K. (Eds.). (1995). *Breastfeeding: Biocultural perspectives.* Hawthorne, NY: Aldine de Gruyter.

Sundby, J. (1997). Infertility in The Gambia: Traditional and modern health care. *Patient Education and Counseling, 31,* 29–37.

Turiel, J. S. (1998). *Beyond second opinions: Making choices about fertility treatment.* Berkeley: University of California Press.

United Nations. (1995). *The world's women 1995: Trends and statistics.* New York: United Nations.

van Balen, F., & Trimbos-Kemper, T. C. M. (1993). Long-term infertile couples: A study of their well-being. *Journal of Psychosomatic Obstetrics and Gynecology, 16,* 137–144.

van Balen, F., & Trimbos-Kemper, T. C. M. (1995). Involuntary childless couples: Their desire to have children and their motives. *Journal of Psychosomatic Obstetrics and Gynecology, 16,* 137–144.

van Balen, F., Verdurmen, J. E. E., & Ketting, E. (1995). *Caring about infertility: Main results of the national survey about behavior regarding infertility.* Delft: Eburon.

van der Ploeg, I. (1995). Hermaphrodite patients: In vitro fertilization and the transformation of male infertility. *Science, Technology and Human Values, 20,* 460–481.

WHO (World Health Organization). (1975). *The epidemiology of infertility: Report of a WHO scientific group.* World Health Organization Technical Report Series No. 582.

WHO (World Health Organization). (1987a). Infections, pregnancies, and infertility: Perspectives on prevention. *Fertility and Sterility, 47,* 964–968.

WHO (World Health Organization). (1987b). *World Health Organization manual for the examination of human semen and semen-cervical mucus interaction.* Cambridge: Cambridge University Press.

WHO (World Health Organization). (1989). *Guidelines on diagnosis and treatment of infertility.* Copenhagen: World Health Organization Regional Office for Europe.

WHO (World Health Organization) (1993). *Manual for the standard investigation and diagnosis of the infertile couple.* Geneva: World Health Organization/Cambridge University Press.

TWO

The Uses of a "Disease"
Infertility as Rhetorical Vehicle

Margarete Sandelowski and Sheryl de Lacey

Infertility is a topic that evidently offers something for everyone. Since the advent in the late 1970s of in vitro fertilization (IVF) techniques to enhance fertility and to bypass physical and biological impediments to procreation, infertility has increasingly attracted the attention of a diverse and growing constituency, including behavioral, biological, and social scientists; scholars from the practice disciplines; ethicists, theologians, lawyers, and legislators; social activists and cultural critics; and journalists and television commentators. Indeed, the interest in infertility has engendered some strange bedfellows; for example, feminists have found themselves allied with pro-family (and often antifeminist) activists to denounce assisted reproductive techniques as alternatively antiwoman and antinature (e.g., Farquhar, 1996).

As both infertile and fertile women increasingly have been used as "test sites" for new drugs and surgeries (Klein & Rowland, 1989), infertility has itself become a discursive site for the examination and critique of a wide variety of phenomena, including human agency and objectification (Cussins 1996, 1998a); the culture of risk (Becker & Nachtigall, 1994); the politics of gender (Lorber, 1987); "genealogical bewilderment" (Humphrey & Humphrey, 1986); class, capitalism, and the commodification of human life (Raymond, 1993); deviance and stigma (Whiteford & Gonzalez, 1994); hegemony and concordance (Condit, 1994); and even discourse itself (Lloyd, 1997; van der Ploeg, 1995). More specifically, these scholars have found infertility fertile ground for exploring whether and how Western[1] (largely biomedical and media) constructions and management of infertility have contributed to alterations in the self and personal volition, women's heightened perceptions of risk for infertility and their continuing willingness to take risks to reverse infertility, and to the recirculation of gender and social class inequalities. They have also found in the various discourses on infertility cause to be concerned over the resurgence of eugenic imperatives, the renewed emphasis on the importance of biological (especially genetic) kinship and the bewilderment experienced when these ties are disrupted, and the role that media play in a hypermediated culture in disseminating dominant ideology. Infertile couples, especially the Western white and socioeconomically advantaged couples able to afford high-priced medical and adoption services, have provided much material and data—not only for commercial, but also for academic, exchange. Indeed, infertility has come to exemplify what Lather (1995, p. 51) described in another context as the "violence of objectification required by turning another's life into information for academic trade."

But what is it about infertility that has made it so interesting, so valuable as Western currency? And is infertility per se even the real concern? As Brumberg (1988, p. 1) asked in relation to anorexia, why does a "disease" like infertility become more prominent in one time period than in another, especially when its overall incidence in the West has changed very little (Mosher and Pratt, 1990; Sandelowski, 1993). In this chapter, we draw from biomedical, social science, and popular literature, as well as our own research with infertile couples, to explore the uses of infertility as a "rhetorical vehicle," "rallying point" (Brandt, 1987, p. 6), and "frame" (Rosenberg, 1989) for a variety of Western concerns and the impact of this use on infertile couples themselves. Although there is arguably no real infertility epidemic in the West, there is certainly—what Treichler (1990) discussed in the context of HIV/AIDS—an "epidemic of signification," or a proliferation of meanings of infertility. Like all persons directly affected by or afflicted with newsworthy, ambiguous, or controversial diseases (Sandelowski, 1993), infertile couples are in "double jeopardy" (Brandt, 1987, p. 5). They bear the burdens not only of infertility and its varied medical and social treatments but also of ideas about infertility: its various "constructions" (e.g., Scritchfield, 1989a, b) and the varied and often conflicting (mis)representations of the infertile. Like HIV/AIDS, infertility has a "dual life—as both a material and linguistic entity" (Treichler, 1990, p. 287). We recognize that by describing the "uses" (Sicherman, 1977) of infertility, we, too, are *using* infertility and infertile couples for our own discursive ends.

THE INVENTION OF *IN*-FERTILITY

Arguably, infertility was "invented" with the in vitro conception and birth in 1978 of Baby Louise. That is, in the spirit and language of the Foucauldian-inspired "genealogical method" (Armstrong, 1990), infertility was discovered—or, more precisely, discursively created (Armstrong, 1986; Arney & Bergen, 1984)—when *in*-fertility became possible. Whereas *barrenness* used to connote a divine curse of biblical proportions and *sterility* an absolutely irreversible physical condition, infertility connotes a medically and socially liminal state in which affected persons hover between reproductive incapacity and capacity: that is, "not yet pregnant" (Greil, 1991) but ever hopeful of achieving pregnancy and having a baby to take home. The betwixt-and-between condition of infertility emerged when both infertile couples and their physicians began to expect that virtually any kind of biological or physical impediment to reproduction could eventually be bypassed, even if not removed or cured.

Although the infertility that has been the object of so much attention in the past two decades has similarities to the historical entities of barrenness and sterility that preceded it, it is also different from them. Post-1978 infertility is a product of the technology that has made it possible even to think about circumventing virtually any obstacle to procreation, including advancing age. Women in their forties, fifties, and even sixties (e.g., Paulson, Thornton, Francis, & Salvador, 1997) have been made to conceive and carry pregnancies successfully to term, thereby calling into question the physiological status of both menopause and the infertility normally associated with it. Midlife infertility is thus another condition once considered normal and natural but now treated as pathological or at least pathogenic (Brett & Niermeyer, 1998). Post-1978 infertility is a chronic condition now extending well into middle age and newly distinguished by the infertility "career" (Conrad, 1987, p. 9), or the public, no-holes-barred, concentrated, and frequently never-enough pursuit of a baby of one's own. New assisted reproductive techniques (including refinements of such old techniques as donor insemination) are, arguably, less a response to infertility than a precursor of it. Barrenness and sterility may have been among the reasons for the interest in developing these techniques, but infertility is a consequence of them.

By virtue of its in-between state, the new infertility has become a place where people with competing interests and claims meet (Clarke & Montini, 1993) and a discursive site where language and practices intended to expose, deconstruct, and to make sense of ambiguity and contradiction converge (Powers, 1996). Infertility triggers grave anxieties about how far human beings can and should go to circumvent nature, fate, and divine will in the pursuit of health and happiness. Infertility remains ambiguous medically as it is variously conceptualized as itself a disease, a symptom of disease, a cause of disease, a consequence of disease, and as not a disease at all. The etiology of infertility remains uncertain as biological, behavioral, psychological, and sociocultural factors continue to be variously implicated and as the actual causes of infertility in any one case are often difficult to discern, even when specific medical disorders are identified (Sandelowski, 1993). Also contributing to the ambiguity of infertility is that it is biologically located and, in the West, culturally located, not in individuals, but rather between them. Infertility is here typically treated as a problem in a reproductive partnership: that is, in "a couple." In cases of "male" infertility, in which females are generally the objects of treatment because of the dearth of treatments to apply to male bodies, the infertility patient is often not a typical man at all but rather a hermaphrodite: a technologically constructed and linguistically deployed entity (van der Ploeg, 1995). This entity first appears to be a typical male with a sperm defect who subsequently appears as a not so typical (fe)male, as s/he is said to have succeeded or failed to become pregnant after undergoing in vitro procedures. In short, infertility may be usefully studied as a Western culture-specific disorder, as conceptions of what is included in this category of disorder and of how it is manifested, discovered and diagnosed, and treated reflect and depend on culture-specific technologies and ideologies. Treating infertility as a cultural disorder does not deny the organic pathologies, symptoms, or suffering in individuals associated with it but rather emphasizes how such conditions can serve as "mirrors" of cultural norms and "'barometers'" of cultural change (Johnson, 1987, p. 351).

(MIS)REPRESENTATIONS OF THE INFERTILE

A by-product of the new infertility and the technology that made it possible has been a profusion of representations of the infertile—as objects of sympathy, pity, curiosity, and even condemnation. The infertile appear in contemporary Western professional and popular discourse in various guises—as patients, as emotionally distressed, as socially handicapped, as consumers, as cultural dupes and foils, and as cultural heroes. These guises are neither mutually exclusive nor uniformly tied to any one constituency but rather complement or compete with each other and variously lend themselves to strategic uses by different constituencies. Moreover, they are largely guises of white, married, and socioeconomically advantaged persons, as members of poor and minority groups are seen to be hyperfertile and single persons and gay and lesbian couples to be "dysfertile," that is, as unsuitable for parenthood no matter what their fertility status (e.g., de Lacey, 1998; Ikemoto, 1996; Somerville, 1982).

As Patients

When infertility is problematized as a disease or symptom of one or more organic dysfunctions or hormonal aberrations, the infertile are viewed as patients, that is, as persons in need of medical diagnosis and treatment. Failed body functions are the targets of intervention, and the infertile are categorized by diagnosis (e.g., ovarian failure, semen deficiency), treatment (e.g., in vitro patient), or physical response to treatment (e.g., "poor responder").

The representation of the infertile as patients is arguably the least objectionable (cf. Becker & Nachtigall, 1992), most culturally resonant, and most useful—to Western infertile couples themselves—of any of the depictions we describe here. This view of the infertile is based on the assumption that infertility is a disease entity, which, like cancer and heart disease, profoundly undermines health and well-being and is, therefore, deserving of public support for treatment, including insurance coverage and sick leaves. Those designated as patients tend also to be largely relieved of most of the responsibility for causing or curing their disease (Brickman et al., 1982; Sontag, 1990).

Yet, unlike cancer and heart disease, infertility still needs to be justified as worthy of public expenditures (e.g., Drewett, 1994). Infertile couples, most notably members of the self-help groups RESOLVE in the United States and ACCESS in Australia, are prominent among activists seeking to secure the designation of infertility as a disease and of themselves as patients, as the status of infertility as disease remains controversial. Most infertile couples in public view[2] want to be seen as having a medical disorder, but they are still often denied patient status as infertility is not generally considered to pose physical harm and therefore is not seen as requiring treatment. Moreover, unlike cancer and heart disease, infertility is often seen less as a body failure than as a failure to satisfy a desire. The desire for a child is here likened to the desire for a straighter nose or slimmer hips. That is, although they are medical treatments, in that only physicians can offer them, neither infertility treatments nor cosmetic surgery are seen to address truly or wholly medical problems.

As Emotionally Distressed

In contrast to the view of infertility as a medical problem, where the target concern is the bodily failure itself, is the view of infertility as largely a psychological problem. In the psychological model, the problem or target of intervention is the behavioral or emotional response to both body and recurring treatment failures. Infertility is problematized as a constellation of negative or unhealthful behavioral and/or emotional responses to the inability to reproduce and, more often, to the medical means to resolve it. Indeed, in much of the contemporary psychologically oriented literature on infertility, the focus is less on responses to infertility per se than on responses to its medical treatment. That is, the psychological or emotional response to the treatment-become-disease (see Peitzman, 1989) is the treatable problem.

The infertile are persons in need of counseling or other psychological therapies aimed at helping them to understand and then to modify aberrant feelings or behaviors or "purge" emotions (Hunt & Meerabeau, 1993). The infertile are variously depicted as potentially or actually (dis)stressed, depressed, anxious, hostile, and ineffective copers as a consequence of their failure to reproduce and therefore as in danger of long-term psychic damage, sexual dysfunction, marital disruption, or poor pregnancy and parenting outcomes, should they achieve pregnancy and parenthood (e.g., Berg & Wilson, 1995; Domar, Broome, Zuttermeister, Seibel, & Friedman, 1992; Golombok, Cook, Bish, & Murray, 1995; Halman, Oakley, & Lederman, 1995; Hirsch & Hirsch, 1995). Foci of the now vast psychological literature on infertility (e.g., Greil, 1997) include adjustment and coping: after both treatment failure and success, during different stages of infertility treatment, and in relation to gender and specific therapies, such as donor insemination and IVF (e.g., Beaurepaire, Jones, Thiering, Saunders, & Tennant, 1994; Berg & Wilson, 1991; Carmeli & Birenbaum-Carmeli, 1994; Edelmann, Connolly, & Bartlett, 1994; Hynes, Callan, Terry, & Gallois, 1992; Laffont & Edelmann, 1994; Litt, Tennen, Affleck, & Klock, 1992; Nachtigall, Becker, & Wozny, 1992; Prattke & Gass-Sternas, 1993; van Balen, Naaktgeboren, & Trimbos-Kemper, 1996; Weaver, Clifford, Hay, & Robinson, 1997; Wright et al., 1991).

Perhaps even more significantly, the future success of medical treatment is seen as in jeopardy should the unhealthful responses of the infertile continue without appropriate psychological intervention (e.g., Demyttenaere, Nijs, Evers-Kieboom, & Koninckx, 1992; Facchinetti, Matteo, Artini, Volpe, & Genazzani, 1997; Takefman, Brender, Boivin, & Tulandi, 1990). In contrast to the medical model of infertility, in the psychological model at least some of the responsibility for causing infertility is returned to infertile couples. The continuing failure to adjust and to adapt is seen as interfering with medical treatment and, later on, with positive pregnancy outcomes and parental competence. Although cause and consequence in the matter of the emotional distress of infertile couples have yet to be disentangled (e.g., Schover, 1997; Stoleru, Teglas, Spira, Magnin, & Fermanian, 1996; Wasser, Sewall, & Soules, 1993; Wright, Allard, Lecours, & Sabourin, 1989), stress and emotions are currently seen in this model less as primary causes of infertility than as consequences of infertility that may, in turn, act as secondary causes of the continuing failure to reproduce. They are also seen as causes, paradoxically, of infertile couples' failures to adjust to *success*, which is typically defined as the achievement of pregnancy and parenthood. A more recent focus of psychological research is to discern whether there are differences in the way infertile (as opposed to normally fertile) couples experience pregnancy and parenting after infertility (e.g., Golombok et al., 1995; McMahon, Ungerer, Beaurepaire, & Tennant, 1995; McMahon, Ungerer, Tennant, & Saunders, 1997).

The depiction of the infertile as in need of psychological counseling and emotional support legitimates the need for not just any counselors but experts in infertility counseling (Covington, 1995). Indeed, a significant component of the "professionalization of infertility" (Cussins, 1998b, p. 97) has occurred not just in the domain of medicine but also outside it, in the areas of psychology and the emotions. An array of experts has emerged to compete for the care of infertile couples: to appraise their feelings toward infertility; their readiness and suitability for medical and alternative treatments, including adoption; and, to reduce their distress.

Moreover, in the depiction of infertile couples as psychologically distressed or emotionally needy lie explanations not only for treatment failures but also for why they do not seek counseling in numbers these new experts deem sufficient. Although the infertile display a range of behavioral and emotional responses, studies have increasingly demonstrated that they are largely within the range of normal psychological functioning (e.g., Berg & Wilson, 1990; Bringhenti, Martinelli, Ardenti, & La Sala, 1997; Edelmann et al., 1994; Weaver et al., 1997). The emphasis on emotions, but the failure to show serious consequences from them in the majority of infertile couples, has led some clinicians to question the call for counseling (e.g., Boivin, 1997) and some scholars to wonder whether the representation of infertile couples' emotions may not be more a product of the discourse of emotions than of infertility itself (Hunt & Meerabeau, 1993). The discourse of emotions may thus be less about validating the emotions of the infertile than legitimating the need for emotion experts.

Indeed, there is some evidence that infertile couples resist the psychological model. Although they want others to be sympathetic to the difficulties of infertility and generally view the availability of psychological services for those who need them as positive, infertile couples often do not avail themselves of these services (Boivin, 1997). Moreover, they often decline to participate in psychologically oriented research studies. Yet their nonparticipation is made "meaningful" (Lloyd, 1996) by explanations that suggest serious maladjustment (e.g., Weaver et al., 1997). This is particularly evident in the case of men who, more than women, have been reluctant to become research subjects in infertility studies (Lloyd, 1996).

As Socially Handicapped

Whereas the views of the infertile as patients in need of medical treatment or as clients in need of psychological counseling emphasize the infertile themselves, the view of the infertile as socially disabled emphasizes them in social interaction. When infertility is problematized as a social disability, the infertile are viewed as socially handicapped by virtue of their childlessness and therefore in need of social supports for adoption or living without children. Adoption is still generally regarded in the West as a second-best solution to infertility. It requires would-be adoptive parents to accept a biologically unrelated child as their own in a social milieu that favors biology as the proper basis for parental ties and birth mothers to choose relinquishment over abortion as the resolution to an unintended or otherwise "problem" pregnancy.

An alternative social solution to adoption is "childfree living" (Carter & Carter, 1989, p. 29), a new designation for a state of being and resolution to infertility in couples wanting children that is intended to stand in sharp contrast to the negative or lesser state of child*less*ness for couples when they decide against adoption. Whereas involuntary childlessness signifies a deficit, a life lived in default, or a third-best solution to infertility, childfree living signifies a proactive choice freely made. The discursive intent is to make the "childfree" couple over to resemble more closely the voluntarily childless couple who, although never wanting children, freely chose this option.

In the social model, the social and the natural are conflated as infertility appears as the fact of nature that, paradoxically, both imposes social obligations on the infertile and makes them socially suspect. Viewed as socially disabled by virtue of their childlessness, infertile couples are often also seen as the solution to the problem of another socially disabled group: namely, unwanted children or children without parents of their own. Indeed, those who criticize reproductive techniques for being antiwoman, antifamily, or antinature or anti-God implicate infertile couples for relentlessly pursuing biological parenthood when so many children have no parents. For these critics, infertility is nature's remedy for parentless children. This so-called natural remedy becomes a social remedy entailing little social change. That is, fertile couples are hardly ever asked to (and hardly ever) forgo biological reproduction in favor of adopting a child and therefore remain absolved of the responsibility for such children. Moreover, no new model of parenting is endorsed, other than the one whereby children are raised by a mother and a father who alone are considered their parents.

Yet, paradoxically, infertile couples' reproductive impairments also make them suspect as potential parents; their infertility may be seen as nature's way of signaling that they should not have children. Infertile couples may be subject to appraisal of their future parental competence as a condition for acceptance into medical treatment programs; they are always subject to appraisal before being considered acceptable adoptive parents. Infertile couples, by virtue of requiring assistance to have children, are thus subject to a kind of public scrutiny and to designations as socially "deviant"[3] that their fertile counterparts tend to escape by virtue of their not requiring such aid (de Lacey, 1998; Somerville, 1982; Steinberg, 1997).

As Consumers

In contrast to, but coexisting with, views of the infertile as medically, psychologically, or socially disabled is the view of the infertile as customers. When infertility is problematized as a consumer issue, the infertile are viewed as buyers in need of customer satisfaction. The infertile appear here as consumers in a service industry where "coitus," procreation, and "commerce" meet (Hollinger, 1985). Having a DINK (dual income, no kids), yuppie, or socioeconomically privileged couple in mind as the stereotypical consumer of infertility services, some popular media commentators and feminist writers have compared the inability of couples to have a baby to the inability to purchase other prestige commodities, such as houses and cars (e.g., Chesler, 1988; Gibbs, 1989; Quindlen, 1987). Indeed, the pursuit of these other commodities is sometimes depicted as the reason for infertility; that is, their pursuit of careers and merchandise caused the infertile to delay pregnancy too long. In a more complimentary variant of the consumer model, researchers have explored women's and couples' motivations for choosing, continuing, or stopping treatments, appropriate advertising and marketing strategies, and whether and how couples can be satisfied, even when they have failed to achieve pregnancy (e.g., Halman, Abbey, & Andrews, 1993; Sabourin, Wright, Duchesne, & Belisle, 1991; Special issue, 1997; van Balen, Verdurmen, & Ketting, 1997).

In contrast to other representations of the infertile that variously acknowledge a serious problem or need, the depiction of the infertile as consumers tends to trivialize their plight, cheapen their motivations, transform infertility into a marketing problem, or reduce having a baby to a matter of dollars and cents. As consumers, the infertile appear acquisitive, bent on satisfying only a desire, or even just plain selfish. The consumer model also masks the role that the marketing, commercialization, and professionalization of infertility have played in creating customer demand for services and in transforming conceptive techniques into "consumer products" (Condit, 1996, p. 345) for infertile couples to buy.

As Cultural Dupes and Foils

While the representations of the infertile as patients, as emotionally distressed, as socially disabled, and as customers all foreground infertility or the infertile themselves (albeit with varying degrees of sympathy and blame), there is yet another depiction of the infertile as dupes of and foils for cultural norms that are seen to require changing. When infertility is problematized as a cultural problem, both infertility and the infertile almost completely recede from view as pronatalism, patriarchalism, capitalism, and the technological imperative take center stage and are targeted for harsh criticism and reform. Problem and solution are reversed here as reproductive technology itself and the cultural norms it sustains are viewed as the problem—not infertility per se (Scritchfield, 1989a; Strickler, 1992).

An illustration of the convergence of these norms in the cultural model is the discourse—on the discourse—on "desperation" (Crowe, 1985; Franklin, 1990; Gerson, 1989; Williams, 1990). In this largely feminist discourse, infertile couples' desperation to conceive a biologically related child is constructed—by those feminists wary of or frankly opposed to assisted reproductive techniques—*as constructed* by advocates of these techniques to justify their continued use, despite their high failure and medical complication rates. What remains ambiguous in this discourse-on-discourse is whether those seeking to illuminate or to deconstruct it view desperation as "social product" or "social construct" (cf. Busfield, 1988). Infertile women in particular are presented as truly suffering from their inability to have a child, their desperation viewed as a by-product of largely antiwoman pronatalist and patriarchal norms compelling women to want to have babies at any cost to themselves and to other women. Yet infertile women are also presented as not truly desperate at all, or as not having to be desperate, but rather made to appear, or encouraged to be, desperate by physicians, drug companies, and other marketers of infertility services and products. While the *truly desperate* rendering of infertile women's experiences presents them as cultural dupes, the *not-truly-desperate* rendering presents them as cultural foils (e.g., for capitalism and technology). In both renderings, infertile women—as real and living individuals with varying responses to infertility—are hard to find.

In the largely "fundamentalist" feminist critiques (Farquhar, 1996)[4] of conceptive techniques, infertility is depicted as a patriarchally induced condition whereby women are pitted against each other by their drive to have babies (e.g., Arditti, Klein, & Minden, 1984; Corea, 1985; Raymond, 1993; Rothman, 1989; Spallone & Steinberg, 1987). In this discourse, infertile women are the privileged but not wholly rational (e.g., Koch, 1990) exploiters of often profoundly underprivileged women, wresting their babies from them via expensive traditional adoption and new surrogacy arrangements. Infertile women's ability to pay for what these critics view as unnecessary and dangerous medical treatments is pitted against other women's inability to obtain even the most basic health care services. These condemnatory depictions of infertile women have engendered, in turn, a feminist discourse critical of representations that denigrate these women, rest on unwarranted generalizations about women's experiences of infertility, and essentialize women as mothers or as patriarchal victims (e.g., Birke, Himmelweit, & Vines, 1990; Donchin, 1996; Farquhar, 1996; St. Peter, 1989; Sandelowski, 1990). Variously inhabiting all of these ostensibly pro-woman but competing discourses, infertile women appear less as agents deciding their fates than as trapped among a host of cultural and specifically feminist contradictions concerning the benefits or liabilities of both technology and motherhood for women.

As Heroic Sufferers

While the infertile are often denied the privileges of patient status and infertile women are often denied the privilege of naming their own experiences, they are accorded a privileged status as heroic sufferers when infertility is conceived as an illness. In the illness model, a product of the recent discovery in the 1980s of the person as narrating subject and of illness as narrative (e.g., Frank, 1995; Hyden, 1997; Sandelowski, 1991b), the infertile are viewed as suffering "disrupted lives" (Becker, 1994) and in need of narrative repair and reconstruction (Williams, 1984). Infertility is variously viewed as what Conrad (1987, pp. 24–27) described in a general illness context as a "lived-with," "at-risk," "stigmatizing," or "invisible" illness and as a narrative response to bodily, social, and cultural failure. That is, infertile women undergoing infertility treatments are at risk for medical complications and for feelings of failure. Although the biological factors impeding reproduction are invisible, the social fact of childlessness is visible and thereby stigmatizing. Moreover, the infertile often experience their infertility as a chronic illness because of the availability of new techniques that infertile couples may feel recurringly "compelled to try" (Sandelowski, 1991a) or because, in the case of women in particular, they feel emotionally damaged for life.

The representation of the infertile as narrating sufferers, best exemplified in ethnographic and other qualitative studies with infertile women and couples (e.g., Greil, 1991; Sandelowski, 1993), acknowledges the profound "biographical disruption" (Bury, 1982) engendered by the failure to have children and permits an aesthetic and ordered presentation of lives lived as infertile or with infertility. In the narrative-illness model, infertile couples are neither patients nor dupes but protagonists encountering the greatest obstacle of their lives and seeking to resolve the contradictions of their culture (e.g., concerning who can be a legitimate patient, who can be a legitimate parent, and the utility and morality of conceptive technology) with courage and even daring.

CONCLUSION: THE END OF INFERTILITY OR SIMPLY THE DISAPPEARANCE OF THE INFERTILE?

An effect of the invention of infertility has been the many faces of infertility. This is not surprising given the new status of infertility as a liminal phenomenon and the multiple identities and selves said to be engendered, in part, by new reproductive (and other media or medical) technologies (Cussins, 1996; Sharp, 1995; Timmermans, 1996). Yet the paradox in these multiple guises of infertility is the virtual disappearance of infertility as a phenomenological event (Riessman, 1989, p. 749), or an event that individuals experience uniquely. The "deflective power" (Woliver, 1989) of reproductive technology has shifted attention not only from how to prevent infertility and from pursuing nontechnological options for it but also from infertility and the infertile themselves. As in vitro techniques have made way for ever more spectacular reproductive and genetic feats, infertility—the ostensible reason for in vitro techniques—has increasingly been replaced as the "attention-getter" (Condit, 1996, p. 342): the target of interest and concern. Infertile couples now compete with octuplets, cloned sheep, and fantastic manipulations of egg and sperm as objects of attention and subjects for study. Reproductive technology may be putting an end to infertility as a problem of the body by circumventing impediments to procreation and by extending the "natural" end of fertility well into middle age. But by virtue of its being a necessary prelude to other technological marvels in the genetic domain, this technology is also putting an end to infertility as an experience that can be understood out of the realm of new and ever more spectacular technology.

Ethnographic and other qualitative studies of infertile couples have arguably been the most successful in maintaining the focus on individual infertile persons and in offering more nuanced descriptions of their experiences. But ethnographers, too, run the risk of using "diseases" and those affected by them for purposes that serve the ethnographic enterprise, as opposed to the affected persons themselves. For example, ethnographers have become increasingly interested in "intervening" in scientific, technological, and medical practices (e.g., Downey & Dumit, 1997) and with "defamiliarizing" taken-for-granted cultural norms and prescriptions (e.g., Franklin & Ragone, 1998, p. 5) in the health care arena. Their project is to expose the *culture* in science and technology, two entities conventionally seen as outside of culture, and thereby to "trouble" (Downey & Dumit, 1997, p. 28) their status as real and natural. Topical, or currently fashionable, diseases, especially those that permit entrée into the current "attractions" (Downey & Dumit, 1997, p. 28) of science, technology, and medicine, are an important currency in serving interests that may be far removed from those of the persons most affected by them.

In short, newsworthy diseases, such as infertility, provide a means to showcase not only the culture in every human activity but also ethnography as an action-oriented practice and ethnographers as deserving of a prominent role in making policy decisions concerning those diseases. Thus all of us, ethnographers included, who have "traded" on infertility in the hope of intervening on behalf of infertile couples must, at the very least, acknowledge the benefits we also accrue from our various "uses" of this "disease."

NOTES

1. "Western" here refers largely to Australia, western Europe, and North America.

2. These "visible" infertility patients stand in sharp contrast to those individuals, who are unmarried, and to couples, who are lesbian, from lower socioeconomic classes, or from minority groups, who want children, cannot have them on their own, but are virtually invisible as infertile. We still know much less about them and their desires.

3. The invisible infertile persons mentioned in note 2 become visible when they seek infertility services. They are conceived as doubly deviant, infertile or childless and unsuitable for parenthood or infertility services.

4. Farquhar usefully contrasted the primarily feminist but also secular "fundamentalist" discourse with the primarily medical and popular "liberal" discourse on new conceptive technology, in which these technologies are generally positively depicted as offering women new options for controlling their reproductive futures.

REFERENCES

Arditti, R., Klein, R. D., & Minden, S. (Eds.). (1984). *Test-tube women: What future for motherhood?* London: Pandora Press.

Armstrong, D. (1986). The invention of infant mortality. *Sociology of Health & Illness, 8,* 211–232.

Armstrong, D. (1990). Use of the genealogical method in the exploration of chronic illness: A research note. *Social Science & Medicine, 30,* 1225–1227.

Arney, W. R., & Bergen, B. J. (1984). Power and visibility: The invention of teenage pregnancy. *Social Science & Medicine, 18,* 11–19.

Beaurepaire, J., Jones, M., Thiering, P., Saunders, D., & Tennant, C. (1994). Psychosocial adjustment to infertility and its treatment: Male and female responses at different stages of IVF/ET treatment. *Journal of Psychosomatic Research, 38,* 229–240.

Becker, G. (1994). Metaphors in disrupted lives: Infertility and cultural constructions of continuity. *Medical Anthropology Quarterly, 8,* 383–410.

Becker, G., & Nachtigall, R. D. (1992). Eager for medicalization: The social production of infertility as a disease. *Sociology of Health & Illness, 14,* 456–471.

Becker, G., & Nachtigall, R. D. (1994). "Born to be a mother": The cultural construction of risk in infertility treatment in the U.S. *Social Science & Medicine, 39,* 507–518.

Berg, B. J., & Wilson, J. F. (1990). Psychiatric morbidity in the infertile population: A reconceptualization. *Fertility and Sterility, 53,* 654–661.

Berg, B. J., & Wilson, J. F. (1991). Psychological functioning across stages of treatment for infertility. *Journal of Behavioral Medicine, 14,* 11–26.

Berg, B. J., & Wilson, J. F. (1995). Patterns of psychological distress in infertile couples. *Journal of Psychosomatic Obstetrics and Gynecology, 16,* 65–78.

Birke, L., Himmelweit, S., & Vines, G. (1990). *Tomorrow's child: Reproductive technology in the 1990s.* London: Virago Press.

Boivin, J. (1997). Is there too much emphasis on psychosocial counseling for infertile patients? *Journal of Assisted Reproduction and Genetics, 14,* 184–186.

Brandt, A. M. (1987). *No magic bullet: A social history of venereal disease in the United States since 1880.* New York: Oxford University Press.

Brett, J. A., & Niermeyer, S. (1998). Neonatal jaundice: The cultural history of the creation and maintenance of a "disease" of newborns. In N. Scheper-Hughes & C. Sargent (Eds.), *Small wars: The cultural politics of childhood* (pp. 111–129). Berkeley: University of California Press.

Brickman, P., Rabinowitz, V. C., Karuza, J., Coates, D., Cohn, E., & Kidder, L. (1982). Models of helping and coping. *American Psychologist, 37,* 368–384.

Bringhenti, F., Martinelli, F., Ardenti, R., & La Sala, G. B. (1997). Psychological adjustment of infertile women entering IVF treatment: Differentiating aspects and influencing factors. *Acta Obstetricia et Gynecologica Scandinavica, 76,* 431–437.

Brumberg, J. J. (1988). *Fasting girls: The emergence of anorexia nervosa as a modern disease.* Cambridge, MA: Harvard University Press.

Bury, M. (1982). Chronic illness as biographical disruption. *Sociology of Health & Illness, 4,* 167–181.

Busfield, J. (1988). Mental illness as social product or social construct: A contradiction in feminists'arguments? *Sociology of Health & Illness, 10,* 521–542.

Carmeli, Y. S., & Birenbaum-Carmeli, D. (1994). The predicament of masculinity: Towards understanding the male's experience of infertility treatments. *Sex Roles, 30,* 663–677.

Carter, J. W., & Carter, M. (1989). *Sweet grapes: How to stop being infertile and start living again.* Indianapolis, IN: Perspectives Press.

Chesler, P. (1988). *Sacred bond: The legacy of Baby M.* New York: Time Books.

Clarke, A., & Montini, T. (1993). The many faces of RU486: Tales of situated knowledges and technological contestations. *Science, Technology, and Human Values, 18,* 42–78.

Condit, C. M. (1994). Hegemony in a mass-mediated society: Concordance about reproductive technologies. *Critical Studies in Mass Communication, 11,* 205–230.

Condit, C. M. (1996). Media bias for reproductive technologies. In R. L. Parrott & C. M. Condit (Eds.), *Evaluating women's health messages: A resource book* (pp. 341–355). Thousand Oaks, CA: Sage.

Conrad, P. (1987). The experience of illness: Recent and new directions. *Research in the Sociology of Health Care, 6,* 1–31.

Corea, G. (1985). *The mother machine: Reproductive technologies from artificial insemination to artificial wombs.* New York: Harper & Row.

Covington, S. N. (1995). The role of the mental health professional in reproductive medicine. *Fertility and Sterility, 64,* 895–897.

Crowe, C. (1985). "Women want it": In vitro fertilization and women's motivations for participation. *Women's Studies International Forum, 8,* 547–552.

Cussins, C. (1996). Ontological choreography: Agency through objectification in infertility clinics. *Social Studies of Science, 26,* 575–610.

Cussins, C. (1998a). Ontological choreography: Agency for women patients in an infertility clinic. In M. Berg & A. Mol (Eds.), *Differences in medicine: Unraveling practices, techniques, and bodies* (pp. 166–201). Durham, NC: Duke University Press.

Cussins, C. (1998b). Producing reproduction: Techniques of normalization and naturalization in infertility clinics. In S. Franklin & H. Ragone (Eds.), *Reproducing reproduction: Kinship, power, and technological innovation* (pp. 66–101). Philadelphia: University of Pennsylvania Press.

de Lacey, S. (1998). Assisted reproduction: Who qualifies? *Collegian, 5,* 28–36.

Demyttenaere, K., Nijs, P., Evers-Kiebooms, G., & Koninckx, P. R. (1992). Coping and the ineffectiveness of coping influence on the outcome of in vitro fertilization through stress responses. *Psychoneuroendocrinology, 17,* 655–665.

Domar, A. D., Broome, A., Zuttermeister, P. C., Seibel, M., & Friedman, R. (1992). The prevalence and predictability of depression in infertile women. *Fertility and Sterility, 58,* 1158–1163.

Donchin, A. (1996). Feminist critiques of new fertility technologies: Implications for social policy. *Journal of Medicine & Philosophy, 21,* 475–498.

Downey, G. L., & Dumit, J. (1997). Locating and intervening: An introduction. In G. L. Downey & J. Dumit (Eds.), *Cyborgs and citadels: Anthropological interventions in emerging sciences and technologies* (pp. 5–29). Santa Fe, NM: School of American Research Press.

Drewett, R. F. (1994). Uncertain comforts: The justification for treating infertility. *Journal of Reproductive & Infant Psychology, 12,* 173–178.

Edelmann, R. J., Connolly, K. J., & Bartlett, H. (1994). Coping strategies and psychological adjustment of couples presenting for IVF. *Journal of Psychosomatic Research, 38,* 355–364.

Facchinetti, F., Matteo, M. L., Artini, G. P., Volpe, A., & Genazzani, A. R. (1997). An increased vulnerability to stress is associated with a poor outcome of in vitro fertilization transfer treatment. *Fertility and Sterility, 67,* 309–314.

Farquhar, D. (1996). *The other machine: Discourse and reproductive technologies.* New York: Routledge.

Frank, A. W. (1995). *The wounded storyteller: Body, illness, and ethics.* Chicago: University of Chicago Press.

Franklin, S. (1990). Deconstructing "desperateness": The social construction of infertility in popular representations of new reproductive technologies. In M. McNeil, I. Varcoe, & S. Yearley (Eds.), *The new reproductive technologies* (pp. 200–229). New York: St. Martin's Press.

Franklin, S., & Ragone, H. (1998). Introduction. In S. Franklin & H. Ragone (Eds.), *Reproducing reproduction: Kinship, power, and technological innovation* (pp. 1–14). Philadelphia: University of Pennsylvania Press.

Gerson, D. (1989). Infertility and the construction of desperation. *Socialist Review, 19,* 45–64.

Gibbs, N. (1989). The baby chase. *Time, 134,* pp. 86–89.

Golombok, S., Cook, R., Bish, A., & Murray, C. (1995). Families created by the new reproductive technologies: Quality of parenting and social and emotional development of the children. *Child Development, 66,* 285–298.

Greil, A. L. (1991). *Not yet pregnant: Infertile couples in contemporary America.* New Brunswick, NJ: Rutgers University Press.

Greil, A. L. (1997). Infertility and psychological distress: A critical review of the literature. *Social Science & Medicine, 45,* 1679–1704.

Halman, L. J., Abbey, A., & Andrews, F. M. (1993). Why are couples satisfied with infertility treatment? *Fertility and Sterility, 59,* 1046–1054.

Halman L. J., Oakley, D., & Lederman, R. (1995). Adaptation to pregnancy and motherhood among subfecund and fecund primiparous women. *Maternal-Child Nursing Journal, 23,* 90–100.

Hirsch, A.M., & Hirsch, S. M. (1995). The long-term psychosocial effects of infertility. *Journal of Obstetric, Gynecologic, & Neonatal Nursing, 24,* 517–522.

Hollinger, J. H. (1985). From coitus to commerce: Legal and social consequences of noncoital reproduction. *Journal of Law Reform, 18,* 865–932.

Humphrey, M., & Humphrey, H. (1986). A fresh look at genealogical bewilderment. *British Journal of Medical Psychology, 59,* 133–140.

Hunt, M., & Meerabeau, L. (1993). Purging the emotions: The lack of emotional expression in subfertility and in the care of the dying. *International Journal of Nursing Studies, 30,* 115–123.

Hyden, L.-C. (1997). Illness and narrative. *Sociology of Health & Illness, 19,* 48–69.

Hynes, G. J., Callan, V. J., Terry, D. J., & Gallois, C. (1992). The psychological well-being of infertile women after a failed IVF attempt: The effects of coping. *British Journal of Medical Psychology, 65,* 269–278.

Ikemoto, L. C. (1996). The in/fertile, the too fertile, and the dysfertile. *Hastings Law Journal, 47,* 1007–1061.

Johnson, T. M. (1987). Premenstrual syndrome as a Western culture-specific disorder. *Culture, Medicine and Psychiatry, 11,* 337–356.

Klein, R., & Rowland, R. (1989). Hormone cocktails: Women as test-sites for fertility drugs. *Women's Studies International Forum, 12,* 333–348.

Koch, L. (1990). IVF: An irrational choice? *Issues in Reproductive and Genetic Engineering, 3,* 235–242.

Laffont, I., & Edelmann, R. J. (1994). Psychological aspects of in vitro fertilization: A gender comparison. *Journal of Psychosomatic Obstetrics and Gynecology, 15,* 85–92.

Lather, P. A. (1995). The validity of angels: Interpretive and textual strategies in researching the lives of women with HIV/AIDS. *Qualitative Inquiry, 1,* 41–68.

Litt, M. D., Tennen, H., Affleck, G., & Klock, S. (1992). Coping and cognitive factors in adaptation to in vitro fertilization failure. *Journal of Behavioral Medicine, 15,* 171–187.

Lloyd, M. (1996). Condemned to be meaningful: Non-response in studies of men and infertility. *Sociology of Health & Illness, 18,* 433–454.

Lloyd, M. (1997). The language of reproduction: Is it doctored? *Qualitative Health Research, 7,* 184–201.

Lorber, J. (1987). In vitro fertilization and gender politics. *Women and Health, 13,* 117–133.

McMahon, C. A., Ungerer, J. A., Beaurepaire, J., & Tennant, C. (1995). Psychosocial outcomes for parents and children after in vitro fertilization: A review. *Journal of Reproductive & Infant Psychology, 13,* 1–16.

McMahon, C. A., Ungerer, J. A., Tennant, C., & Saunders, D. (1997). Psychosocial adjustment and the quality of the mother-child relationship at four months post-partum after conception by in vitro fertilization. *Fertility and Sterility, 68,* 492–500.

Mosher, W. D., & Pratt, W. F. (1990). Fecundity and infertility in the United States, 1965–1988: Advance data. *Vital and Health Statistics of the National Center for Health Statistics, 192,* 1–8.

Nachtigall, R. D., Becker, G., & Wozny, M. (1992). The effects of gender-specific diagnosis on men's and women's response to infertility. *Fertility and Sterility, 57,* 113–120.

Paulson, R. J., Thornton, M. H., Francis, M. M., & Salvador, H. S. (1997). Successful pregnancy in a 63-year-old woman. *Fertility and Sterility, 67,* 949–951.

Peitzman, S. J. (1989). From dropsy to Bright's disease to end-stage renal disease. *Milbank Quarterly, 67,* 16–32.

Powers, P. (1996). Discourse analysis as a methodology for nursing inquiry. *Nursing Inquiry, 3,* 207–217.

Prattke, T. W., & Gass-Sternas, K. A. (1993). Appraisal, coping, and emotional health of infertile couples undergoing donor artificial insemination. *Journal of Obstetric, Gynecologic, & Neonatal Nursing, 22,* 516–527.

Quindlen, A. (1987, June). Baby craving. *Life,* pp. 23–42.

Raymond, J. G. (1993). *Women as wombs: Reproductive technologies and the battle over women's freedom.* New York: HarperCollins.

Riessman, C. K. (1989). Life events, meaning and narrative: The case of infidelity and divorce. *Social Science & Medicine, 29,* 743–751.

Rosenberg, C. E. (1989). Disease in history: Frames and framers. *Milbank Quarterly, 67(suppl. 1),* 1–15.

Rothman, B. K. (1989). *Recreating motherhood: Ideology and technology in a patriarchal society.* New York: W. W. Norton.

Sabourin, S., Wright, J., Duchesne, C., & Belisle, S. (1991). Are consumers of modern fertility treatments satisfied? *Fertility and Sterility, 56,* 1084–1090.

St. Peter, C. (1989). Feminist discourse, infertility, and reproductive technologies. *NWSA Journal, 1,* 353–367.

Sandelowski, M. (1990). Fault lines: Infertility and imperiled sisterhood. *Feminist Studies, 16,* 33–51.

Sandelowski, M. (1991a). Compelled to try: The never-enough quality of conceptive technology. *Medical Anthropology Quarterly, 5,* 29–47.

Sandelowski, M. (1991b). Telling stories: Narrative approaches in qualitative research. *Image: Journal of Nursing Scholarship, 23,* 161–166.

Sandelowski, M. (1993). *With child in mind: Studies of the personal encounter with infertility.* Philadelphia: University of Pennsylvania Press.

Schover, L. R. (1997). Recognizing the stress of infertility. *Cleveland Clinic Journal of Medicine, 64,* 211–214.

Scritchfield, S. A. (1989a). The infertility enterprise: IVF and the technological construction of reproductive impairments. *Research in the Sociology of Health Care, 8,* 61–97.

Scritchfield, S. A. (1989b). The social construction of infertility: From private matter to social concern. In J. Best (Ed.), *Images of issues: Typifying contemporary social problems* (pp. 99–114). New York: Aldine de Gruyter.

Sharp, L. A. (1995). Organ transplantation as a transformative experience: Anthropological insights into the restructuring of the self. *Medical Anthropology Quarterly, 9,* 357–389.

Sicherman, B. (1977). The uses of a diagnosis: Doctors, patients, and neurasthenia. *Journal of the History of Medicine and Allied Sciences, 32,* 33–54.

Somerville, M. A. (1982). Birth technology, parenting and "deviance." *International Journal of Law & Psychiatry, 5,* 123–153.

Sontag, S. (1990). *Illness as metaphor and AIDS and its metaphors.* New York: Anchor Books.

Spallone, P., & Steinberg, D. L. (Eds.). (1987). *Made to order: The myth of reproductive and genetic progress.* Oxford: Pergamon Press.

Special Issue on Advertising and Marketing Infertility Services. (1997). *Women's Health Issues, 7(3).*

Steinberg, D. (1997). A most selective practice: The eugenics logics of IVF. *Women's Studies International Forum, 20,* 33–48.

Stoleru, S., Teglas, J.-P., Spira, A., Magnin, F., & Fermanian, J. (1996). Psychological characteristics of infertile patients: Discriminating etiological factors from reactive changes. *Journal of Psychosomatic Obstetrics and Gynecology, 17,* 103–118.

Strickler, J. (1992). The new reproductive technology: Problem or solution? *Sociology of Health & Illness, 14,* 111–132.

Takefman, J. E., Brender, W., Boivin, J., & Tulandi, T. (1990). Sexual and emotional adjustment of couples undergoing infertility investigation and the effectiveness of preparatory information. *Journal of Psychosomatic Obstetrics and Gynecology, 11,* 275–290.

Timmermans, S. (1996). Saving lives or saving multiple identities? The double dynamic of resuscitation scripts. *Social Studies of Science, 26,* 767–797.

Treichler, P. A. (1990). AIDS, homophobia and biomedical discourse: An epidemic of signification. *Cultural Studies, 1,* 263–305.

van Balen, F., Naaktgeboren, N., & Trimbos-Kemper, T. C. (1996). In vitro fertilization: The experience of treatment, pregnancy, and delivery. *Human Reproduction, 11,* 95–98.

van Balen, F., Verdurmen, J., & Ketting, E. (1997). Choices and motivations of infertile couples. *Patient Education & Counseling, 31,* 19–27.

van der Ploeg, I. (1995). Hermaphrodite patients: In vitro fertilization and the transformation of male infertility. *Science, Technology and Human Values, 20,* 460–481.

Wasser, S. K., Sewall, G., & Soules, M. R. (1993). Psychosocial stress as a cause of infertility. *Fertility and Sterility, 59,* 685–689.

Weaver, S. M., Clifford, E., Hay, D. M., & Robinson, J. (1997). Psychosocial adjustment to unsuccessful IVF and GIFT treatment. *Patient Education & Counseling, 31,* 7–18.

Whiteford, L. M., & Gonzalez, L. (1994). Stigma: The hidden burden of infertility. *Social Science & Medicine, 40,* 27–36.

Williams, G. (1984). The genesis of chronic illness: Narrative re-construction. *Sociology of Health & Illness, 6,* 175–200.

Williams, L. S. (1990). Wanting children badly: A study of Canadian women seeking in vitro fertilization and their husbands. *Issues in Reproductive and Genetic Engineering, 3,* 229–234.

Woliver, L. R. (1989). The deflective power of reproductive technologies: The impact on women. *Women & Politics, 9,* 17–47.

Wright, J., Allard, M., Lecours, A., & Sabourin, S. (1989). Psychosocial distress and infertility: A review of controlled research. *International Journal of Fertility, 34,* 126–142.

Wright, J., Duchesne, C., Sabourin, S., Bissonnette, F., Benoit, J., & Girard, Y. (1991). Psychosocial distress and infertility: Men and woman respond differently. *Fertility and Sterility, 55,* 100–108.

THREE

Fertile Ground

Feminists Theorize Infertility

Charis M. Thompson

Infertility poses a prima facie tension for feminists. On the one hand, even in an age of decreasing birthrates, voluntary childlessness, and increasing rates of infertility, involuntary childlessness is recognized as one of the greatest forms of unhappiness and loss an adult woman might endure. Infertility is frequently experienced by would-be fathers as a source of deep sorrow and as a threat to desired kinship roles and masculinity. Nevertheless, the burden of involuntary childlessness is considered especially heavy for women, and prominent feminists have long called for it to be taken seriously as a feminist issue (Birke, Himmelweit, & Vines, 1990; Pfeffer & Woollet, 1983; Stolcke, 1986). On the other hand, feminists are also interested in disrupting the gendered role expectations and the essentialist connection between motherhood and women's identity that greatly intensify infertile women's suffering. Contemporary infertility and its treatment are conceptualized and structured on a strongly coupled, ultraheterosexual, consumer-oriented, normative nuclear family scenario. When successful, treatment enables women to reinscribe themselves into that logic. The paradox of infertility for feminism, then, is this: feminists are well placed to understand the special burden involuntary childlessness places on women, but they are ambivalent about supporting women who seek infertility treatments because it seems to lend implicit support to conventional gender roles and gendered stratification. Not surprisingly, the relationship between infertility treatment advocates (including infertile patients, medical personnel, and some social science researchers) and feminists has been strongly marked by this tension.

In this chapter I trace the evolution of views evident in the explosion of feminist work on infertility in the age of new reproductive technologies. I argue that the high-tech medicalization of infertility combines or has been presented as combining the economic, technical, rhetorical, personal, legal, and political elements through which the phases and conflicts of recent feminism have been articulated. In other words, infertility in the age of reproductive technologies has been performed as the perfect feminist text. From early feminist writings denouncing the infertility business through increasingly sensitive work on the experience and consequences of infertility, feminist treatments of infertility have come increasingly to embrace both sides of the feminist tension. Understanding the trajectory of infertility as a feminist text should go a long way toward improving the strained relations between advocates for the infertile and some feminist scholars and activists.

To advance this argument, I use a crude but handy more or less chronological distinction between phase 1 (roughly 1984–1991) and phase 2 (roughly 1992–1999) of feminist writings on reproductive technologies and infertility. Phase 1 scholarship includes the work on infertility and new reproductive technologies representative of the initial galvanization of feminists on the topic. Phase 2 includes work that has not only continued but also been critical of work in phase 1. As part of the overarching argument that infertility has been performed as the perfect feminist text, I hold that these phases have much in common with the distinction sometimes made between second and third wave feminism. Second wave feminist concerns were exemplified in the first phase of writing about infertility in the age of reproductive technologies. Just as materialist and structural-functionalist feminists were vying with mainstream liberal feminists in second wave feminism writ large, radical feminist critiques of infertility and reproductive technologies challenged liberal accounts of the technologies in the first phase of feminist engagement. The argument is even stronger regarding the second phase of writing about infertility and reproductive technologies. Not only did this phase exemplify emerging third wave, or poststructuralist, feminist concerns, such as the recasting of agency, but, in addition, the writings in this phase represented one of the sites of feminist activism and scholarship that precipitated third wave feminism.

PHASE 1: FEMINISTS ENGAGE
NEW REPRODUCTIVE TECHNOLOGIES

Shortly after the birth in England in 1978 of Louise Brown, the world's first test-tube baby, feminist theorists and activists seized on the new medicalization of infertility as an issue of special concern to women. A number of factors contributed to the rise of feminist concern about reproductive technologies. While mainstream or liberal Western feminists tended then, as they still do, to broadly support the development of biomedical reproductive techniques, on the grounds that they augment reproductive choice, the techniques acquired a resonance with the more technophobic, antieugenicist, and antipatriarchal sentiments of radical feminism. Feminist utopic longing during the 1970s for a world in which technological progress would free women from their reproductive biologies (Firestone, 1970) was all but dead among academic feminists and others by the pronatalist 1980s, and reproductive technologies were interpreted as increasing, not decreasing, subservience to one's biological destiny (Spallone, 1989). Despite the conventional antipathy between many feminists and the religious Right and antiabortion activists, that opposition to reproductive technologies might add support to these groups' agendas did not deter many feminists from decrying the procedures.

Feminist Critiques of Science, Technology, and Medicine Applied to New Reproductive Technologies

Feminist writings critical of reproductive technologies must be understood as having grown out of and in turn developing several themes that were core parts of second wave feminist scholarship on science, medicine, childbirth, and reproductive rights. First, from the mid-1970s a number of influential feminists have written about the crisis for women posed by the excessive medicalization of reproduction in the West (canonical works include Arms, 1975; Bernard, 1974; Donnison, 1977; Ehrenreich & English, 1978; Homans, 1986; Kitzinger, 1978; Martin, 1987; Oakley, 1984; O'Brien, 1981; Rich, 1976; Rothman, 1982, 1986, 1989). As they saw it, pregnancy and childbirth had become mechanized and pathologized by a patriarchal and increasingly interventionist medical establishment, such that, as Kitzinger (1978, p. 74) expressed it, many women were led to believe that if only that establishment were not around, "the pregnancy could progress with more efficiency." Their agenda was simple: a rejection of masculinist technologization and a reclaiming of "natural" childbirth by and for women. As the 1980s progressed, the use of women, particularly women of color and of the working classes, as victims of medical experimentation and the veritable litany of atrocities and absurdities women have faced at the hands of doctors throughout history were beginning to be revealed (Axelson, 1985; Davis, 1983; Ehrenreich & English, 1973; Jordanova, 1989). The connections among eugenics, medicine, and the control of women's reproduction were being patched together by a new generation of feminist scholars and activists (Ginsburg, 1989; Gordon, 1977; Luker, 1984; Petchesky, [1984], 1990). And the use of reproductive medicine to subject women to ever greater surveillance was also thematized (Terry, 1989). Likewise, by the beginning of the 1980s, feminists made up a significant contingent of the various critical science and technology movements (Bleier, 1984; Bordo, 1986; Cockburn, 1982; Cowan, 1983; Easlea,

1981, 1983; Fausto-Sterling, 1985; Fee, 1979; Hubbard, 1982; Hubbard, Henifin, & Fried, 1979; Keller, 1985; Longino and Doel, 1983; Martin, 1991; Merchant, 1980; Moscucci, 1990; Rose, 1982; Sawicki, 1991; Schiebinger, 1989; Wacjman, 1991).

The various feminist concerns were brought to bear on infertility and its supposed treatment in phase 1. Contributors to the first wave of important feminist anthologies and monographs on new reproductive technologies addressed these issues critically as they resonated with infertility medicine (Arditti, Klein, & Minden, [1984], 1989; Corea, 1985; Holmes, 1992; Holmes, Hoskins, & Gross, 1981; Klein, 1989; McNeil, Varcoe, & Yearley, 1990; Raymond, 1993; Rothman, 1986; Rowland, 1992; Scutt, 1990; Spallone, 1989; Spallone & Steinberg, 1987; Stanworth, 1987). In vitro fertilization (IVF, the making of so-called test-tube babies) was the most common aspect of infertility treatment to provoke commentary, but "artificial" or therapeutic donor insemination was also addressed. Writers warned about the technological push or momentum of the new technologies and the apparent lag in legal and social means for incorporating them responsibly. They noted the technological imperative on women to resort to expensive high-tech procedures, exerted by the mere existence of prenatal screening and infertility treatments and their "never-enough" quality (Sandelowski, 1991). The charge was renewed against reproductive technologies that patriarchal control of women's bodies was achieved through medicine. In a small number of notorious cases of infertility treatment, women taking hormones to stimulate their ovaries to produce lots of eggs at one time had died or almost died from ovarian hyperstimulation syndrome (Solomon, 1989). These cases and the physically demanding and experimental nature of the new medical infertility procedures prompted alarm that women's bodies were becoming experimental sites (Klein & Rowland, 1989). The extremely low and often misleadingly presented success rates of infertility clinics were cited as evidence of the emptiness of the promise of technological salvation for involuntary childlessness (Marcus-Steiff, 1991). As was often pointed out, treatments such as in vitro fertilization did not cure infertility even when they were successful; rather, they alleviated the condition of involuntary childlessness.

The search for safe, affordable, appropriate, and available contraceptives continued to unite liberal and radical feminists. Feminist consensus on and technological optimism about any of the new reproductive technologies, however, was hard to find in phase 1. Genetic screening and prenatal testing reeked of the potential for eugenic abuse and seemed a largely inappropriate technology in the absence of research to improve understanding of and infrastructure for disability (Rapp, 1987; Roggencamp [1984], 1989; Saxton [1984], 1989; Spallone, 1989). IVF was too expensive, dangerous, and ineffective to give many women increased reproductive choice that could then offset the patriarchal control of women's bodies enabled by the new technologies. The resolution passed at the Feminist International Network of Resistance to Reproductive and Genetic Engineering (FINRRAGE) conference in Sweden (see more on this group below), while not officially "Luddite," nonetheless called for "a different kind of science and technology that respects the dignity of womankind and all life on earth" (Spallone and Steinberg, 1987, p. 212). The dominant message was that it was "not too late to say 'no' to these technologies" (Arditti et al., [1984], 1989, p. xxi).

As far as I can tell, there were only two possible sources of optimism for new reproductive technologies among feminists in this period. The first was that of socialist feminists, for whom the march of history includes the inevitability of technological developments. Their optimism, if it can be called that, derived from the desire to direct the use of reproductive technologies toward improving women's lives by alleviating class differences. Their argument was this. Reproductive technology now exists. It cannot be undiscovered by turning back the clock. Fears about the misuse of these techniques cannot be answered by banning them but only by their being democratically controlled. Either they are going to be controlled by us for our own benefit, or they will be used by private businesses to make money from us and threaten our well-being. They cannot be independent of class society (Seal, 1990, p. 21). A number of radical feminists espoused a second possibility: namely, subverting the technologies to break down compulsory heterosexuality and facilitate lesbian parenting, either through self-insemination or through the development of parthenogenesis (Arditti et al. [1984], 1989, pp. 371–456).

Infertility and Stratification

In addition to having roots in and becoming part of second wave feminist arguments about science, medicine, and reproduction, phase 1 writings on infertility and reproductive technologies were interpolated with more overtly political feminist conversations about privacy, the family, and stratification. Stratification has always been at the heart of feminist analysis, with gender being the basis of stratification constitutive of and most consistently investigated in feminist theory. Even among nonfeminist writings, gender roles and expectations loom large when talking about infertility, so for feminist analyses of infertility, gender is of heightened significance. Stratification by class, race, age, country of origin, and able-bodiedness has also loomed large (Ginsburg & Rapp, 1995).

Interestingly, though, insofar as phase 1 writings had any global dimension at all, they tended to deal with contraceptive and prenatal technologies for the non-Western fertile Other while examining conceptive techniques for infertility only in the West. FINRRAGE, an international group that first convened in 1985, articulated the transnational reproductive politics and feminist struggles that are illustrative of this period (Franklin & McNeil, 1988). German sensitivity to the eugenic resonances of genetic engineering was evident, as were South Asian critiques of the use of prenatal testing for female feticide and other writings on son preference (Kaupen-Haas, 1988; Patel, 1987; Williamson, 1976). There was also international concern with abuses of sterilization, contraceptives testing and dumping, and access to family planning and abortion (Mies, 1987). Together, these international issues modulated the predominantly North American, Australian, and western European feminists' associations of technology and medicine with patriarchal and capitalist expansion (Spallone & Steinberg, 1987, pp. 211–212).

Furthermore, early phase 1 writings were notable for placing considerably more emphasis on concerns of structural stratification than on acknowledging or alleviating negative experiences of infertility. Toward the end of phase 1, feminist ethnography began to take women's experiences of infertility seriously for purposes other than criticizing the technologies (Modell, 1989; Stacey, 1992). In the earlier part of this period, however, some feminists went as far as to attempt to deconstruct women's desire for children and their desire for access to assisted reproductive technologies as the result of ideological duping (Crowe, 1985; see chap. 2, this volume). Because of the overwhelming focus on the perpetuation of systematic structural discrimination, feminist work in phase 1 exhibited overall a denunciatory and morally unambiguous "just say no" tone. Thus critics argued in response that feminists in this period were asking women dealing with infertility to give up their individual desire to have children in the name of the general goals of feminism.

A number of more liberally inclined feminists and other social analysts of the new reproductive technologies tried to answer these critiques with a more balanced or mainstream approach. A second round of anthologies and monographs came out that were not exactly in the genre of self-help but self-consciously addressed and included active infertility patients. These works recommended judicious stewardship of the deployment of the technologies; they suggested such commonsense correctives as better information about treatments, including the alternatives of adoption or "child-free living," better clinical standards and results, and proper discussion of and regulatory attention to discrepancies in access to treatment (Bartels, Priester, Wawter, & Caplan, 1990; Birke et al., 1990; Lasker & Borg, 1989; Rodin & Collins, 1991; Wymelenberg, 1990). Collected volumes on the ethics of reproductive technologies began to appear in this period, too, suggesting that the mainstreaming of the critique and reform of infertility medicine was in full swing (Purdy, 1989; Singer & Wells, 1985; Whiteford

& Poland, 1989). Similarly, books summarizing current and pending laws, legal precedent, and landmark cases gave order to the public's and the media's speculations about the new technical and social situations the technologies permitted (Cohen & Taub, 1989).

From the mid-1980s patients, activists, drug company representatives, professional organizations, and governments in a number of countries forged criticism and reform in a progressive, commonsense, educational idiom. There are many reasons for this, one of which was that there was wide recognition of the inevitably public and contentious nature of the issues. The market for new reproductive technologies, atypical in medicine, was also crucial. Most patients were high-paying consumers not suffering life-threatening conditions but pursuing life-defining goals. Given a patient population many of whom had the buying power to go elsewhere and had equal or greater social status than their treating physicians, the cutting edge of the field developed more like a consumer-oriented business than a state-sponsored social service (see chap. 2, this volume). Transparency and reform were market strategies.

Patient activism coordinated through organizations such as RESOLVE waged legislative battles for standards and patient information in several countries (see chap. 4, this volume). The charismatic and mediaphilic Robert Edwards met criticisms of the technologies head-on and began what has now become a characteristic of the field of infertility medicine: preemptive popular books and journal articles by prominent physicians addressing the legal and ethical issues sparked by the technologies (Edwards, 1989; see Casper [1998] for a comparison with the almost contemporaneous fetal surgery whose practitioners went out of their way to shun publicity and critique). Professional organizations such as the American Society for Reproductive Medicine (ASRM) and hormonal drug companies such as Serono began an extraordinarily efficient effort to colonize the information gap. Balanced, informative, women-friendly publications on every aspect of assisted conception from stress to donor eggs to electroejaculation to surrogacy to fibroids to adoption to the ardors of sex-on-schedule are now features of every infertility doctor's office. One result of this remarkable mainstreaming of criticism and reform was that to some extent the industry stole the ground out from under the feet of the radical critics.

This liberal, ameliorist approach seemed too complacent to many radical feminists. Had reproductive technologies simply raised the debate as to whether or not they benefited women, it is unlikely that many theorists would have advocated a simple prelapsarian rejection of them. The strength of the fear and revulsion the technologies evoked for some has to be understood in terms of the multiple systems of stratification potentially reinforced by reproductive technologies. Concerns were raised about gender, class, age, race, nationality, and species stratification, as well as the newly growing opposition between the mother-to-be and the fetus. Normalizing the technologies, as implicitly or explicitly recommended by the liberal and mainstream trends, risked rendering each of these dimensions of the technologies invisible. To many, that removal of fundamentally political matters of distributive justice from the political realm to the medicotechnical realm was simply unacceptable.

The class dimensions of reproductive technologies remained a major concern that the liberal approach could only hope to address by trickledown. The parents of the first test-tube baby, Louise Brown, were working class, and it is possible for some infertility patients to receive treatment paid for by the National Health Service at a few facilities in the U.K. and by state-subsidized health care systems in other countries. Options vary greatly by region, however, and waits for appointments are often long, which can be disastrous for older women (Seal, 1990, pp. 70–73). Disparity in access is even more striking in countries such as the United States that do not have universal health care. The cost of infertility procedures varies between countries and regions, over time, by procedure, and within procedure according to characteristics of the individuals involved. Nonetheless, a cycle of IVF, if paid for out of pocket, costs patients the equivalent of several thousand U.S. dollars. This is obviously prohibitive for most people in the world. It means that wealthy people have much better access to the procedures than do poor people. This, in turn, means that the technologies only selectively increase reproductive choice.

Given that there are limited resources for medical and other social services (cf. Ansprach, 1989) and that even those resources are unevenly distributed, some feminists questioned the spending of resources—both personal and public—on treatments like IVF. Adoption was advocated as a preferable alternative, because it spreads scarce resources better throughout society (Klein,1989, pp.18, 33–34, 109, 192–197). Some feminists noted the interconnections between race and class and argued that basic child and maternal health services for poor women and children and women and children of color should be a greater funding priority than techniques of assisted reproduction (Coalition to Fight Infant Mortality, [1984], 1989).

The other infertility practice that raised economic and cultural issues of class in an especially poignant way was conventional commercial surrogacy (Ince, [1984], 1989; Scutt, 1990). As Corea sarcastically expressed it:

> Women's bodies are not only the *recipients* of so-called treatments for infertility like *in vitro* fertilization. In the institution of surrogate motherhood, our bodies actually *become* infertility treatments. Women are hired to be artificially inseminated, to gestate a child, and then to turn that child over to the sperm donor, thereby "treating" the infertility of the sperm donor's wife. (1989, p.133; emphasis in original)

The infamous cases of surrogates Mary Beth Whitehead, who fought an unsuccessful custody battle for "Baby M," and Alejandra Munoz, who was tricked into coming to the United States from Mexico and being a surrogate for a Mexican-American couple in the belief that she was having "embryo flushing," brought the class issues to the fore. Paid surrogates are typically of considerably lower socioeconomic status than the commissioning couple, and the payment they receive for conceiving and gestating a child, together with the signed contract of intention to give up the child, is usually sufficient to override the surrogate's claim to custody. Surrogates have to make themselves somehow exempt from the general trend to the genetically based sentimentalization and decommodification of the value of children that has existed during the last century in the West (Zelizar, 1985). Drawing on class-based stereotypes, commercial surrogacy presupposes that lower-class women either have less strong sentimental ties to children to start with, are hardier and can endure their rupture more easily, are happy to give to others what comes so naturally to them (pregnancy and childbirth), or simply have greater need and so are willing to withstand the commercialization of feeling (Hochschild, 1983). While feminists in this phase generally concluded that surrogacy was not the same as slavery or baby selling (Allen, 1990), many lamented the increase in the commodification of reproduction facilitated by reproductive technologies, including surrogacy.

There were other bases of stratification that feminists feared would be exacerbated by encouraging new reproductive technologies. Age-based exploitation made the news as teenagers struggled for privacy and reproductive rights and as postmenopausal grandmothers were recruited as gestational surrogates (Cannell, 1990; Corea, 1989, p. 137). Religion continued to be a bugbear for some feminists, as it restricted many women's access to birth-preventing or birth-enabling technologies and increased pressure on infertile women by socially condemning anything other than monogamous and childbearing roles for women. There was a great deal of enthusiasm for the subversive use of reproductive technologies to enable single and lesbian women to become mothers, but feminists noted that most clinics implicitly or explicitly restricted services to heterosexual, married couples (Feminist Self Insemination Group, 1980). A less common concern was the species-ism of reproductive technologies. Nonhuman animals, including primates, were used for such routine infertility procedures as testing hormonal drugs, and the hamster test for sperm viability required superovulated mother hamsters to be sacrificed (Klein, 1989, p. 245).

This was also the period during which feminist scholars began to notice the ideological wedge being driven between a pregnant woman and her fetus. With the help of the technologies of visualization and prenatal screening that had been developed with the new infertility treatments and

fueled by antiabortion politics, a hierarchy was being set up between pregnant woman and fetus. The trend was toward considering a fetus as separate
and distinct from the woman on whose body it was dependent. This was
interpreted as an assault on the bodily integrity, right to choose, and privacy
of women (Baruch, D'Adamo, & Seager, 1988; Franklin, 1991; Ginsburg
& Tsing, 1990; Petchesky, 1987).

Thus, while in some ways the time period covered by phase 1 saw the
mainstreaming of feminist critiques of reproductive technologies, many of
the social justice issues of radical feminists remained unaddressed by
greater public accountability. The expression of these concerns sustained
the impasse between the infertile and radical feminists, because solutions
to inequalities seemed to require that infertile couples suffer personally so
as to prevent the perpetration of public wrongs for which they were hardly
responsible.

THE TRANSITION TO PHASE 2

The break between feminist theorizing in phase 1 and phase 2 was not a
clean one, and many of the major participants of the first phase continued
to be among the most significant theorists of the second. Toward the end
of phase 1, developments in the feminist literature on infertility and reproductive technologies began to reflect and add to changes that had been
occurring in feminist theory. Ways to move beyond the "just say no" politics
of the early work and address the "paradox of infertility" for feminism were
developed that did not require more radical feminists to drop their interests in stratification (Franklin & Ragone, 1998). Feminist theory in the
1970s and 1980s tended to be concerned with large-scale, structural-
functionalist explanations for gender stratification (Rosaldo & Lamphere,
1974; Rubin, 1975), but there were a few highly influential feminist texts
that offered explanations based on the psychological internalization of
learned gender-differentiated roles (Chodorow, 1978; Ortner, 1974). With
a number of theorists explicitly building on these works, a whole genre of
feminist writing appeared that valorized womanhood itself, equating it with
motherhood or using maternalist metaphors (Gilligan, 1982; Griffin, 1978;
Treblicot, 1984). Womanhood, essentialized on caring, connected, au-
thentic, antiviolent stereotypes of motherhood, was proposed as the surest
spiritual, moral, and epistemological basis for feminist change in the world
(Daly, 1978; McMillan, 1982; Ruddick, 1983). This writing valorizing
women's experience, which itself had come out of structuralist understandings of gender, paradoxically gave analysts of infertility medicine the means
to argue for the return of agency to infertile women. The argument was
made that radical feminist critics had been mistaken to deny the authen-
ticity of the maternal instinct. Whether it was socially conditioned or innate

was irrelevant; infertile women's desire to have children was more important and more substantial than simply a patriarchal mandate to reproduce (Sandelowski, 1990, 1993). This step opened feminist writing on infertility and reproductive technologies to developments in feminist poststructuralism, feminist science and technology studies, and feminist anthropology that together cemented the transition to phase 2.

Feminist poststructuralism and feminist science and technology studies galvanized the thinking on reproductive politics by the late 1980s. Poststructuralists were showing the interdependence of what I have here been calling "stratification" or "structure" and "agency" and "experience." While no one in fact wrote as if they were completely separate, many treated them for analytic purposes as being governed by different causal logics. By showing that bases for stratifying people such as gender, race, class, and sexuality are intertwined with (instead of being caused by or being the cause of) the culture, identity, and experience of group members, poststructuralists liberated feminist thinking about the problem of infertility (cf. Butler, 1990). If poststructuralism blended material and ideal, structure and agency, in ways that were stimulating for understanding the experience of infertility, the exciting new genre of feminist science and technology studies made the technologies come alive by insisting that analysts pay attention to their technical and material specificity (Haraway, 1989).

The feminist anthropologists Marilyn Strathern and Sarah Franklin and others of Strathern's colleagues and students simultaneously transformed both feminist scholarship on the new reproductive technologies and the anthropological study of kinship (Edwards, Franklin, Hirsch, Price, & Strathern, 1993; Franklin, 1997; Strathern, 1992). The very word *kinship* had come to sound primitive, and a biological understanding of descent had become thoroughly naturalized in mainstream thinking (Yanagisako & Delaney, 1995). In infertility treatments the dissociation of childbirth from biological motherhood and the polygyny involved in gestational surrogacy and egg donation sounded like exotic forms of kinship indeed, and yet they were coming out of the cutting edge of Western scientific and medical practice (Strathern, 1992). New reproductive technologies and the court cases prompted by custody battles over resultant children made biological motherhood uncertain just as DNA testing was beginning to make the notoriously uncertain facts of paternity more certain. Perhaps of even greater significance to the broader shape of feminist theory, these anthropologists embarked on a program exploring how biological narratives of the facts of life become fundamental, how and when they remain stably thus, and under what circumstances they can be denaturalized. They were joined in their endeavor to revitalize kinship studies and interrogate the multiple meanings of blood and biology in designating kin by an increasingly sophisticated anthropology of families that did not conform to the linear cognatic model. Gay parenting, families formed by public, private, and transnational adoption, ethnically based and state-sponsored initiatives to remove children from their biological parents, and circumstances under which shared blood did and did not confer kinship were all thematized (e.g., Gailey, 1998; Howell, 1998; Lewin, 1993; Modell, 1994; Strong, 1998; Weston, 1991).

Taking these strands together, the early 1990s saw a shift from the moral certainty that marked phase 1 to a tone of moral ambivalence that became the hallmark of phase 2. This change in tone in part reflected the sheer amount of public debate on new developments and the activist "biosociality" that blurred boundaries between groups that had been considered in phase 1 to have distinct interests, such as doctors and patients (cf. Epstein, 1995; Rabinow, 1992). Historians of infertility in the United States and Britain also did much to disrupt the tone and content of the phase 1 paradigm, showing the continuity of old and new reproductive technologies (Pfeffer, 1993), the existence among the poor as well as the rich of involuntary childlessness (May, 1995; Rainwater, 1960), and the surprising degree of agency exercised historically by infertile women patients (Marsh & Ronner, 1996).

The shift to phase 2 sensibilities also reflected other changes in feminist scholarship on infertility. Among other things, anthropologists and interdisciplinary feminist scholars (coming from cultural studies, science and technology studies, and women's studies) were beginning to pay close attention to the lived worlds of infertility and reproductive medicine (Becker, 1994; Cussins, 1996, 1998; Franklin, 1997; Inhorn, 1994, 1996; Layne, 1994; McNeil & Franklin, 1993; Sandelowski, 1993). From the perspective of "the belly of the beast," it turned out, for example, that doctors were and always had been a mixed bunch, at least some of whom were interested at least some of the time in the same goals as feminists; indeed, several of them were feminists, and several of them had endured personal struggles with infertility. Actors' motives, insofar as intentionality and internal states could be inferred or imputed to anyone, and the distribution of power appeared more diffuse, more mundane, more up for grabs, less conspiratorial, and more contingent than they had been portrayed in phase 1.

Science, Medicine, Technology, and Infertility

Many of the issues raised in phase 1 continued to concern writers in phase 2, but the tone had changed. A new generation of feminist scholars documented the pathologization and technologization of reproduction (Akrich & Pasveer, 1997; Davis-Floyd, 1992; Todd, 1998; van der Ploeg, 1998) but with an eye as much to examining the active role of technology in determining the semiotics of reproduction as to denouncing the adverse effects of technology for women (Clarke & Montini, 1993; Davis-Floyd & Dumit, 1998; Hartouni, 1997; Oudshoorn, 1994). Meanwhile, in the United States, for example, physicians and regulatory bodies (including the National Institutes of Health, the American Bar Association, the National Advisory Board on Ethics and Reproduction [NABER], the Society for Assisted Reproductive Technologies [SART], and ASRM) collaborated on laboratory standards, implementation of the Fertility Clinc Success Rate and Certification Act (Wyden Law) of 1992, and production of major ethics reports (Hogden, Wallach, & Mastroianni, 1994; National Institutes of Health, 1994). ASRM also supported RESOLVE in its argument to the insurance companies and to legislators that infertility should be covered as a disease or illness that needed treatment and not be considered an elective condition like cosmetic surgery. The major Anglophone journals, *Fertility and Sterility* (ASRM's official journal) in the United States and *Human Reproduction* in Britain, continued to publish timely opinions on controversial topics, often written by leaders in the field (Chung, Yeko, Meyer, Sanford, & Maroulis, 1995; Collins, 1995; Duka & DeCherney, 1994; Edwards, 1993; Egozcue, 1993; Katz, 1995; Robertson, 1996; Schenker, 1996; Seibel, Glazier Seibel, & Zilberstein, 1994; Shenfield, 1994; also see Farquhar [1996] for comment on this). Likewise, clinics (on the whole, as there are huge discrepancies between clinics) improved their understanding of the broader meanings of infertility for their patients and began to offer psychological and even debt counseling (!) (Pfeffer, 1993, p. 230). From the patients' point of view, success rates were improving from the 5 to 10 percent "take-home-baby rate" per treatment cycle, the best that could be expected in the mid-1980s, to at least double that a decade later. And by the end of the 1990s, serious attention finally began to be paid to the possible connection between superovulation and ovarian cancer and to the health, financial, and emotional burdens that typically result from high-order multiple births (Finkel, 1999).

Phase 2 writings did not exhibit a light-headed technophilia as regards the medical, scientific, and technical aspects of infertility in the age of reproductive technologies. They did not even express a liberal or socialist feminist faith in technological progress and reproductive choice. Nonetheless, they granted the technologies a much less monolithic, oppositional, and inhuman role and a much more mediating and active role than their predecessors had. They saw in the development of reproductive technologies the potential to articulate new ways of embodying reproduction, some of which would disrupt conventional families and gender stereotypes, and they refused to read new reproductive technologies as simply signing and sealing preexisting oppressive social orders. The catchphrase "every technology's a reproductive technology" was commonly cited, and captured the dual sense of the birth of new possibilities inherent in technology and the belief that women and members of historically oppressed groups should not reject but entangle themselves with "the most powerful games in town": science, technology, and medicine (Haraway, 1995, 1997). Among some, there was a sense that the fragility of the reigning social order and the potential for social change were never so great as at times of great biological innovation. The new front line was inside, not outside, the laboratory and clinic.

Stratification and Difference: Gender, Race, Class, Sexuality, Nation, Religion

If the front line was now inside the clinic and the laboratory, in terms of the medicalization of infertility, what was happening to feminist theorizing about infertility on questions of stratification and difference? Given the faltering moral certainty that came to dominate in this period, one might expect injustice and inequality to have taken a backseat to the cultural and ontological arguments that were preoccupying theorists. To some extent this was true. As we shall see, some work emphasizes "horizontal" difference (things like race and sexuality) because it is easier to conceptualize in the cultural poststructuralist terms of phase 2; thus it disproportionately ignores "vertical" stratification (primarily social and economic class) because it smacks too much of structure and phase 1 moral certainty. As in feminist theory more generally, then, phase 2 work increased sophistication on matters of "difference," but to its own detriment it lost some of its critical hold on socioeconomic status. Nonetheless, these apolitical and politically correct antidotes to the structural black-and-whiteness of phase 1 were but one manifestation, destabilized by the same observations that precipitated them: the interdependence of biological and social systems of classification and the interdependence of experience and stratification. These observations—made ethnographically, archivally, and theoretically—showed that exploring the experience of infertility and reproductive technologies revealed as much about how society is stratified as it does about what it is like to be infertile "from the inside," because the two depend on each other.

Findings about gender in feminist works written in phase 2 focused more on the mundanity of gendered orderings of the world and the extent to which we are all instinctively highly adept at complying with those orderings. Infertility patients display exaggerated stereotypical gender attributes at appropriate times during treatment, perhaps to signal their fitness to become heterosexual nuclear parents and perhaps also to rescue gender and sexual identities compromised by the lack of fertility. Patients had to act out these roles emotionally, economically, and legally to have access to treatments, which if successful allow them to reassert their station in this normative social order (Cussins, 1998; Pfeffer, 1993, p. 216). Although much remains to be done, men's role in infertility also finally began to be pried apart from an unexamined assumption of "hegemonic masculinity" (Cussins, 1999b; Schmidt & Moore, 1998). These changes in theorists' emphasis from systematic to mundane aspects of gender roles with regard to infertility were echoed in feminist theory more generally.

During the 1990s, motherhood (increasingly called "mothering," to make it an activity and not a state of being) was still very important in feminist theory, but it enjoyed neither the valorizing, essentializing kind of attention nor the denigrating, rejecting kind that it had experienced in feminist theory in the 1970s and 1980s. Instead, writers were often curious about ways women and men work with and against mothering stereotypes, are liberated and oppressed by them, and change them as they go (Chang & Forcey, 1994; Ladd-Taylor & Umansky, 1998). Writing on patriarchy and infertility no longer ignored experience but precisely found the expression of the one through the other (Inhorn, 1996). More conventional gender equality battles arising from developments in reproductive technologies, such as whether or not postmenopausal women should be allowed to have children at ages at which men still frequently become fathers, received much more coverage in mainstream venues than in feminist theory.

The discussions of both class and race in phase 2 writings about infertility and reproductive technologies focused on prenatal screening and surrogacy. Rapp's (1999) work, for one, insisted on class, race, and religion, as well as individual life experiences, as essential to the meanings and uses of prenatal screening and disability. Her empirical research left no doubt that race and class determine not just access to and uses of technology but its meaning, too, and she showed the ambivalence women often feel regarding the availability and use of reproductive technologies, which they simultaneously want and fear. Thus wholesale condemnations or promotions of the technologies are misguided; instead, political action needs to be embedded in a greater level of context specificity.

Writings about conventional surrogacy in phase 2 also continued to raise issues of class in a poignant manner. Ragone's (1994) monograph on the experiences of conventional surrogates confirmed the observations of phase 1 writers about the class dimensions of commercial surrogacy, but it also paid attention to the nonmonetary motivations surrogates had for participating and the pleasures and frustrations of the class mobility associated with being pregnant for a couple of a higher socioeconomic status.

In addition, perhaps the signature legal case taken up by phase 2 feminists interested in stratification as evidenced in assisted reproductive technologies was a gestational surrogacy case: the so-called Calvert and Johnson case. Feminist scholars took up the case to illustrate the way in which race is used as a marker of hierarchies of fit motherhood (Grayson, 1998; Hartouni, 1997, pp. 85–98). This work critically interpolated race into the question of whose body can be hired for reproductive labor, and it brought out the connections exemplified in the case among racial classification, alienated reproductive labor, perceived phenotypic resemblance, and natural descent (see Collins, 1990; Ikemoto, 1995).

Feminist theorists in phase 2 continued to be very concerned about the growing conflict between mother and fetus in industrialized countries, evidenced by increased social, legal, and medical salience and rights being accorded to fetuses (Adams, 1994; Cartwright, 1992; Casper, 1998; Daniels, 1993; Duden, 1993, 1997; Hartouni, 1997; Morgan & Michaels, 1999; Squier, n.d.; Taylor, 1992). This was part and parcel of a new and theoretically important emphasis on the question of privacy evident in this period, merging general feminist theory with feminist scholarship on infertility and the new reproductive technologies. These works plotted the relations between technologies that permit knowledge of infertility and pregnancy and the ways in which that knowledge inevitably changes which aspects of a women's body and experience are private and protected as such and which aspects are subject to public legal or medical intervention. Berlant (1997) argued that fetal personhood has become vital to contemporary U.S. ideas of citizenship and that this public fetus has paradoxically privatized, and rendered intimate and apolitical, the prevalent form of citizenship. In one way or another, many phase 2 feminists were questioning what is sometimes taken to be fundamental to feminist reproductive politics in the West: namely, the desirability of making reproduction a private matter. Some were noting that the 1980s shift in reproductive responsibility toward women was not simply a result of a feminist victory in establishing the principle of a woman's right to control her own body (Morantz-Sanchez, 1997). They argued that privatized and medicalized reproductive services were still tied into broader state policies of selective pro- and antinatalism. For example, those in the middle classes are encouraged or at least not discouraged in their efforts to have children, whereas those without work have the opposite fate (King & Harrington Meyer, 1997).

Pfeffer and others have shown that state concern about infertility and the medicalization of childlessness have been at the heart of twentieth-century politics, nationally and internationally (Dixon-Mueller, 1993; Pfeffer, 1993). Non-Western feminists writing during phase 2 have also emphasized "the relation between the order of the family and the order of the state" (Das, 1995, p. 232). It could even be argued that state concern about infertility flows from the idea of population, which is the basis of political power in the modern nation-state (Foucault, 1978; Sawicki, 1991). Phase 2 feminists have begun to show that modern nation-states still take an interest in reproduction, despite the framing of infertility in the quasi-private realms of medicine, reproductive choice, and the market.

In some ways, then, the culminating achievement of phase 2 feminist scholarship on infertility and reproductive technologies was to bring work on infertility into the framework of the transnational politics of reproduction (Ginsburg & Rapp, 1995). The extent to which reproductive labor, despite occurring in the private realm of the family and home, is nonetheless part of the broader systems of meaning and stratification that make up a given society had become increasingly apparent (Dikötter, 1998; Greenhalgh, 1995; Kanaaneh, 1997; Lurhmann, 1996; Morgan, 1997). A number of studies dealing specifically with infertility in non-Western countries showed that these dynamics also held for infertility. Thus, for example, in patriarchal societies, infertility deprives women of access to the public goods of economic protection and status because they are unable to produce children (Bledsoe, 1995, p. 133; Inhorn, 1996, pp. 1–50). Others showed the ways in which state, religious, and ethnonationalist aspirations and anxieties play themselves out on the bodies of the infertile (Feldman-Savelsberg, 1999, chap. 11, this volume; Handwerker, 1995, chap. 16, this volume; Horn, 1994; Inhorn, 1994, 1996; Kahn, 1998, chap. 15, this volume; Lurhmann, 1997). The advent of so-called procreative tourism also brought to light the need for transnational analysis of infertility in Western liberal democracies (Birenbaum-Carmeli, 1998). Such issues of reproduction and transnationalism were brought together in 1995 with the publication of Ginsburg and Rapp's pioneering edited volume, *Conceiving the New World Order* (1995), which integrated essays on transnational reproductive politics based on the notion of "stratified reproduction."

CONCLUSION: DIRECTIONS FOR THE NEW MILLENNIUM?

As evidenced by this volume, the framing of infertility in terms of the global politics of reproduction has been achieved by the end of phase 2 and has brought together recalcitrant feminist worries about stratification, the experience of infertility, and social theory in a global context. This marks a great improvement in our understanding of infertility. It also lessens the antipathy between feminists and advocates for the infertile, because it sees the experience of infertility and stratification produced by the politics of reproduction as inextricably connected and as two sides of the same feminist coin. It has also become clear that feminist theorizing about infertility does not just reflect concerns being pioneered in other areas of feminist thought and action. The cumulative feminist work on infertility and the new reproductive technologies has become one of the most fertile places for the production of new feminist theory (see Browner & Sargent, 1996).

I anticipate that these budding efforts to understand infertility and the new reproductive technologies within a framework of the stratified transnational politics of reproduction will flourish in the new millennium. I would also expect work on the relations between biology and culture to be of great help in understanding the impending genetic revolution (Andrews, 1999; Cussins, 1999a; Franklin, 1999; Nussbaum & Sunstein, 1998; Squier & Kaplan, 1999). Likewise, tracking the changing landscape of reproductive science and its effects on our ideas of personhood will aid in evolving concepts of legal and political citizenship. In short, I expect infertility to continue to be a most fertile topic for feminist action and scholarship.

REFERENCES

Adams, A. (1994). *Reproducing the womb: Images of childbirth in science, feminist theory, and literature.* Ithaca: Cornell University Press.
Akrich, M., & Pasveer, B. (1995). *De la conception à la naissance: Comparaison France / Pays-Bas des réseaux et des pratiques obstétriques.* Paris: École Nationale Supèrieure des Mines.
Allen, A. (1990). Surrogacy, slavery, and the ownership of life. *Harvard Journal of Law and Public Policy, 13,* 139–149.
Andrews, L. B. (1999). *The clone age: Adventures in the new world of reproductive technology.* New York: Henry Holt.
Anspach, R. (1989). From principles to practice: Life-and-death decisions in the intensive-care nursery. In L. Whiteford & M. Poland (Eds.), *New approaches to human reproduction* (pp. 53–69). Boulder, CO: Westview Press.
Arditti, R., Klein, R. D., & Minden, S. (Eds.). (1984, 1989). *Test-tube women: What future for motherhood?* London: Pandora Press.
Arms, S. (1975). *Immaculate deception: A new look at women and childbirth in America.* Boston: Houghton Mifflin.
Axelson, D. (1985). Women as victims of medical experimentation. *Scholarly Journal of Black Women 2(2),* 10–13.
Bartels, D., Priester, R., Wawter, D., & Caplan, A. (Eds.). (1990). *Beyond Baby M.: Ethical issues in new reproductive techniques.* Clifton, NJ: Humana Press.
Baruch, E., D'Adamo, A., & Seager, J. (Eds.). (1988). *Embryos, ethics, and women's rights: Exploring the new reproductive technologies.* New York: Harrington Park Press.
Becker, G. (1994). Metaphors in disrupted lives: Infertility and cultural constructions of continuity. *Medical Anthropology Quarterly 8,* 383–410.
Berlant, L. (1997). *The Queen of America goes to Washington City: Essays on sex and citizenship.* Durham, NC: Duke University Press.
Bernard, J. (1974). *The future of motherhood.* New York: Dial Press.
Birenbaum-Carmeli, D. (1998). Reproductive partners: Doctor-woman relations in Israeli and Canadian IVF contexts. In N. Scheper-Hughes & C. Sargent (Eds.), *Small wars: The cultural politics of childhood* (pp. 75–92). Berkeley: University of California Press.
Birke, L., Himmelweit, S., & Vines, G. (1990). *Tomorrow's child: Reproductive technologies in the 1990s.* London: Virago Press.
Bledsoe, C. (1995). Marginal members: Children of previous unions in Mende households in Sierra Leone. In S. Greenhalgh (Ed.), *Situating fertility: Anthropology and demographic inquiry* (pp. 130–153). Cambridge: Cambridge University Press.

Bleier, R. (1984). *Science and gender: A critique of biology and its theories on women*. New York: Pergamon Press.

Bordo, S. (1986). The Cartesian masculinization of thought. *Signs 11*, 439–456.

Browner, C. H., & Sargent, C. F. (1996). Anthropology and studies of human reproduction. In C. F. Sargent & T. M. Johnson (Eds.), *Medical anthropology: Contemporary theory and method* (pp. 219–234). Westport, CT: Praeger.

Butler, J. (1990). *Gender trouble: Feminism and the subversion of identity*. New York: Routledge.

Cannell, F. (1990). Concepts of parenthood: The Warnock Report, the Gillick debate, and modern myths. *American Ethnologist 17*, 667–688.

Cartwright, L. (1992). Women, X-rays, and the public culture of prophylactic imaging. *Camera Obscura, 29*, 19–56.

Casper, M. (1998). *The making of the unborn patient: A social anatomy of fetal surgery*. New Brunswick, NJ: Rutgers University Press.

Chang, G., & Forcey, L. R. (Eds.). (1994). *Mothering: Ideology, experience, and agency*. New York: Routledge.

Chodorow, N. (1978). *The reproduction of mothering: Psychoanalysis and the sociology of gender*. Berkeley: University of California Press.

Chung, P., Yeko, T., Meyer, J., Sanford, E., & Maroulis, G. (1995). Assisted fertility using electroejaculation in men with spinal cord injury: A review of literature. *Fertility and Sterility, 64*, 1–9.

Clarke, A., & Montini, T. (1993). The many faces of RU486: Tales of situated knowledges and technological contestations. *Science, Technology and Human Values, 18*, 42–78.

Coalition to Fight Infant Mortality. (1984, 1989). Equal opportunity for babies? Not in Oakland! In R. Arditti, R. D. Klein, & S. Minden (Eds.), *Test-tube women: What future for motherhood?* (pp. 391–396). London: Pandora Press.

Cockburn, C. (1982). *Brothers: Male dominance and the new technology*. London: Pluto Press.

Cohen, S., & Taub, N. (Eds.). (1989). *Reproductive laws for the 1990s*. Clifton, NJ: Humana Press.

Collins, J. (1995). An estimate of the cost of in vitro fertilization on services in the United States in 1995. *Fertility and Sterility, 64*, 538–545.

Collins, P. H. (1990). *Black feminist thought: Knowledge, consciousness, and the politics of empowerment*. New York: Routledge.

Corea, G. (1985). *The mother machine: Reproductive technologies from artificial insemination to artificial wombs*. New York: Harper & Row.

Corea, G. (1989). Surrogacy: Making the links. In R. Klein (Ed.), *Infertility: Women speak out about their experiences of reproductive medicine* (pp. 133–166). London: Pandora Press.

Cowan, R. S. (1983). *More work for mother: The ironies of household technology from the open hearth to the microwave*. New York: Basic Books.

Crowe, C. (1985). "Women want it": In vitro fertilization and women's motivations for participation. *Women's Studies International Forum, 8*, 547–552.

Cussins, C. (1996). Ontological choreography: Agency through objectification in infertility clinics. *Social Studies of Science, 26*, 575–610.

Cussins, C. (1998). Producing reproduction: Techniques of normalization and naturalization in an infertility clinic. In S. Franklin & H. Ragone (Eds.), *Reproducing reproduction* (pp. 66–101). Philadelphia: University of Pennsylvania Press.

Cussins, C. T. (1999a). Confessions of a bioterrorist: Subject position and the valuing of reproductions. In S. Squier & A. Kaplan (Eds.), *Reproductive technologies and representation* (pp. 189–219). New Brunswick, NJ: Rutgers University Press.

Cussins, C. T. (1999b). Is man to father as woman is to mother? Masculinity in contemporary U.S. infertility clinics. Paper prepared for the Unit for Criticism, University of Illinois at Urbana-Champaign, February.

Daly, M. (1978). *Gyn/ecology: The metaethics of radical feminism.* Boston: Beacon Press.

Daniels, C. R. (1993). *Women's expense: State power and the politics of fetal rights.* Cambridge, MA: Harvard University Press.

Das, V. (1995). National honor and practical kinship: Unwanted women and children. In F. Ginsburg & R. Rapp (Eds.), *Conceiving the new world order: The global politics of reproduction* (pp. 212–233). Berkeley: University of California Press.

Davis, A. (1983). *Women, race, and class.* New York: Vintage Books.

Davis-Floyd, R. (1992). *Birth as an American rite of passage.* Berkeley: University of California Press.

Davis-Floyd, R., & Dumit, J. (Eds.). (1998). *Cyborg babies: From techno-sex to techno-tots.* New York: Routledge.

Dikötter, F. (1998). *Imperfect conceptions: Medical knowledge, birth defects, and eugenics in China.* New York: Columbia University Press.

Dixon-Mueller, R. (1993). *Population policy and women's rights: Transforming reproductive choice.* Westport, CT: Praeger.

Donnison, J. (1977). *Midwives and medical men: A history of interprofessional rivalry and women's rights.* London: Heinemann.

Duden, B. (1993). *Disembodying women: Perspectives on pregnancy and the unborn.* Cambridge, MA: Harvard University Press.

Duden, B. (1997). The history of security in the knowledge of pregnancy. Paper prepared for Max Planck Institute for the History of Science workshop on epistemological security.

Duka, W. E., & DeCherney, A. H. (1994). *From the beginning: A history of the American Fertility Society.* Birmingham, AL: American Fertility Society.

Easlea, B. (1981). *Science and sexual oppression: Patriarchy's confrontation with women and nature.* London: Weidenfeld and Nicholson.

Easlea, B. (1983). *Fathering the unthinkable: Masculinity, scientists and the nuclear arms race.* London: Pluto Press.

Edwards, J., Franklin, S., Hirsch, E., Price, F., & Strathern, M. (1993). *Technologies of procreation: Kinship in the age of assisted conception.* Manchester: Manchester University Press.

Edwards, R. (1989). *Life before birth: Reflections on the embryo debate.* London: Hutchinson.

Edwards, R. (1993). Pregnancies are acceptable in post-menopausal women. *Human Reproduction, 8,* 1542–1544.

Egozcue, J. (1993). Sex selection: Why not? *Human Reproduction, 8,* 1777.

Ehrenreich, B. & English, D. (1973). *Complaints and disorders: The sexual politics of sickness*. Old Westbury, NY: Feminist Press.

Ehrenreich, B., & English, D. (1978). *For her own good: 150 years of the experts' advice to women*. New York: Doubleday.

Epstein, S. (1995). The construction of lay expertise: AIDS activism and the forging of credibility in the reform of clinical trials. *Science, Technology and Human Values, 20*, 408–437.

Farquhar, D. (1996). *The other machine: Discourse and reproductive technologies*. New York: Routledge.

Fausto-Sterling, A. (1985). *Myths of gender: Biological theories about women and men*. New York: Basic Books.

Fee, E. (1979). Nineteenth-century craniology: The study of the female skull. *Bulletin of the History of Medicine, 53*, 415–433.

Feldman-Savelsberg, P. (1999). *Plundered kitchens, empty wombs: Threatened reproduction and identity in the Cameroon Grassfields*. Ann Arbor: University of Michigan Press.

Feminist Self Insemination Group (1980). *Self insemination*. P.O. Box 3, 190 Upper Street, London N1.

Finkel, D. (1999). A human toll in the battle on infertility. *Washington Post, March 21*, p. A1.

Firestone, S. (1970). *The dialectic of sex: The case for feminist revolution*. New York: Morrow.

Foucault, M. (1978). *The history of sexuality, volume 1*. Trans. R. Hurley. New York: Pantheon.

Franklin, S. (1991). Fetal fascinations: New medical constructions of fetal personhood. In S. Franklin, C. Lury, & J. Stacey (Eds.), *Off-centre: Feminism and cultural studies* (pp. 190–206). London: Unwin Hyman.

Franklin, S. (1997). *Embodied progress: A cultural account of assisted conception*. London: Routledge.

Franklin, S. (1999). Kinship, genes and cloning: Life after Dolly. Paper prepared for Wenner Gren Foundation for Anthropological Research Symposium 124, Anthropology in the age of genetics: Practice, discourse, critique, Teresopolis, Brazil, June 11–19.

Franklin, S., & McNeil, M. (1988). Reproductive futures: Recent feminist debate of new reproductive technologies. *Feminist Studies, 14(3)*, 545–574.

Franklin, S., & Ragone, H. (Eds.). (1998). *Reproducing reproduction*. Philadelphia: University of Pennsylvania Press.

Gailey, C. W. (1998). The search for Baby Right: Race, class, and gender in U.S. international adoptive kinship. Paper prepared for the conference New directions in kinship study: A core concept revisited. Wenner-Gren Foundation for Anthropological Research, Illetas, Majorca, March 24–April 4.

Gilligan, C. (1982). *In a different voice: Psychological theory and women's development*. Cambridge, MA: Harvard University Press.

Ginsburg, F. (1989). *Contested lives: The abortion debate in an American community*. Berkeley: University of California Press.

Ginsburg, F., & Rapp, R. (Eds.). (1995). *Conceiving the new world order: The global politics of reproduction*. Berkeley: University of California Press.

Ginsburg, F., & Tsing, A. L. (Eds.). (1990). *Uncertain terms: Negotiating gender in American culture.* Boston: Beacon Press.

Gordon, L. (1977). *Woman's body, woman's rights: A social history of birth control in America.* New York: Penguin.

Grayson, D. (1998). Mediating intimacy: Black surrogate mothers and the law. *Critical Inquiry, 24,* 525–546.

Greenhalgh, S. (Ed.). (1995). *Situating fertility: Anthropology and demographic inquiry.* Cambridge: Cambridge University Press.

Griffin, S. (1978). *Woman and nature: The roaring inside her.* New York: Harper & Row.

Handwerker, L. (1995). The hen that can't lay an egg (*Bu xia dan de mu ji*): Conceptions of female infertility in China. In J. Terry & J. Urla (Eds.), *Deviant bodies: Critical perspectives on difference in science and popular culture* (pp. 358–386). Bloomington: Indiana University Press.

Haraway, D. (1989). *Primate visions: Gender, race and nature in the world of modern science.* New York: Routledge.

Haraway, D. (1991). *Simians, cyborgs and women: The reinvention of nature.* New York: Routledge.

Haraway, D. (1995). Universal donors in a vampire culture. It's all in the family: Biological kinship categories in the twentieth-century United States. In W. Cronon (Ed.), *Uncommon ground: The reinvention of nature* (pp. 321–366). New York: W. W. Norton.

Haraway, D. (1997). *Modest Witness@Second Millennium.FemaleMan© Inc. Meets Oncomouse: Feminism and technoscience.* New York: Routledge.

Hartouni, V. (1997). *Cultural conceptions: On reproductive technologies and the remaking of life.* Minneapolis: University of Minnesota Press.

Hochschild, A. R. (1983). *The managed heart: Commercialization of human feeling.* Berkeley: University of California Press.

Hogden, G., Wallach, E., & Mastroianni, L. (1994). Ethical considerations of assisted reproductive technologies. Paper prepared on behalf of the Ethics Committee of the American Fertility Society. Birmingham, AL: American Fertility Society.

Holmes, H. B. (Ed.). (1992). *Issues in reproductive technology: An anthology.* New York: Garland.

Holmes, H., Hoskins, B., & Gross, M. (Eds.). (1981). *The custom-made child? Woman-centered perspectives.* Clifton, NJ: Humana Press.

Homans, H. (1986). *The sexual politics of reproduction.* Aldershot, UK: Gower.

Horn, D. (1994). *Social bodies: Science, reproduction, and italian modernity.* Princeton, NJ: Princeton University Press.

Howell, S. (1998). Is blood thicker than water? Some issues derived from transnational adoption in Norway. Paper presented at the conference New directions in kinship study: A core concept revisited. Wenner-Gren Foundation for Anthropological Research, Illetas, Majorca, March 24–April 4.

Hubbard, R. (1982). *Biological woman, the convenient myth.* Cambridge, MA: Schenkman.

Hubbard, R., Henifin, M. S., & Fried, B. (Eds.). (1979). *Women look at biology looking at women: A collection of feminist critiques.* Cambridge, MA: Schenkman.

Ikemoto, L. (1995). The code of perfect pregnancy: At the intersection of the ideology of motherhood, the practice of defaulting to science, and the interventionist mindset of the law. In R. Delgado (Ed.), *Critical race theory: The cutting edge* (pp. 478–497). Philadelphia: Temple University Press.

Ince, S. (1984) 1989. Inside the surrogate industry. In R. Arditti, R. D. Klein, & S. Minden (Eds.), *Test-tube women: What future for motherhood?* (pp. 99–116). London: Pandora Press.

Inhorn, M. C. (1994). *Quest for conception: Gender, infertility, and Egyptian medical traditions.* Philadelphia: University of Pennsylvania Press.

Inhorn, M. C. (1996). *Infertility and patriarchy: The cultural politics of gender and family life in Egypt.* Philadelphia: University of Pennsylvania Press.

Jordanova, L. (1989). *Sexual visions: Images of gender in science and medicine between the eighteenth and twentieth centuries.* London: Routledge.

Kahn, S. (1998). Gentile sperm and rabbinic uses of non-Jewish bodies for Jewish reproduction. Paper presented at the annual meeting of the American Anthropological Association, Philadelphia, December 2–6.

Kanaaneh, R. A. (1997). Conceiving difference: Birthing the Palestinian nation in the Galilee. *Critical Public Health, 3–4,* 64–79.

Katz, M. (1995). Federal Trade Commission staff concerns with assisted reproductive technology advertising. *Fertility and Sterility, 64,* 10–12.

Kaupen-Hass, H. (1988). Experimental obstetrics and national socialism: The conceptual basis of reproductive technology. *Reproductive and Genetic Engineering: Journal of International Feminist Analysis, l,* 127–132.

Keller, E. F. (1985). *Reflections on gender and science.* New Haven, CT: Yale University Press.

King, L., & Meyer, M. H. (1997). The politics of reproductive benefits: U.S. insurance coverage of contraceptive and infertility treatments. *Gender & Society, ll,* 8–30.

Kitzinger, S. (1978). *Women as mothers: How they see themselves in different cultures.* New York: Vintage Books.

Klein, R. (Ed.). (1989). *Infertility: Women speak out about their experiences of reproductive technologies.* London: Pandora Press.

Klein, R., & Rowland, R. (1989). Hormone cocktails: Women as test-sites for fertility drugs. *Women's Studies International Forum, 12,* 333–348.

Ladd-Taylor, M., Umansky, L. (Eds.). (1998). *"Bad mothers": The politics of blame in twentieth-century America.* New York: New York University Press.

Lasker, J., & Borg, S. (1989). *In search of parenthood: Coping with infertility and high tech conception.* London: Pandora Press.

Layne, L. (1994). "Never such innocence again": Irony, nature, and technoscience in narratives of pregnancy loss. In R. Cecil (Ed.), *The anthropology of pregnancy loss* (pp. 131–152). Oxford: Berg.

Lewin, E. (1993). *Lesbian mothers: Accounts of gender in American culture.* Ithaca: Cornell University Press.

Longino, H., & Doel, R. (1983). Body, bias, and behavior: A comparative analysis of reasoning in two areas of biological science. *Signs, 9,* 207–227.

Luker, K. (1984). *Abortion and the politics of motherhood.* Berkeley: University of California Press.

Lurhmann, T. (1996). *The good Parsi: The fate of a colonial elite in a postcolonial society.* Cambridge, MA: Harvard University Press.

Marcus-Steiff, J. (1991). Les taux de 'succès' de FIV-Fausses transparences et vrais mensonges. *La Recherche, 20, 25.*

Marsh, M., & Ronner, W. (1996). *The empty cradle: Infertility in America from colonial times to the present.* Baltimore: Johns Hopkins University Press.

Martin, E. (1987). *The woman in the body: A cultural analysis of reproduction.* Boston: Beacon Press.

Martin, E. (1991). The egg and the sperm: How science has constructed a romance based on stereotypical male-female roles. *Signs, 16, 485–501.*

May, E. (1995). *Barren in the promised land: Childless Americans and the pursuit of happiness.* New York: Basic Books.

McMillan, C. (1982). *Women, reason, and nature.* Princeton, NJ: Princeton University Press.

McNeil, M., & Franklin, S. (Eds.). (1993). Procreation stories. Special issue of *Science as Culture, 3(4).*

McNeil, M., Varcoe, I., & Yearley, S. (Eds.). (1990). *The new reproductive technologies.* London: Macmillan.

Merchant, C. (1980). *The death of nature: Women, ecology, and the scientific revolution.* San Francisco: Harper & Row.

Mies, M. (1987). Sexist and racist implications of new reproductive technologies. *Alternatives, 12, 323–342.*

Modell, J. (1989). Last chance babies: Interpretations of parenthood in an IVF program. *Medical Anthropology Quarterly, 3, 124–138.*

Modell, J. (1994). *Kinship with strangers: Adoption and interpretations of kinship in American culture.* Berkeley: University of California Press.

Morantz-Sanchez, R. (1997). Coming to grips with the limitations of science: Infertility and heredity in American history. *Reviews in American History, 25, 207–212.*

Morgan, L. (1997). Ambiguities lost: Fashioning the fetus into a child in Ecuador and the United States. In C. Sargent & N. Scheper-Hughes (Eds.), *The cultural politics of child survival* (pp. 58–74). Berkeley: University of California Press.

Morgan, L., & Michaels, M. W. (Eds.). (1999). *Fetal subjects, feminist positions.* Philadelphia: University of Pennsylvania Press.

Moscucci, O. (1990). *The science of woman: Gynaecology and gender in England, 1800–1929.* Cambridge: Cambridge University Press.

National Institutes of Health. (1994). *Final report of the Human Embryo Research Panel (Muller panel).* Bethesda, MD: National Institutes of Health.

Nussbaum, M., & Sunstein, C. R. (Eds.). (1998). *Clones and clones: Facts and fantasies about human cloning.* New York: W. W. Norton.

Oakley, A. (1984). *The captured womb: A history of the medical care of pregnant women.* Oxford: Blackwell.

O'Brien, M. (1981). *The politics of reproduction.* London: Routledge & Kegan Paul.

Ortner, S. (1974). Is female to nature as male is to culture? In M. Rosaldo & L. Lamphere (Eds.), *Women, culture and society* (pp. 67–96). Stanford, CA: Stanford University Press.

Oudshoorn, N. (1994). *Beyond the natural body: An archaeology of sex hormones.* New York: Routledge.

Patel, V. (1987). Eliminate inequality, not women. *Connexions, 25,* 2–3.

Petchesky, R. P. (1984, 1990). *Abortion and women's choice: The state, sexuality, and reproductive freedom.* Boston: Northeastern University Press.

Petchesky, R. P. (1987). Foetal images: The power of visual culture in the politics of reproduction. In M. Stanworth (Ed.), *Reproductive technologies: Gender, motherhood, and medicine* (pp. 57–80). Cambridge: Polity Press.

Pfeffer, N. (1993). *The stork and the syringe: A political history of reproductive medicine.* Cambridge: Polity Press.

Pfeffer, N., & Woollett, A. (1983). *The experience of infertility.* London: Virago.

Purdy, L. (Ed.). (1989). *Hypatia: Special Issue on Ethics and Reproduction, 4(3).*

Rabinow, P. (1992). Artificiality and enlightenment: From sociobiology to biosociality. In J. Crary & S. Kwinter (Eds.), *Incorporations* (pp. 234–252). New York: Zone.

Ragone, H. (1994). *Surrogate motherhood: Conception in the heart.* Boulder, CO: Westview Press.

Rainwater, L. (1960). *And the poor get children: Sex, contraception and family planning in the working class.* With K. K. Weinstein. Chicago: Quadrangle Books.

Rapp, R. (1987). Moral pioneers: Women, men and fetuses on a frontier of reproductive technology. *Women and Health, 13,* 101–116.

Rapp, R. (1999). *Testing women, testing the fetus: The social impact of amniocentesis in America.* New York: Routledge.

Raymond, J. (1993). *Women as wombs: Reproductive technologies and the battle over women's freedom.* San Francisco: Harper.

Rich, A. (1976). *Of woman born: Motherhood as experience and as institution.* New York: W. W. Norton.

Robertson, J. (1996). Legal troublespots in assisted reproduction. *Fertility and Sterility, 65,* 11–12.

Rodin, J., & Collins, A. (Eds.). (1991). *Women and new reproductive technologies: Medical, psychosocial, legal and ethical dilemmas.* Hillside, NJ: Lawrence Erlbaum Associates.

Roggencamp, V. (1984, 1989). Abortion of a special kind: Male sex selection in India. In R. Arditti, R. D. Klein, & S. Minden (Eds.), *Test-tube women: What future for motherhood?* (pp. 266–277). London: Pandora Press.

Rosaldo, M., & Lamphere, L. (Eds.). (1974). *Women, culture and society.* Stanford, CA: Stanford University Press.

Rose, S. (Ed.). (1982). *Towards a liberatory biology: The dialectics of biology group.* London: Allison & Busby.

Rothman, B. K. (1982). *In labor: Women and power in the birthplace.* New York: W. W. Norton.

Rothman, B. K. (1986). *The tentative pregnancy: Prenatal diagnosis and the future of motherhood.* New York: Viking Press.

Rothman, B. K. (1989). *Recreating motherhood: Ideology and technology in a patriarchal society.* New York: W. W. Norton.

Rowland, R. (1992). *Living laboratories: Women and reproductive technologies.* Bloomington: Indiana University Press.

Rubin, G. (1975). The traffic in women: Notes on the "political economy" of sex. In R. Reiter (Ed.), *Toward an anthropology of women* (pp.157–210). New York: Monthly Review Press.

Ruddick, S. (1983). Maternal thinking. In J. Treblicot (Ed.), *Motherhood: Essays in feminist theory.* Totowa, NJ: Rowman & Allenheld.

Sandelowski, M. (1990). Failures of volition: Female agency and infertility in historical perspective. *Signs, 15,* 475–499.

Sandelowski, M. (1991). Compelled to try: The never-enough quality of conceptive technology. *Medical Anthropology Quarterly, 5,* 29–40.

Sandelowski, M. (1993). *With child in mind: Studies of the personal encounter with infertility.* Philadelphia: University of Pennsylvania Press.

Sawicki, J. (1991). *Disciplining Foucault: Feminism, power, and the body.* London: Routledge.

Saxton, M. (1984, 1989). Born and unborn: The implications of reproductive technologies for people with disabilities. In R. Arditti, R. D. Klein, & S. Minden (Eds.), *Test-tube women: What future for motherhood?* (pp. 298–312). London: Pandora Press.

Schenker, J. (1996). Religious views regarding gamete donation. In M. Seiber & S. Crockin (Eds.), *Family building through egg and sperm donation* (pp. 238–250). Sudbury: Jones and Bartlett.

Schiebinger, L. (1989). *The mind has no sex? Women in the origins of modern science.* Cambridge, MA: Harvard University Press.

Schmidt, M., & Moore, L. J. (1998). Constructing a "good catch," picking a winner: The development of technosemen and the deconstruction of the monolithic male. In R. Davis-Floyd & J. Dumit (Eds.), *Cyborg babies: From techno-sex to techno tots* (pp. 21–39). New York: Routledge.

Scutt, J. (Ed.). (1990). *The baby machine: Reproductive technology and the commercialization of motherhood.* London: Green Print.

Seal, V. (1990). *Whose choice? Working class women and the control of fertility.* London: Fortress Books.

Seibel, M. M., Glazier Seibel, S., & Zilberstein, M. (1994). Gender distribution— not sex selection. *Human Reproduction, 9,* 569–570.

Shenfield, F. (1994). Sex selection: A matter for "fancy" or the ethical debate? *Human Reproduction, 9,* 569.

Singer, P., & Wells, D. (1985). *Making babies: The new science and ethics of conception.* New York: Charles Scribner's Sons.

Solomon, A. (1989). Sometimes Perganol kills. In R. Klein (Ed.), *Infertility: Women speak out about their experiences of reproductive technologies* (pp. 46–50). London: Pandora Press.

Spallone, P. (1989). *Beyond conception: The new politics of reproduction.* London: Macmillan.

Spallone, P., & Steinberg, D. (Eds.). (1987). *Made to order: The myth of reproductive and genetic progress.* London: Pergamon Press.

Squier, S. (N.d.). Fetal subjects and maternal objects: Reproductive technology and the new fetal/maternal relation. Unpublished manuscript.

Squier, S., & Kaplan, A. (Eds.). (1999). *Reproductive technologies and representation.* New Brunswick, NJ: Rutgers University Press.

Stacey, M. (Ed.). (1992). *Changing human reproduction: Social science perspectives.* London: Sage.

Stanworth, M. (Ed.). (1987). *Reproductive technologies: Gender, motherhood, and medicine.* Cambridge: Polity Press.

Stolcke, V. (1986). New reproductive technologies: Same old fatherhood. *Critique of Anthropology, 6,* 5–31.

Strathern, M. (1992). *Reproducing the future: Anthropology, kinship, and the new reproductive technologies.* Manchester: Manchester University Press.

Strong, P. T. (1998). To forget their tongue, their name, and their whole relation: The contest of kinship in North America. Paper prepared for the conference New directions in kinship study: A core concept revisited. Wenner-Gren Foundation for Anthropological Research, Illetas, Majorca, March 24–April 4.

Taylor, J. (1992). The public fetus and the family car. *Public Culture, 4,* 67–80.

Terry, J. (1989). The body invaded: Medical surveillance of women as reproducers. *Socialist Review, 19,* 13–43.

Todd, A. D. (1998). *Intimate adversaries: Cultural conflict between doctors and women patients.* Philadelphia: University of Pennsylvania Press.

Treblicot, J. (1984). *Mothering: Essays in feminist theory.* Totowa, NJ: Rowman & Allanheld.

van der Ploeg, I. (1998). *Prosthetic bodies: Female embodiment in reproductive technologies.* Maastricht: Maastricht University Press.

Wacjman, J. (1991). *Feminism confronts technology.* Cambridge: Polity Press.

Weston, K. (1991). *Families we choose: Lesbians, gays, kinship.* New York: Columbia University Press.

Whiteford, L., & Poland, M. (Eds.). (1989). *New approaches to human reproduction: Social and ethical dimensions.* Boulder, CO: Westview Press.

Williamson, N. (1976). *Sons of daughters: A cross-cultural survey of parental preferences.* London: Sage.

Wymelenberg, S. (1990). *Science and babies: Private decisions, public dilemmas.* Washington, DC: National Academy Press.

Yanagisako, S., & Delaney, C. (Eds.). (1995). *Naturalising power: Feminist cultural analysis.* New York: Routledge.

Zelizar, V. (1985). *Pricing the priceless child.* New York: Basic Books.

FOUR

The Psychologization of Infertility

Frank van Balen

One of the most intriguing aspects of the study of infertility is its relationship with psychology, in particular, the various contrasting ways in which the causality of the relationship between psychological problems and infertility has been interpreted. Since biblical times, it has been noted that involuntarily childless women, such as Sarah, the wife of Abraham, frequently showed behavior that would be interpreted today as a sign of psychological problems. As there was in the past little knowledge about the process of human reproduction, various ideas about the origin of infertility have existed throughout Western history. One of these was the idea that, in one way or another, the woman caused her own infertility—for instance, through bad behavior or a disturbed mind. And in many parts of the world these ideas are still shared by a considerable segment of the population (cf. Inhorn, 1994).

In the past five decades, modern biomedicine as it pertains to infertility has taken amazing steps forward. In the early 1950s, almost no cures existed, except for artificial insemination with donated sperm (AID), and many mechanisms of infertility were not understood. The most important breakthrough regarding female infertility was the introduction in the 1950s of oocyte induction by hormonal or chemical treatment. Then, in 1977, in vitro fertilization (IVF) was first applied successfully, leading to the birth in 1978 of Louise Brown in Britain. Initially, IVF was a solution for women with tubal blockage, who before that time were mostly treated surgically (a form of treatment that generally was not very successful). Later on, IVF was also applied for many other indications, such as unexplained infertility and male infertility. During the past decade, the spectacular breakthrough of intracytoplasmic sperm injection (ICSI), a variant of IVF in which one sperm is injected directly into the oocyte, has provided a real opportunity to overcome what were once considered untreatable male infertility problems.

These advances in modern biomedicine are impressive, and, as a consequence, we know much more about the mechanisms of infertility, including its somatic and genetic causes. Nonetheless, psychological explanations of infertility linger in the literature and are reminiscent of ideas that were put forward nearly a half century ago.

In this chapter I trace the ideas about the relationship between infertility and psychological problems as they developed in the past half century within Western culture. For this analysis, I restrict myself to scientific papers and volumes in social science and medicine. I classify the explanations about the relationship between infertility and psychological problems according to four models and discuss the main line of argument of each. The four models are (1) the full psychogenic model; (2) the model that postulates the psychogenesis of unexplained infertility; (3) the psychological consequences model; and (4) the cyclical model. Although I have discerned these models based on analysis of the infertility literature, I must note a major problem with that literature: namely, many of the publications dealing with infertility and psychological problems do not clearly state the supposed direction of the relationship. In these cases I have attempted to uncover the implicit assumptions of the authors.

I also discuss the adherence to and influence of these various models since the end of World War II. For the sake of clarity, it must be stated that the rise and fall in popularity of the models cannot be demarcated clearly; thus different models have coexisted for some time. However, I try to relate the influence of the various explanatory models to important changes that were taking place in the last five decades, especially concerning new biomedical discoveries and the patient empowerment movement.

I must emphasize here my own view that research regarding the psychological causation of somatic conditions such as infertility is valid and may improve our understanding of the intricate relationships between mind and body. However, as will be clear in the following sections, my intention is to put forward a challenging critique of the often unquestioned assumption of the psychological origin of infertility, as found in the scientific literature over the past fifty years.

FULL PSYCHOGENIC INFERTILITY

In the full psychogenic model, it is supposed that all cases of infertility or sterility[1] are basically caused by psychological problems or psychological mechanisms (see fig. 1). Psychological disturbances of various kinds are perceived as generating infertility. Generally, only the female mind and body are considered to be the vehicles for this causal relationship. A potential male factor in psychological etiology is seldom discussed.

The idea that infertility is caused by psychological mechanisms within the woman may seem rather odd and outdated, but especially in the immediate postwar years, this line of thinking was very popular. As described by Ford and his coworkers, rather rapidly "a considerable literature ha[d] accumulated on the subject of psychogenic sterility." This way of thinking was not specific for infertility, for it could be said that there was "a growing awareness of the influence of the psyche on all kinds of somatic dysfunctions and disease" (Ford et al., 1953, p. 456).

An important authoritative source for the psychogenic model can be found in the extensive works of the American Freudian psychoanalyst Helene Deutsch. In her widely published books on the psychology of women (1st ed., 1945), infertility was considered. Her works appeared in several reprints, and a French translation was published in 1962. In her opinion, cases of organic infertility were in essence based on disturbed psychological functioning: "When we refer to psychological difficulties of conception, we mean that the given woman's inability to become a mother has psychic causes that have disturbed some part of the physiologic process" (Deutsch, 1947, p. 93).

Deutsch stated that unconscious anxieties over motherhood and sexuality were the underlying mechanisms leading to infertility, or, as she put it, "[T]he most frequent cause of sterility is unconscious fear." She discerned six types of women for which this situation would lead to infertility: (1) "the physically and psychologically infantile woman"; (2) "the woman who spends her rich motherliness on love for her husband"; (3) "the feminine-erotic woman, who fears the competition of motherhood with her warm, rich erotic life"; (4) "the woman who devotes her life to an ideology or another emotionally determined interest"; (5) "the masculine-aggressive woman"; and (6) "the emotionally disturbed woman" (Deutsch, 1947, pp. 99–102). Deutsch argued that although many women could be categorized into these six types, many "mixed" types also existed. Moreover, many other types of sterile women would eventually be established. Thus, according to this theory, almost every case of infertility could be related to psychogenic causes. Adding fuel to this theory, Theresa Benedek (1952), another leading psychoanalyst, pointed to a "hostile mother identification" as a distinctive form of psychopathology among infertile women.

Two points are especially surprising. First, given that women psychoanalysts initiated this psychological model, it is interesting that the psychological functioning of the male is not taken into account at all. Second, at that time the idea of psychogenic infertility was even applied to cases in which physical obstructions existed. According to Deutsch, physical ob-

1. Psychogenic model

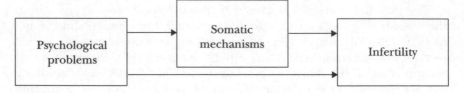

2. Psychogenic explanation of unexplained infertitlity

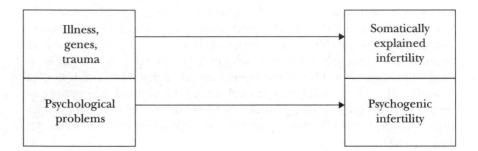

3. Psychological-effect model

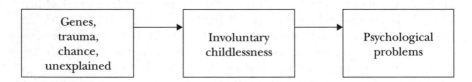

4. Cyclical model

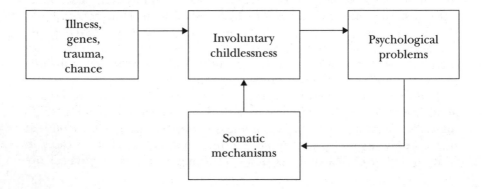

structions were secondary causes. For example, even in the case of blocked fallopian tubes, a somatic origin was questioned and a psychogenic explanation was proposed (Ford et al., 1953). As late as 1979, Foldes and Foldes (1979) described tubal occlusion as generated by spasms or temporary occlusions that, in turn, had a psychogenic origin.

This psychodynamic perspective, in which unconscious drives and unresolved psychological problems generate infertility, was prominent in Western psychological and medical thinking after World War II. Many psychiatrists and clinical medical specialists supported these ideas, and in a large number of studies, it was implicitly assumed that psychogenic and social factors were the causes for infertility. For example, the prominent gynecologist, Kroger (1963), stated that hidden anxieties of pregnancy and motherhood are the essential causes of infertility and that resolving these problems would lead to pregnancy. He suggested that infertile women renunciate their careers in order to free their feelings of motherliness, which in turn might bring about the long-desired pregnancy. In addition, a wide range of symptoms were thought to indicate a psychosomatic problem leading to infertility; stuttering was perceived as one of these symptoms (Schellen, 1960).

A telling illustration of the significant influence of the psychogenic model is evident in the proceedings of the congresses of the International Society of Psychosomatic Obstetrics and Gynecology, a large international organization that was initiated by psychologically minded gynecologists. The society holds triannual congresses attended by many hundreds of physicians and psychologists. In the proceedings during the 1970s and early 1980s (Carenza & Zichella, 1979; Dennerstein & De Senarclens, 1983; Hirsch, 1975; Morris, 1972), about half of the contributions covering infertility or sterility adopted a full psychogenic model, whether explicit or implicit. Even as late as 1988, Bydlowski and Dayan-Lintzer (1988) presented a study, based on psychodiagnostic interviews with one hundred infertile women, in which they concluded that an unresolved psychological problem was the fundamental cause of infertility in all cases. Although they discarded Deutsch's idea about the psychological profiling of the "sterile" woman, their central thesis was that "a latent psychological conflict always underlies complaints of infertility" (Bydlowski & Dayan-Lintzer, 1988, p. 139).

THE PSYCHOGENIC DEFINITION OF UNEXPLAINED INFERTILITY

In the decades after Deutsch forwarded her ideas about psychogenic infertility, many somatic causes of infertility were definitively proven. For example, it became widely acknowledged that genetic factors, certain illnesses, and infections could result in infertility, without the involvement of any psychological factors. However, initially at least, there were a large percentage of infertility cases in which no somatic cause could be found. These cases were often deemed "unexplained infertility," the term I use here, and were often perceived as having psychogenic origins. For example, in the 1960s, 40 to 50 percent of infertility cases were unexplained and were hence deemed the result of emotional factors (Eisner, 1963). By the early 1980s, it was still estimated that about 15 percent of cases were unexplained and hence psychologically implicated (Templeton & Penney, 1982).

It is important to note that the very act of measuring the percentage of unexplained infertility cases is a difficult task. For instance, the moment of measurement influences the magnitude of the percentage, as more difficult cases take longer to diagnose. To make things even more confusing, the terms "functional infertility" and "idiopathic infertility" have both been used as synonyms for unexplained infertility, meaning that no clear-cut causal factor for the infertility has been found. In addition to these three purportedly neutral terms, "psychogenic infertility" and "psychosomatic infertility" have also been used. Clearly, these latter two terms suggest psychogenic causality.

Until the beginning of the 1980s, when studies of IVF took off and rapidly became the major topic, almost all of the nonmedical studies of infertility were aimed at discovering the relationship between psychological problems and infertility, particularly of the unexplained type. Often the direction of the causal relationship between these two variables was not stated at all or was left implicit. However, according to Bell (1981), most of the studies suggested psychological factors in the etiology of infertility rather than psychological consequences *of* infertility (the model described below). Indeed, a large number of studies considered unexplained infertility psychogenic, even though the existence of somatically explained infertility was also recognized (see fig. 1; e.g., Demyttenaere, Nijs, Steeno, Koninckx, & Evers-Kieboom, 1988; Kemeter & Eder, 1982; Kemeter, Eder, & Springer-Kremser, 1985; Kipper, Zigler-Shani, Zerr, & Insler, 1977; Nijs, Koninckx, Verstraete, Mullens, & Nicany, 1984; Pesch, Weyer, & Taubert, 1989; Sandler, 1965; Sandler, 1968; Stolevic, Hajdukovic, & Markovic, 1979).

In some of these studies, the psychoanalytic typecasting first developed by Deutsch can be discerned. For instance, Kemeter et al. (1985, p. 527) describe "an ambivalent, symbiotic mother-daughter relationship of the 'clinging type' " (similar to Deutsch's type one), which proves to be a "pathogenetic concept" resulting in female sterility. However, it is clear that during the 1980s, the focus of the papers on infertility at the congresses of the International Society of Psychosomatic Obstetrics and Gynecology shifted from a full psychogenic model (described above) to a model concerning the psychogenic origins of unexplained infertility.

Today, the psychogenic model of unexplained infertility still has some supporters. One possible way to support this view scientifically would be to find that unexplained infertile persons display higher levels of psychological problems when compared with infertile persons for whom a somatic cause has been established. Indeed, Wasser and coworkers (Wasser, Sewall, & Soules, 1993) concluded on the basis of such an empirical study that conflict with father, hostility, anxiety, and phobic anxiety were more pronounced among infertile individuals for whom anatomic causes of infertility were less evident. They advised, therefore, that "if the body has evolved to respond to certain stressors by temporarily suppressing reproductive processes," then there should be "therapeutic removal or modifications of those stressors" (Wasser et al., 1993, p. 689). However, many other empirical studies have not shown significant differences regarding various psychological indicators between persons with unexplained infertility and persons with somatically explained infertility (Brand, Roos, & van den Merwe, 1982; Daniluk, 1988; Domar, Seibel, Broome, Friedmann, & Zuutermeister, 1992; Kipper et al., 1977; Mai, Munday, & Rump, 1972; Paulson, Haarman, Salerno, & Aimar, 1988; van Balen & Trimbos-Kemper, 1994).

Recently, a series of papers with a psychogenic orientation appeared in the major biomedical journal *Human Reproduction* (Christie 1998; Sanders & Bruce, 1997). The tone of some of these advocates of psychogenesis is much more modest and tentative than before. Nonetheless, Sanders and Bruce (1997) postulated that psychosocial stress could inhibit conception and conducted a study among thirteen women, using a large number of independent psychological variables. They found a significant difference regarding two variables (mood state and day-to-day vexations); and although this result may well be a "chance effect," they concluded that relief from stress indeed promotes fertility. Christie (1998, p. 232), furthermore, lamented the "failure to accept the importance of psychological and psycho-social influences upon human fertility" and acknowledged that "[t]here has been a tendency on our part to support an assumption that this will require proving the infertile are more psychiatrically ill or psychologically disturbed than their fertile counterparts." Nonetheless, he states that "[c]linical experience also suggests that a link can exist between unexplained infertility and a deep sensitivity within the individual, at an unconscious level, to some situation rendering it an unsuitable time or place to allow the arrival of a baby" (1998, pp. 232).

This kind of reasoning, however, has been thrown into question by the significant increase in somatic explanations for infertility that has taken place in recent years. Indeed, as more insight has been gained into the workings of the human body and the processes of fertilization and implantation, the percentage of unexplained infertility cases has steadily decreased over time. In particular, knowledge regarding genetic defects of oocytes and semen—for instance, deletions on the Y chromosome—has expanded. In addition, the intricacies of fertilization and nidation (the grafting of the embryo in the lining of the uterus), as well as problems in these areas, have become the subject of intensive research, and since the 1980s a great deal of attention has been given to the influence of hormones on pregnancy chance (Dennerstein & De Senarclens, 1983; Dennerstein & Fraser, 1986; van Hall & Everaerd, 1989).

It is also important to note that one explanation of unexplained infertility is based on a chance model. According to this model, (almost) every couple has a certain chance to reach a pregnancy during each cycle. For normal fertile couples, this chance, depending on female age, varies from 15 to 25 percent. In other words, the chance of becoming pregnant is compared to throwing dice with the odds of 15/100 and 25/100, respectively. Following this model, some couples will always, or at least over a very long period, have bad luck. According to this model, in the case of an odds ratio of 20/100, 4.3 percent of couples will remain childless after two years (Leridon & Spira, 1982). So, to summarize, this model suggests that part of the incidence of unexplained infertility can simply be explained by bad luck.

As more and more becomes known about human fertility and infertility, the percentage of cases of unexplained infertility will decrease even further. However, the complex influence of hormones and other fluids on the process of fertilization, nidation in the uterus, and embryonic growth are still not completely clear. Therefore, this leaves room for theories about potential psychological stressors in unexplained infertility.

THE PSYCHOLOGICAL CONSEQUENCES MODEL

The theory of psychological consequences has been dominant during the past decade, but can be traced back to the early 1980s (Domar et al., 1992). In this model, causality is reversed. It is assumed that infertility—rather than being caused by psychological stressors—may instead lead to psychological problems, such as stress, anxiety, depression, low self-esteem, sexual dysfunction, and other health complaints. Infertility itself is perceived as something that is caused by genetic, somatic, or traumatic (such as accidental) factors. Psychological distress, in turn, is supposedly caused by infertility, its treatment, or the resulting state of childlessness (see fig. 1).

Indeed, Brkovich and Fisher (1998, p. 218) conclude in a short review of studies about psychological distress and infertility that "[m]ost physicians today agree that infertility may cause depression and anxiety, but few are convinced that the opposite is true." Furthermore, Greil (1997, p. 1682) argues on the basis of an extensive and thorough review of the literature on infertility and psychological distress that "[m]ost contemporary studies assume that infertility is the source, rather than the cause, of psychological distress." As most of the studies reviewed by Greil show, there are no significant differences in psychological distress among persons with unexplained infertility and persons with somatically explained infertility.

Nonetheless, the number of empirical studies that have been carried out according to the psychological consequences model among couples with infertility problems is relatively small. There are many more studies on IVF and the various psychological aspects of that treatment than on the psychological consequences of infertility per se. Most of these studies, furthermore, use a cross-sectional design, in which an infertile group is compared with a control group (e.g., Abbey, Andrews, & Halman, 1991). Or some studies of infertile couples have compared their responses to standard values on indicators of psychological problems, such as anxiety scales, depression scales, and measures of physical well-being (e.g., Daniluk, 1988; Freeman, Boxer, Rickels, Tureck, & Mastroianni, 1985; Stanton, Tennen, Affleck, & Mendola, 1991; van Balen & Trimbos-Kemper, 1993). These studies have shown significant differences between infertile women and fertile women regarding various indicators of psychological and physical well-being. Differences among men were far less pronounced.

Although Greil (1997) has demonstrated that a large number of these studies have methodological shortcomings, the evidence is still so robust that he reaches two major conclusions. The first is that infertility itself is a stressful and identity-threatening experience. The second is that infertile persons, especially women, show a raised level of distress but that this distress does not normally extend into the clinically significant range. Taken together, these conclusions do not lend support to the psychogenic model, insofar as it may be supposed that a "mild" level of distress is not serious enough to bring about infertility. A light or moderately raised level of stress is more in line with the psychological consequences model. On the other hand, the psychological consequences model is not entirely supported. For one, the various studies show "effects" on different subsets of indicators of psychosocial stress. Furthermore, a few of the studies do not show any significant differences between fertile and infertile persons on various psychological measures.

To date, what is still lacking is a methodologically rigorous longitudinal study of women and men who are followed from well before their attempts to have a child to well after—the only way the psychological consequences model can truly be "proven." If such a study were to be conducted, psychological indicators measured before starting these attempts should demonstrate approximately equal values between two groups: namely, those who later prove to be fertile and those who later prove to have an infertility problem. However, the latter group should have raised values once their infertility is discovered when compared with fertile men and women.

THE CYCLICAL MODEL

Old ideas sometimes reappear in new guises. Such is the case with the fourth and final model, which I call the cyclical model.

It is now generally accepted that infertility is a negative life event and therefore may result in a raised level of stress. For example, a representative Dutch national study investigated the public attitude toward involuntary childlessness. It appeared that 73 percent of the women and 50 percent of the men questioned considered childlessness to be one of the most serious, negative experiences facing an individual (NIPO, 1996). Some researchers suppose that the levels of stress that arise as a consequence of childlessness may have an influence on the final outcome: that is, of having a child. In this way, a cyclical model can be envisioned in which infertility leads to stress and the resulting stress influences the chance of a pregnancy, whether or not medical technology is used (see fig. 1).

The cyclical model can be discerned in studies by O'Moore and coworkers. They postulate that whether or not psychological factors are the cause or the effect of infertility, "the psychological disturbance is likely a source of stress which may interfere with the hormonal balance" (O'Moore, O'Moore, Harrison, Murphy, & Carruthers, 1983). It is tacitly assumed that there are individual differences in stress levels, which lead to differences in levels of hormones, such as prolactin. Next it is assumed that these different hormone levels have a significant influence on pregnancy chance and, more specifically, that high stress levels eventually lead to a lower chance of pregnancy.

Since the beginning of the 1980s, a large number of studies have been carried out from the premise that high stress levels influence hormone levels and other relevant bodily fluids in a negative way with respect to fertility (e.g., Demyttenaere, 1990; Ehlert, Heim, & Rösner, 1995; Harper, Lenton, & Cooke, 1985; Jürgesen & Bardé, 1983; Pepperell, 1981; Sobrinho, Nunes, Calhaz-Jorge, Santos, & Sousa, 1983). In a sense, through such studies, the theory of psychogenic causation of infertility has been resurrected. Various attempts are being undertaken to measure both psychological and physiological stress values and to connect these with pregnancy chance. The chance of success of IVF outcome has become an especially important area of research. For instance, Stoléru and coworkers (1997) explored various independent variables and concluded that female perception of marital harmony, which plausibly is influenced by the partner's support in experiencing childlessness, is a statistically significant predictor of successful in vitro fertilization.[2]

The relationship between stress and IVF outcome is the subject of much medical-psychological research and can now be considered a separate and specific field within infertility studies. However, these studies have yet to prove unambiguously that psychogenic mechanisms exist to influence pregnancy chance. It appears that this research often "capitalizes on chance findings" (i.e., using a large number of independent, sometimes post hoc, composed variables). Moreover, there are large contradictions regarding the proposed psychogenic mechanism (e.g., about the causative hormone and about the relevant moment of influence). In almost all the published studies, furthermore, the specific IVF-treatment stressors are not analyzed in their relationship to general psychological aspects of infertility and childlessness.

It is also important to point out that the potential influence of male stress on the vitality of the sperm is seldom considered in such IVF stress studies. Interesting in this regard are emerging contradictory findings about raised stress levels and semen. At least one study established a positive relationship between high stress and high semen quality and quantity (Poland, Giblin, Ager, & Moghissi, 1986). This result raises two salient issues that are not discussed by proponents of the cyclical model: First, does male stress matter? And, second, is a (moderately) raised level of stress counterproductive in all cases? For instance, in a recent study on the possible positive effects of sodium restriction on anxiety during IVF, it was reported as an "aside" that increase in anxiety was significantly higher among women who conceived as compared to those who did not (Beerendonk et al., 1999). (The sodium restriction itself did not have any influence, interestingly.)

THE PSYCHOLOGIZATION OF INFERTILITY AND ITS CONSEQUENCES

Psychological theory over the past fifty years has given strong credence to the idea of psychogenic origins of infertility. Regardless of the direction of causality, infertility and psychic stress, in Western culture at least, are perceived to be strongly associated. Strikingly, the psychologization of infertility has been focused almost exclusively on the female patient, although a relationship between stress and infertility may also be operative within the male partner.

What are the repercussions of this psychologization for infertility patients themselves? I argue here that there are a number of important consequences.

Psychogenic Diagnosis

First, because of ongoing psychologization, a considerable number of physicians still approach infertility as psychogenic, although in a more veiled way. Today, these physicians usually do not explicitly follow a psychogenic model but still often advise patients (mostly women) to "have a rest," "take a vacation," or "come to terms with your personal problems." Advice to relax, not to ponder one's condition, and not to be concerned is regularly given, at least in the first stages of infertility treatment. From letters to the magazine of the Dutch patient organization (*Freya,* 1985–1999), it appears that physicians still regularly call on psychogenic diagnoses in advising their patients to postpone and avoid medical treatment.

Furthermore, in the leading gynecological journal *Fertility and Sterility,* Domar, Seibel, and Benson (1990, p. 246) reported a "role for stress reduction in the long-term treatment of infertility" and proposed "that behavioural treatment should be considered for couples with infertility." In the same journal, Wasser, Sewall, and Soules (1993, p. 689) proposed that "therapeutic removal or modifications of those stressors should be among the most effective ways of reversing this [negative: FvB] reproductive response." Again in a recent study, Domar et al. (2000) concluded that psychological group therapy raises the chance of viable pregnancies.

Such psychogenic diagnosis of infertility by physicians in clinical settings, as well as proposals for psychological therapy, may have important consequences for the patient, usually the female partner. The patient may feel that she is to blame for the infertility. Hence, she may experience decreased self-respect and self-esteem, which may already be diminished by the inability to bear children. It may also make it more difficult for the patient to come to terms with childlessness. Indeed, continuing psychogenic diagnosis of infertility could be considered a source of "iatrogenic" stress in and of itself.

Psychological Research

A second and at present more frequent source of possible iatrogenic stress for the infertile patient is probably the pressure to participate in various psychological research projects. Infertility patients undergoing treatment are desired subjects for psychological research. In many infertility centers, couples are asked, and often gently pressed, to fill in all kinds of questionnaires or participate in semistructured or in-depth interviews about their well-being and associated subjects.

There are several reasons for this. First, evaluation programs concerning new reproductive technologies are initiated by the clinic or by government agencies. Women and sometimes men are interrogated about physical and psychological burdens of the treatment, as well as the psychological consequences of failed treatment. Because of fears about the well-being of children born following these treatment protocols, these children are also extensively investigated and followed, to establish whether they show genetic defects or any other physical or psychological disturbances during their later development (for a review, see van Balen [1998]). Second, a considerable number of studies are carried out regarding psychological, somatic, and demographic variables that may influence the outcome of the treatment (see also the section on the cyclical model). Clinics want to raise their treatment success rates and are looking for variables that may lead to superior results. Third, there still is some research being conducted that follows a psychogenic orientation, which requires extended psychological questionnaires and in-depth interviews.

These areas of psychological research are steered primarily by medical interests and are carried out in medical centers. Consent for participation in the relevant study is asked by or on behalf of the treating medical doctor; questionnaires are handed out and even answered in a clinic or hospital; observations are done in a medical setting; and the aims of the studies are set or at least controlled by members of the medical profession. Because patients are dependent on the goodwill of the medical staff who handle their oocytes, sperm, and embryos, they may be reluctant to refuse cooperation.

Thus it appears rather usual that a person in Western society who is undergoing a "modern" infertility treatment is confronted with psychological questionnaires of one kind or another. Being infertile and seeking treatment makes couples already "accountable" to others in their everyday lives. Often, questions are asked by family members, friends, and acquaintances about (1) why they are having so much trouble having a child and then (2) why they are troubling themselves with so much medical intervention to have a child. Added to this is the frank intrusion on the part of researchers in infertility treatment centers.

Patient Empowerment

Although ongoing psychogenic diagnoses and the frequent exposure to psychological research may negatively influence the self-esteem of the infertility patient, two developments have strengthened the patient's position, at least in Western societies. The first is patient organization and empowerment, and the second is the emergence of counseling that is carried out based on the needs and perspectives of infertile persons.

Empowerment of patients suffering from various illnesses has been an important development in recent years. Patients and parents or other family members of patients have frequently organized themselves in influential voluntary societies. Not surprisingly, perhaps, persons with infertility problems have organized in national associations, often with chapters in many regions. These associations fulfill various functions, including providing a supportive environment for infertile people, organizing self-help groups, providing counseling and advice, collecting and giving information, following and monitoring medical developments, reporting on abuses, pressing for easy availability of new medical treatments, and discussing alternatives such as adoption or fostering. Such associations exist today in the United States (since 1974), the U.K. (since 1976), the Netherlands (since 1985), Canada (since 1987), Australia (since 1987), France (since 1988), New Zealand (since 1989), Denmark (since 1990), Iceland (since 1990), Switzerland (since 1992), Germany (since 1995), and Italy (since 1995). These kinds of associations are of enormous influence on the well-being of infertile people, and they can serve to counter negative associations and public images of the childless. They may also be powerful counterweights to the interests of the medical profession and the pharmaceutical industry. Moreover, of special relevance to this discussion, they can change the image of the "helpless, psychologically disturbed patient" and make it more difficult for physicians to present infertility as a kind of self-inflicted psychosomatic disease.

Infertility Counseling

From the 1950s through the early 1970s, professional or specialized counseling regarding infertility was nonexistent. During that era, childlessness was considered a taboo subject in the strict sense: a thing not spoken about with people other than one's partner (Vermeer & Stoeten, 1980). However, since that time, infertile persons have played an important role in stimulating the development of individual and group counseling that is carried out from the subjects' perspective.

At present, there are branches of social services and professional therapists who specialize in this field. For instance, the magazine of the Dutch infertility patient organization carries the advertisements of infertility counselors and psychotherapists of various inclinations. Also, the state-funded Dutch federation of institutes for unwed mothers has for a few years now added counseling and psychotherapy of infertile couples to its core task, partly because of the dwindling number of teenage mothers—and thus babies available for adoption—in the Netherlands. In addition, in cooperation with patient organizations, individual or group information and counseling are offered by various infertility clinics. Finally, and probably most important, patient organizations themselves offer counseling and information (such as telephone helplines) by persons who are "experience-experts," as well as organize self-help groups. An important feature of this kind of information and counseling is that it is done from the perspective of the infertile person.

CONCLUSION

In closing, it is important to point out that models positing a psychological origin for infertility can be considered a traditional "Western" type of explanation. Such models offered a solution for the explanation of infertility at a time when biomedical progress in infertility treatment was still in its inchoate stage of development. The psychogenic model is built on systematic and theoretical grounds, such as psychoanalysis, and therefore is different from old ideas in Europe about the origins of infertility, such as secret relationships with demons and dwarves and the power of witches and sorcerers (Nave-Herz, 1988). Still, the psychogenic model is in some respects reminiscent of the long and steady Western tradition of seeking to have a baby with spiritual help, such as by the use of amulets, magic stones and elixirs, devotion to the holy Anna, the mother of Maria, and by seeking alternative medicine, such as homeopathy and the assistance of various healers such as haptonomists, iriscopists, and hypnotists.[3] In a certain way, the continuing attraction of "New Age" ideas can be perceived as an ongoing sign of such Western "psychospiritual" thinking.

In the past fifty years, the somatic causes of infertility have become increasingly clear and effective treatments have become available. Therefore, psychogenic explanations of infertility have lost ground. However, as I have suggested, they have not disappeared completely, even though the relationship between psychological problems and infertility remains to be proven. In the case of psychogenic infertility, it is plausible that the psychological problems must be rather severe to produce an effect; however, studies have overwhelmingly shown that the intensity of the psychological problems of infertile persons are not in the clinical range.

Proving the direction of causality between psychological factors and infertility will require a costly and large-scale, long-term prospective study. It must be carried out among a representative sample of women and men, of whom the fertile/infertile status is still unknown. In fact, the study must be initiated before the couple attempts to have a child. Psychological variables should be measured at regular time intervals and compared with the occurrence of infertility problems. To reach conclusive results, related psychological variables should show a coherent pattern. Finally, such a study should not only be aimed at establishing significant differences, but also the magnitude of effects, if any.

On the other hand, the idea that the Western biomedical model will in due course "explain away" every case of psychologically induced infertility looks unlikely. Psychological stress may indeed play a role in disturbing hormonal processes, in timing of ovulation, and in influencing other factors of fertility—although these effects appear not to be so decisive, frequent, straightforward, and continuous as formerly expected.

Unfortunately, the ongoing psychologization of infertility evident in treatment centers may reinforce the different status and stigma of infertile couples. Because of the differences in resources and status between the medical and the psychological disciplines (Bourdieu, 1988), it is the medical profession that sets the terms for research in most cases. Most psychological studies in the West in the field of infertility are therefore aimed at answering medically oriented questions. Because IVF centers still have meager success rates, on the average of about 20 percent per cycle, every possibility, including the detrimental effect of various psychological stressors, is being explored in an effort to raise low percentage rates. Often, the infertile person appears to be an "incidental" subject of this medically oriented research. Sociologically or anthropologically motivated studies in which childlessness is investigated for its experiential and social sequelae are not part of the established research agenda.

In summary, over the past fifty years, the psychologization of infertility has been—and continues to be—implicitly accepted by many psychologists and gynecologists, rather than treated as something tentative. Furthermore, the psychogenic model is essentially "victim blaming" and, through its application by various Western biomedical and psychological professionals, unintendedly has served to increase rather than decrease the suffering of infertile women and men. The psychogenic model places the cause of infertility squarely in the mind of the infertile person. This "blame the victim" notion is not specific to infertility. Other illnesses, for instance, cancer and asthma, are also supposed to have a psychological component. It is often suggested that people have to fight these sicknesses through "positive thinking."

Needless to say, the psychological victimization of the infertile has not made psychogenic infertility popular among associations of childless persons. This type of causal argument has become more difficult to sell, given the collective organization of infertile persons in many Western countries. It can now be said that in many Western societies infertile patients are in the process of forming coalitions against the power of the medical establishment and its psychological associates to "psychologize" them as patients. Thus the process of psychologization is changing, and research today is becoming more positively attuned to the needs and interests of childless couples in the forms of counseling and individual support. This transformation has been accomplished in part through the creation and expansion of independent associations of infertile persons, which, in the West at least, have become an immensely important resource in helping to alleviate some of the suffering—psychic and otherwise—associated with infertility.

NOTES

1. In the older literature, the term "sterility" is mostly used; however, in the more recent literature, the term "infertility" dominates. See also chapter 2 in this volume. In this chapter, "infertility" is used.

2. Nonetheless, the results of this study can be criticized for the post hoc definition of the instrument and the unexplained relationship between processes in the human body and their effects in the petri dish, where in vitro fertilization takes place.

3. In a recent Dutch national study, it appeared that about 10 percent of the infertile respondents used alternative medicine (van Balen, Verdurmen, & Ketting, 1995).

REFERENCES

Abbey, A., Andrews, F. M., & Halman, L. J. (1991). Gender's role in response to infertility. *Psychology of Women Quarterly, 15,* 295–316.

Beerendonk, C., Hendriks, J., Scheeper, H., Braat, D., Merkus, J., Oostdam, B., & Van Dop, P. (1999). The influence of dietary sodium restriction on anxiety levels during an in vitro procedure. *Journal of Psychosomatic Obstetrics and Gynecology, 20,* 97–103.

Bell, J. S. (1981). Psychological problems among patients attending an infertility clinic. *Journal of Psychosomatic Research, 25,* 1–3.

Benedek, T. (1952). Infertility as a psychosomatic defense. *Fertility and Sterility, 3,* 80–86.

Bourdieu, P. (1988). *Homo Academicus.* Cambridge: Polity Press.

Brand, H. J., Roos, S. S., & van den Merwe, A. B. (1982). Psychological stress and infertility, part II: Psychometrical test data. *British Journal of Medical Psychology, 55,* 385–388.

Brkovich, A. M., & Fisher, W. A. (1998). Psychological distress and infertility: Forty years of research. *Journal of Psychosomatic Obstetrics and Gynecology, 19,* 218–228.

Bydlowski, M., & Dayan-Lintzer, M. (1988). A psycho-medical approach to infertility: "Suffering from sterility." *Journal of Psychosomatic Obstetrics and Gynecology, 9,* 139–151.

Carenza, L., & Zichella, L. (Eds.) (1979). *Emotion and reproduction: 5th international congress of psychosomatic obstetrics and gynaecology.* London: Academic Press.

Christie, G. L. (1998). Some socio-cultural and psychological aspects of infertility. *Human Reproduction, 13,* 232–242.

Daniluk, J. C. (1988). Infertility, intrapersonal and interpersonal impact. *Fertility and Sterility, 49,* 982–986.

Demyttenaere, K. (1990). *Psychoendocrinological aspects of reproduction in women.* Louvain: Peeters.

Demyttenaere, K., Nijs, P., Steeno, O., Koninckx, P., & Evers-Kieboom, G. (1988). Anxiety and conception rates in donor insemination. *Journal of Psychosomatic Obstetrics and Gynecology, 8,* 174–181.

Dennerstein, L., & De Senarclens, M. (Eds.). (1983). *The young women, psychosomatic aspects of obstetrics and gynaecology, invited papers of the 7th International Congress on Psychosomatic Obstetrics and Gynaecology, Dublin, Ireland, 11–15 September 1983.* Amsterdam: Excerpta Medica.

Dennerstein, L., & Fraser, I. (Eds.). (1986). *Hormones and behaviour, proceedings of the 8th International Congress of the International Society of Psychosomatic Obstetrics and Gynaecology, Melbourne, 10–14 March 1986.* Amsterdam: Excerpta Medica.

Deutsch, H. (1947). *The psychology of women: A psychoanalytical interpretation.* Vol. 2, *Motherhood.* 1st ed. New York: Grune and Stratton; London: Research Books.

Domar, A. D., Clapp, D., Slawsby, E. A., Dusek, J., Kessel, B., & Freizinger, M. A. (2000). Impact of group psychological interventions on pregnancy rates in infertile women. *Fertility and Sterility, 73,* 805–811.

Domar, A. D., Seibel, M. D., & Benson, H. (1990). The mind/body program for infertility: A new behavioral treatment approach for women with infertility. *Fertility and Sterility, 53,* 246–249.

Domar, A. D., Seibel, M. D., Broome, A., Friedmann, R., & Zuutermeister, P. C. (1992). The prevalence and predictability of depression in infertile women. *Fertility and Sterility, 58,* 1158–1163.

Ehlert, U., Heim, C., & Rösner, A. (1995). Behavioral medicine in gynecology: Psychoendocrinological correlates of female infertility. In J. Bitzer & M. Stauber (Eds.), *Psychosomatic obstetrics and gynaecology* (pp. 301–308). Bologna: Monduzzi.

Eisner, B. G. (1963). Some psychological differences between fertile and infertile women. *Journal of Clinical Psychology, 19,* 391.

Foldes, J. J., & Foldes, J. A. (1979). Psychosomatic sterility in a selected group of educated career women. In L. Carenza & L. Zichella (Eds.), *Emotion and reproduction* (pp. 277–281). London: Academic Press.

Ford, E. S. C., Forman, I., Wilson, J. R., Char, W., Mixson, W. T., & Scholz, C. (1953). A psychodynamic approach to the study of infertility. *Fertility and Sterility, 4,* 456–465.

Freeman, E. W., Boxer, A. S., Rickels, K., Tureck, R., & Mastroianni, L., Jr. (1985). Psychological evaluation and support in a program of in vitro fertilization and embryo transfer. *Fertility and Sterility, 43,* 48–53.

Freya (formerly *Nieuwsbrief NVRB*). 1985–1999. Magazine of Freya, the Dutch association of patients with infertility problems, Wijchen.

Gerris, J. M. R. (1998). *A comparative investigation into the real efficacy of conventional therapies versus advanced reproductive technology in male reproductive disorders.* Antwerp: Universiteit van Antwerpen.

Greil, A. L. (1997). Infertility and psychological distress: A critical review of the literature. *Social Science & Medicine, 45,* 1679–1704.

Harper, R., Lenton, E. A., & Cooke, I. D. (1985). Prolactin and subjective reports of stress in women attending an infertility clinic. *Journal of Reproductive & Infant Psychology, 3,* 3–8.

Hirsch, H. (Ed.). (1975). *The family, 4th International Congress of Psychosomatic Obstetrics and Gynaecology, Tel Aviv, October 27– November 2, 1974.* Basel: Karger.

Inhorn, M. C. 1991. Umm Il-Ghayyib, mother of the missing one: A sociomedical study of infertility in Alexandria, Egypt. Ph.D. dissertation, University of California, Berkeley.

Jürgensen, O., & Bardé, B. (1983). Psychodynamic findings in women with elevated prolactin. In L. Dennerstein & M. De Senarclens (Eds.), *The young women: Psychosomatic aspects of obstetrics and gynaecology* (pp. 138–148). Amsterdam: Excerpta Medica.

Kemeter, P., & Eder, A. (1982). A diagnostic instrument to evaluate the psychosomatic background of gynaeco-endocrinal disturbances and functional sterility. In H. J. Prill & M. Stauber (Eds.), *Advances in psychosomatic obstetrics and gynaecology* (pp. 224–226). Berlin: Springer-Verlag.

Kemeter, P., Eder, A., & Springer-Kremser, M. (1985). Psychosocial testing and pretreatment of women for in vitro fertilization. *Annals of the New York Academy of Sciences, 442,* 523–532.

Kipper, D. A., Zigler-Shani, Z., Zerr, D. M., & Insler, V. (1977). Psychogenic infertility, neuroticism and feminine role: A methodological inquiry. *Journal of Psychosomatic Research, 21,* 353–368.

Kroger, W. S. (1962). Evaluation of personality factors in the treatment of infertility. In W. S. Kroger (Ed.), *Psychosomatic obstetrics, gynecology, and endocrinology* (pp. 361–371). Springfield, IL: Charles C. Thomas.

Leridon, H., & Spira, H. (1984). Problems in measuring the effectiveness of infertility therapy. *Fertility and Sterility, 41,* 580–586.

Mai, F. M., Munday, R. N., & Rump, E. E. (1972). Psychosomatic and behavioural mechanisms in psychogenic infertility. *British Journal of Psychiatry, 120,* 199–204.

Morris, N. (Ed.). (1972). *Psychosomatic medicine in obstetrics and gynaecology, third international congress, London, March 29–April 2, 1971.* Basel: Karger.

Nave-Herz, R. (1988). *Kinderlose Ehen: Eine empirische Studie über die Lebenssituation kinderloser Ehepaare und die Gründe für ihre Kinderlosigkeit* (Childless marriages: An empirical study about the life and circumstances of childless couples and the reasons for their childlessness). Weinheim, Munich: Juventa.

Nijs, P., Koninckx, P. R., Verstraete, D., Mullens, A., & Nicany, H. (1984). Psychological factors of female fertility. *European Journal of Obstetrics, Gynaecology and Reproductive Biology, 18,* 3–14.

NIPO. (1996). *Kinderwens in Nederland, een tijdloze wens?* (The desire to have a child in the Netherlands, is it of all times?). Amsterdam: NIPO.

O'Moore, A. M., O'Moore, R. R., Harrison, R. F., Murphy, G., & Carruthers, M. E. (1983). Psychosomatic aspects in idiopathic infertility: Effects of treatment with autogenic training. *Journal of Psychosomatic Research, 27,* 145–151.

Paulson, J. D., Haarman, B. S., Salerno, R. L., & Aimar, P. (1988). An investigation of the relationship between emotional adjustment and infertility. *Fertility and Sterility, 49,* 258–262.

Pepperell, R. J. (1981). Prolactin and reproduction. *Fertility and Sterility, 35,* 267–274.

Pesch, U., Weyer G., & Taubert, H.-D. (1989). Coping mechanisms in infertile women with luteal phase insufficiency. *Journal of Psychosomatic Obstetrics and Gynecology, 10,* 15–23.

Poland, M. L., Giblin, P. T., Ager, J. W., & Moghissi, K. S. (1986). Effects of stress on semen quality in semen donors. *International Journal of Fertility, 31,* 229–231.

Sanders, K. A., & Bruce, N. W. (1997). A prospective study of psychosocial stress and fertility in women. *Human Reproduction, 12,* 2324–2329.

Sandler, B. (1968). Emotional stress and infertility. *Journal of Psychosomatic Research,* *12,* 51–19.

Sandler, D. M. R. (1965). Conception after adoption: A comparison of adoption rates. *Fertility and Sterility, 16,* 313–332.

Schellen, A. M. C. M. (1960). Een onderzoek naar de aanwezigheid van psychogene en sociale factoren als mogelijke oorzaken van primaire dan wel secundaire huwelijksonvruchtbaarheid bij 680 echtparen (A study of psychogenic and social factors as potential causes of primary and secondary infertility within marriage among 680 couples). *Nederlands Tijdschrift voor Verloskunde en Gynaecologie, 60,* 94–117.

Sobrinho, L. G., Nunes, M. C. P, Calhaz-Jorge, C., Santos, M. A., & Sousa, M. F. F. (1983). Psychosomatic component of the pathogenesis of prolactinomas and other hyperprolactinemic conditions. In L. Dennerstein & M. De Senarclens (Eds.), *The young women: Psychosomatic aspects of obstetrics and gynaecology* (pp. 149–157). Amsterdam: Excerpta Medica.

Stanton, A.L, Tennen, H., Affleck, G., & Mendola, R. (1991). Cognitive appraisal and adjustment to infertility. *Women and Health, 17,* 1–15.

Stoléru, S., Cornet, D., Vaugeois, P., Fermanian, J., Magnin, F., Zerah, S., & Spira, A. (1997). The influence of psychological factors on the outcome of the fertilization step of in vitro fertilization. *Journal of Psychosomatic Obstetrics and Gynecology, 18,* 203–212.

Stolevic, E., Hajdukovic, C., & Markovic, M. (1979). Psychological factors and treatment of infertility. In L. Carenza & L. Zichella (Eds.), *Emotion and reproduction* (pp. 327A–329A). London: Academic Press.

Templeton, A. A., & Penney, G. C. (1982). Unexplained infertility: The incidence, characteristics and prognosis of patients whose infertility is unexplained. *Fertility and Sterility, 37,* 175–182.

van Balen, F. (1998). Development of IVF children. *Developmental Review, 18,* 30–46.

van Balen, F., & Trimbos-Kemper, T. C. M. (1993). Long-term infertile couples: A study of their well-being. *Journal of Psychosomatic Obstetrics and Gynecology, 14,* s53–s60.

van Balen, F., & Trimbos-Kemper, T. C. M. (1994). Factors influencing the well-being of long-term infertile couples. *Journal of Psychosomatic Obstetrics and Gynecology, 15,* 157–164.

van Balen, F., Verdurmen, J. E. E., & Ketting, E. (1995). *Zorgen rond onvruchtbaarheid, voornaamste bevindingen van het nationaal onderzoek naar gedrag bij onvruchtbaarheid* (Caring about infertility: Main results of the national survey about behavior regarding infertility). Delft: Eburon.

van Hall, E. V., & Everaerd, W. (Eds.). (1989). *The free woman, women's health in 1990s. Invited papers of the 9th International Congress on Psychosomatic Obstetrics and Gynaecology.* Casterton Hall: Parthenon.

Vermeer, M., & Stoeten, R. (1980). *Het taboe, gesprekken over kinderloosheid* (Taboo, talking about childlessness). Amsterdam: Meulenhoff.

Wasser, S. K., Sewall, S., & Soules, M. R. (1993). Psychosocial stress as a cause for infertility. *Fertility and Sterility, 59,* 685–689.

PART II

Gender and Body Politics

FIVE

Infertile Bodies

Medicalization, Metaphor, and Agency

Arthur L. Greil

From the vantage point of the discourse of medicine, infertility is the failure to conceive a child after twelve months of unprotected intercourse. From the vantage point of American infertile women, however, infertility is a major disruption in one's projected life course, a failure to live up to normative notions about what it means to be an adult woman in American society, and a challenge to the stability and quality of social relationships. Such personal and social tragedies are frequently the occasion for cultural dramas in which important themes and tensions in a society are brought into clear relief (Becker, 1990; Greil, 1991a; Sandelowski, 1993).

The simultaneously biological, personal, and social drama of infertility is played out in the woman's body (Greil, 1991a, p. 65). Regardless of which partner in an infertile couple is ultimately discovered to have the biological "problem," it is the woman who fails to become pregnant. It is in her body that the emotional rollercoaster of midcycle hopefulness followed by end-of-cycle disappointment is played out. Regardless of which partner has a "problem," it is the woman who is the focus of most infertility treatment. Even if a woman's partner has low sperm count, it is her body that is the locus of artificial insemination or in vitro fertilization (IVF). It is her basal body temperature and her blood levels that must be monitored. It is the woman's body, then, that is most often subjected to the medical gaze.

For the middle-class American women discussed in this chapter, the medicalization of infertility is a fait accompli. These infertile women conceptualize infertility as an organic problem susceptible to a technical solution and see their gynecologists as the "natural" people to whom to bring their concerns (Greil, 1991a, p. 74). According to Conrad and Schneider (1980), medicalization occurs at three levels: conceptual, institutional, and doctor-patient interaction. To say that for middle-class

American women infertility has become medicalized is to say that it is conceptualized in conformity with the biomedical model and with American understandings of health, illness, and the sick role. It is to say also that authoritative knowledge concerning infertility has been deemed the province of medical specialists, who have the exclusive right and obligation to treat it in accordance with the institutional constraints of professional medicine. Finally, the medicalization of infertility implies that the infertile take on the role of patients, subject to the conditions of doctor-patient interaction, including a passive role for the patient and physician dominance over face-to-face interaction (Fisher, 1986; Katz, 1984; Mishler, 1984; Waitzkin, 1991; West, 1984).

A number of works in recent decades have pointed to the importance of attending to the metaphors found in medical discourse about bodies, especially women's bodies (Barker-Benfield, 1976; Davis-Floyd, 1992; Ehrenreich & English, 1979; Kahn, 1995; Martin, 1987, 1988, 1994; Rothman, 1989; Young, 1997). The prevalence of mechanical metaphors, inspired by Cartesian dualism, has long been recognized as a fundamental feature of the culture of modern biomedicine (Osherson & Amara-Singham, 1981). In the biomedical model worldview, the body is seen as analogous to a machine made up of interdependent parts, any of which can malfunction. Given this metaphor, the focus of the culture of medicine is not so much on the person considered as a whole as on the diseased organ (Fisher & Todd, 1983; Mizrahi, 1986; Scully, 1980). Causes of disease other than organic ones existing within the individual are not considered worthy of consideration. The focus of treatment is on eliminating, fixing, or bypassing the malfunctioning part. And if bodies appear under the medical gaze as machines, then women's bodies are often viewed as *flawed* machines requiring expert intervention (Davis-Floyd, 1992; Martin, 1987).

Some students of women's health have gone a step farther, arguing that American medicine has based its image of reproduction on metaphors drawn from the realm of *production*. When Clarke (1988) writes that reproduction has become industrialized, she intends to convey that it has become subject to rational control via the same techniques that have been brought to bear in factory production. Childbirth, for example, has become an enterprise of mass production, supervised by trained specialists, dependent on expensive and sophisticated equipment, and managed according to principles of rational efficiency. In similar fashion, Martin (1987) posits that biomedicine views the female body as a factory, with the women as laborers under the supervision of physician-managers. One clear implication of the factory model of reproduction is that it is the physician, not the "woman in the body," who is conceptualized as being in control. In her analysis of American birth practices, Davis-Floyd argues that American ob-stetrics operates with a "technocratic model of birth." According to Davis-Floyd (1992, p. 152), hospital birth rituals convey clear messages "about the necessity for cultural control of natural processes, the untrustworthi-ness of nature and the associated weakness and inferiority of the female body, the validity of patriarchy, the superiority of science and technology, and the importance of institutions and machines."

Although much has been written about the metaphors that inform bi-omedicine and about the messages conveyed by biomedical practices, less has been written about the responses of American women to these messages and metaphors. The works of Davis-Floyd (1992) and Martin (1987) are two well-known attempts to look not just at medical messages and meta-phors but at women's responses to them as well. As described by Davis-Floyd, women's responses range from full acceptance of the technocratic model of birth through full acceptance of the "wholistic" model of birth, with the majority falling somewhere in between. Martin (1987, pp. 184–187) observed six responses to the medical definition of women's bodies: (1) acceptance, (2) lament, (3) nonaction (boycotting), (4) sabotage, (5) resistance, and (6) rebellion.[1]

Although Davis-Floyd and Martin have made significant contributions to the social scientific understanding of the medicalized body, their analyses share a common flaw in that they treat women's responses as an epiphe-nomenon of medical definitions. Both analyses give primacy of place to medical constructions of reality; women's options seem limited to either acquiescing to medical metaphors and interpretations or resisting them. Neither analysis makes enough room for women's creativity and agency in working within the medical framework to achieve their own ends. Missing from Martin's list of responses to medical definitions is the response that seems most striking among the middle-class infertile women who are the subject of this study: working the system. Like the vast majority (70%) of the women Davis-Floyd interviewed, these women were to a greater or lesser degree in "conceptual harmony" with the biomedical model. But at the same time that these women bought in to the biomedical model, they subtly transformed it to better match their own experiences and to better meet their own goals.

I argue here that infertile women do not respond passively to medical definitions of them but react actively and strategically; they work the system and try to push medical treatment in the direction they want it to go. In-fertile women are neither passive victims of biomedicine nor uncritical con-sumers wanting to take advantage of all available medical technology. Rather, they are problem solvers, operating creatively within a system they do not control.

RESEARCH DESIGN

Data for this chapter come from in-depth, tape-recorded interviews conducted with twenty-two married, infertile couples in western New York
State. Husbands and wives were interviewed simultaneously in their homes
by two separate interviewers. This chapter makes use primarily of material
from the wives' interviews.[2]

The couples in the sample were considerably better off than the national
average in terms of annual family income and education.[3] It is clear that
this sample is not representative of the U.S. infertile population as a whole.[4]
These couples can be presumed to have much greater access to medical
and other resources for coping with infertility and greater exposure to
infertility treatment than the infertile population at large.[5]

The sample included couples with a wide range of medical, reproductive, and family growth histories. Infertility was the result of a female reproductive factor in nine cases, of a male reproductive factor in four, and
of a combination of male and female reproductive factors in six. In the
remaining three cases, the source of the couple's infertility had not been
identified.[6] Of nineteen couples who were involuntarily childless at the start
of their infertility treatment, fourteen had achieved some measure of success in their quest for a child by the time of the interview.

Although most of the couples interviewed had children in the home by
the time the interviews were conducted, they generally (excluding, of
course, the three cases of secondary infertility) exhibited a strong tendency
to discuss their "prechild" days at great length. Thus, to the extent that
respondents discussed what they *had* experienced rather than what they
were currently experiencing, these data suffer from some of the drawbacks
that characterize all retrospective data. Furthermore, individuals who survey the past from the vantage point of present success may develop strikingly different accounts from those who view it from the perspective of
continued failure. Like all data collected by interview techniques, the data
reported here must be understood as couples' interpretive *accounts* of their
attitudes and behaviors rather than as objective records of those attitudes
and behaviors.

INFERTILE WOMEN AND THEIR BODIES

Body as Machine

The prominence of the "body as machine" metaphor and the concomitant
mind/body dualism that characterize biomedicine have already been discussed. What, one might ask, do infertile women say about their *own* bodies? Several ethnographic studies have addressed the question of cultural

metaphors concerning infertility in non-Western societies (Feldman-Savelsberg, 1999; Handwerker, 1995; Inhorn, 1994, 1996). Becker (1994, 1997) has analyzed the metaphoric content of infertility narratives in the American context, but her concern has been to explore the role of metaphor in dealing with disruptions to the life course rather than to examine women's responses to culturally available metaphors.

Given that infertility is a failure to achieve a desired biological and social state, one might expect infertile women to describe infertility in terms of the failure of the body. This was, in fact, the case. Talk of infertility as a failure of the body to work properly was common for these women. When Karen[7] was asked about how infertility has affected her relationship with Brett, the body as machine metaphor came through clearly in her answer:

> I mean it's my body that's not working, it's my body we have to fix. His body is working, and I don't resent his body for working. His body has to work for it to work, but my body also has to work.

Karen was virtually unique among the women in this sample in drawing a clear distinction between her body and her self:

> I see myself as separate from my body. I resent my body; I don't resent myself. Right now I feel like I'm a victim of a lousy package. It doesn't mean I'm not a good person, it just means my body's not working.

But the vast majority of these infertile women made no distinction between failed bodies and failed selves. They seem to experience infertility as a generalized role failure, not just as a failure of the body. Barbara, for example, was more typical: "I had this feeling of failure, an overwhelming image of failure as a baby machine and as a woman." Lynn's words reveal that she sees her defective body, not as something she *has,* but as something she *is:* "I would consider that I am subfertile and that I do need correction." Given cultural definitions that define "motherhood" as an essential component of "womanhood," it should not come as a surprise that so many of these women saw infertility in this way.

Barbara and Lynn, like many other infertile women in the sample, have a tendency to mix their metaphors. They speak of their bodies as machines but rarely refer to them *only* as machines. More often they seem to think about their bodies simultaneously as machines in the service of the self and as integral parts of self. Barbara says she has failed as a baby machine *and* as a woman. Lynn uses the technical term "correction" but identifies *herself,* not just her body, as that which is in need of correction. Despite the power of the body as machine metaphor, it is not the only image of the body that operates either in American culture generally or in the culture of medicine specifically. Synott (1992, 1993) has delineated a number of metaphors for understanding the body that have coexisted in the Western cultural tradition. While the machine metaphor may conflict with and often override these other metaphors, one does not obliterate the other. Infertile women live in several metaphoric worlds at once; they can call on different vocabularies, sometimes simultaneously, to express the ways infertility has affected them.

Body as Emblem of the Self

Another powerful metaphor that exists both in medicine and in the general culture is the notion of the body as the emblem of the self (Synott, 1992, 1993). We are routinely held responsible for our bodies: we are praised for their virtues and blamed for their failures. Sandelowski (1990) has made this point specifically with regard to infertility. There exists a large body of social scientific literature attesting to the fact that bodily shortcomings have clear implications for self. This is, after all, at least one of the things we mean in the social sciences when we talk about stigma (Goffman, 1963). A sense of feeling stigmatized comes through loud and clear in the voices of infertile women (Greil, 1991a, 1991b; Miall, 1985, 1986).

The women in this study described themselves as having, not only imperfect bodies, but spoiled identities as well. Rachel said, "[I feel] not as good as anyone else. You know, like everybody else can get pregnant, and I can't." Debby described herself as "feeling real, real, defective." She elaborated on how infertility affected her sense of self:

> It affects your ego. It has an immense effect on self-concept, in all kinds of crazy ways. You ask, How can I be a real woman? By affecting the self-concept, it affects sexuality, and it affected work for me for a while. How can I be good at this; I'm not a normal person.

Lois seemed somewhat embarrassed when she described her reaction to infertility: "I never felt much like a woman, so to speak. I just felt like I was useless. Which is ridiculous. I know that, but there were times when I felt like that."

Considering that infertility is a condition that is neither visibly obvious nor likely to be discovered in the normal course of daily activities, it is striking that the women I spoke to felt the stigma of infertility so strongly. Scambler (1984) has made a distinction between *enacted stigma*—stigma that stems from intentional discrimination against the stigmatized—and *felt stigma*—the shame felt by the stigmatized because of their internalization of societal evaluation of their condition and the resultant sense that they have failed to live up to the standards of "normality." It would seem that for these infertile women, felt stigma was the source of more anguish than enacted stigma. Infertility is, then, a "secret stigma," hidden from outsiders but nonethless deeply felt (Greil, 1991a, 1991b). That this is the case says much both about the power of social expectations about the "normal" life course for women and about the extent to which infertile women see their bodies as integral parts of self.

Implicit in much of the writing about women's bodies is the assumption that wholeness is better than fragmentation, that activity is better than passivity, that it would be more satisfying to identify body and self than it would be to think of mind and body—or self and body—as separate. But how do these assumptions hold up when one looks at infertility, a situation in which the body is not functioning as desired? In such a situation, the body as machine metaphor could actually be *protective* if it were believed. In a study of working-class men, Sennett and Cobb (1972) assert that a division of the self may at least partially protect against the degradations of the workplace. Rather than see fragmentation as a problem for infertile women, one is tempted to say, if only these infertile women *did* think about their bodies as machines.

Body as Property

In *Recreating Motherhood* (1989), Rothman has drawn attention to the power of another metaphor in American society: the body as property. We think of our bodies, Rothman asserts, as being entities we *own*. While the body as machine metaphor may predominate in the culture of medicine, the body as property metaphor, which lies behind the notion of informed consent and other aspects of clinical practice, coexists with it. While the notion of the owned body obviously derives from capitalist ideology and carries with it the implication that women are alienated from their bodies, Rothman has shown that the body as property metaphor can also be used to assert one's autonomy. After all, if the body is our property, then we can claim the right under the capitalist juridical system to exert control over it without interference.

Among this sample of infertile women, two distinct uses of the body as property metaphor may be observed. Some women invoked it to express the sense that their bodies had betrayed them. These women described their bodies as possessions they had nurtured and cared for and which now owed them something in return. Sally expressed this theme:

> I got angry at my body for having turned on me. In my head that's how it was. I had always been real conscious of what I ate and what I didn't drink, what I didn't smoke, and all that kind of stuff. I had always been pretty good about that stuff and I always got angry at the powers that be for having this happen to me.

Barbara described herself as having reached a state where she no longer trusted her body. She elaborated:

How can my body do this? I had been taking marvelous care of it and feeding it right, getting enough sleep, exercising at the pool and I would go swimming in it daily. Followed just about everything to a T.

Other women invoked the body as property metaphor as a way of claiming the autonomy to make their own decisions in attempting to overcome their infertility. Most frequently, this use of the metaphor surfaced as women spoke about being more involved than their husbands in the treatment process. Rachel saw her right to do what she wanted with her body as justification for pursuing a more activist approach to treatment than her husband, Tom, might have preferred:

It was very much my problem. I mean, it was our problem, but it was my problem. And in a way that made it a little bit easier for me, because he was reluctant to get into it and do stuff. I knew it was my body, and I could go and have as many tests as I wanted to. So, it was easy, and it was harder, because it pulled us apart as a couple, but, yet, I had control over my body. I could go and do whatever I wanted to medically myself.

Dee, too, made it clear that she was in charge of her own treatment decisions, because she had the right to exercise control over her own body.

I discussed the surgery with Paul. I discussed what the doctor said, and Paul was very supportive through it, but he wanted it to be my decision. Because it was my body and my time out of work, and it was my choice. Once I made the decision, he supported me and he was there and all that stuff, but it was my decision.

Focusing on several different metaphors leads to a somewhat different portait of infertile women than would be obtained by concentrating on a single metaphor. Concentrating on the body as machine metaphor can result in a view of infertile women as passive products of medical definitions. Dwelling on the body as the emblem of the self metaphor can lead to seeing infertile women as passive victims of social norms. The body as property metaphor, however, seems to lend itself more to expressions of agency and self-assertion. Paying attention to the range of metaphors infertile women use in speaking of their bodies leads to the suggestion that they are powerfully influenced by medical definitions and normative expectations but that they are not the passive creatures of such definitions and expectations.

PARADOXES OF INFERTILITY TREATMENT

Implicit in the body as machine metaphor is the notion that the body *ought* to be under control. Machines, after all, can be manipulated by their operators. When machines malfunction, operators try to fix them. If they cannot fix them, they feel helpless and out of control. This is what many of the infertile women reported feeling. Cathy expressed it this way:

> I guess loss of control is going to have to come in here. That I didn't have any control over my destiny. It was a real shock to me to find something that I couldn't do anything about.

Teri spoke in similar terms: "There's just this feeling of being so out of control of a situation and so helpless to change the situation and so vulnerable."

The loss of control theme is especially important in understanding infertile women's experience. White middle-class women in the United States supposedly have the ability to determine the number of children they want, to limit the number of children they have, and to plan the spacing of these children. The women in this study are members of a group that has had a high degree of access to and confidence in birth control technology. They grew up believing that the human reproductive process is readily subject to human control. As Lynn put it, "I thought having children would happen when we decided we were going to have them." These women were surprised and demoralized when they realized that birth is not as controllable as they had thought.

The biomedical model and the body as machine metaphor carry with them a clear ideological justification for medical intervention, that is to say, for treatment. If a machine is broken, the natural response is to repair it. The infertile women I spoke with found the medical interpretation of infertility plausible. They saw infertility as a physical problem for which the most appropriate course of action was to search for a physical solution. It is not surprising, then, that they turned to medical treatment as the most promising means of regaining a sense of control. But, because the culture of medicine sees medical personnel as active and patients as passive, entering the medical system placed these women in a paradoxical situation. To regain a sense of control, they found it necessary to place themselves in a situation in which they had very little control indeed. The decision to take action to change their situation necessitated taking on a role in which they were expected to be passive.[8]

But, although these infertile women think of their bodies as machines, they do not think of them only as machines. They also view their bodies as integral to their selves. It was therefore quite common for them to talk about infertility treatment as an invasion of the integrity of the self. This violation of the integrity of the self is what Goffman (1961) called "mortification" in his now-classic study of mental patients.

According to Peg,

> It really wears at you after a while. You have so many doctors poking and prodding you and telling you this and telling you that. You become a specimen almost, rather than a human being. It gets to you.

Lois actually employs a version of the body as machine metaphor to describe the way infertility treatment made her feel:

> By the time I ended up in the hospital—this was after I had probably five or six tests—I'd swear I'd probably pull down my pants for anyone that walked by, because I'd lost all of my dignity. I'm a very modest person, but I began to feel like I was a car being worked on.

There is, then, a second paradox that parallels the paradox of control. Just as the desire for control can lead one to subject oneself to the control of another, so can the desire for bodily integrity lead to mortification.

Because infertility is experienced as a failure both of body and of self, infertile women face a third paradox. Restoring their selves to a sense of wholeness requires participating in a medical system that they feel does not treat them as whole people. Many infertile women were very critical of their physicians for ignoring the human side of healing. Martha described her gynecologist in the following way:

> He's very cold in my opinion, and he doesn't know how to deal with the psychological aspects of it. He never said, Hey, do you have any hangups about this? He just never talked about it. Every month you went in, had the procedure done, went home, waited, and your period came, so you called him up, went back, and . . .

Liz had similar complaints: "Doctor-wise, I just thought it was very much a business. It seemed like they were bored with the people, being interested more in statistics." These infertile women, then, found themselves in a situation in which, to recover their integrity, they were forced to participate in a system they perceived as a threat to that integrity.

RESPONDING TO THE SYSTEM

It is now possible to address the question of how these women responded to the loss of control, mortification, and impersonality they encountered. Because of the inherent power imbalance between doctors and patients, it is sometimes assumed that patients are passive reactors who have no choice but to acquiesce to the demands and definitions of biomedicine. But there is a substantial body of literature that emphasizes the ways in which patients assert agency and autonomy in their interactions with the health care system (Arluke, 1980; Browner & Press, 1996; Chrisman & Kleinman, 1983; Conrad, 1985, 1987; Hayes-Bautista, 1976; McGuire, 1988; Ong, 1995; Roth, 1972; Stimson & Webb, 1975). McGuire (1988, p. 198), noting the way people involved with alternative healing pick and choose when they will and when they will not rely on physicians and follow their advice, describes these individuals as "contractors of their own health care." In a similar fashion, the infertile women in this sample could be described as "infertility contractors."

These women did not simply acquiesce to the medical portrayal of themselves. Rather, they responded actively and strategically. They learned as much as they could about the medical system for treating infertility so as to be better able to move that system in the direction of furthering their own interests. Many of the women said that they read everything they could get their hands on to become more knowledgeable about infertility. Karen describes her reading as a way of taking back control over her own body:

> I do a lot of reading on my own. I've read everything I could find on the subject, and I'm not sure my doctor is real comfortable with that, because I think he likes to be the one in charge. But it's my body, and I want to. I mean, I can feel my body. I can tell when my body's right or wrong. He can't do that. He can take all the tests and things, but I can just feel when my body isn't right. And so I think the more I know about the subject, the more I can help him in the process.

One may observe ambivalence on Karen's part about just who it is that should be in control of her treatment. Karen seems quite deferential to her doctor. She claims to want to know her body better because the more she knows, the better she will be able to help her doctor. At the same time, she invokes the body as property metaphor and claims special access to information about her body as a way of establishing her integral role in the treatment process. Robin, too, talked about reading as a strategy for working the system:

> Well, I had all those routine tests, and I started reading, and I don't think he appreciated my reading. I'd come in, and I'd ask him for the postcoital test, and he'd say, Oh, you don't need the postcoital, because your husband has sperm and you have mucus and things.

It is interesting that both of these women report they feel that active involvement in their treatment put them in conflict with their physicians.

And, in fact, infertile women *did* use their knowledge of infertility to assert their right to influence the course of their medical treatment. These women were often quite ingenious in the strategies they used. Sally provides a striking example:

> Somebody had told me that, if you call your doctor and tell him that you're having problems, he's going to tell you that you have to wait a year and have three months of temperature charts. So I made up some temperature charts. I took my temperature for one month, and then I made up two more. And

then I went to see him. So he took care of everything all at once and didn't say that I had to wait a year or anything.

Cathy, too, used her knowledge to exert some control over her situation:

> I was very well read when we started. I think I just felt extremely confident about my knowledge on how to get pregnant and on recognizing when I was ovulating. After just a few months I was starting to wonder, and after about seven months I was convinced that there was something holding up the show. By seven months, I already had five temperature charts in my hand, and I walked into my doctor's office and said, "I'm not waiting twelve months to start."

Some women made treatment suggestions to their doctors based on their reading. Liz began to suspect that she had tubal problems and insisted that her doctor perform a second hysterosalpingogram. Cathy asked her doctor to test her and her husband, Chip, for a mycoplasma infection. In both of these cases, the suspicions turned out to be justified.

One strategy women commonly used to exert more influence over the treatment process was to change doctors. Barbara called switching physicians a "big step in gaining some control." Women who were unable or unwilling to persuade their physicians to modify the treatment regimen in accordance with their wishes often voted with their feet. One frequently cited reason for switching was dissatisfaction with the slow pace of progress of the treatment process. Mary switched to an infertility specialist because her gynecologist did not seem to accord the same significance to her problem as she did:

> I talked to my gynecologist about it, and he said, "Wait, relax. Sometimes it takes a year, sometimes it takes two years. If nothing happens in a year come back and see me." So we proceeded for another nine months, and then I went back and saw him. And he still said he didn't think there was anything wrong. He just said to continue onward, and if nothing happened we could go and have the sperm test, but he didn't get moving with the testing. That's when we switched to an infertility specialist.

It is worthwhile to note that women tend to take a more active role than men in managing the treatment process. It was virtually always wives, rather than husbands, who initiated treatment, and wives continued to take the leading role throughout the treatment process. Chip made it clear that Cathy was in charge of the infertility treatment process:

> She was the leader. She made the moves. She'd say, Well, I think we should do this now, and I'd say, Okay, what does that mean? And so we'd talk about it. It wasn't my idea to say, Okay, let's go for a laparoscopy. It wasn't my idea to say, Oh, let's do IVF. She kind of led me through the process.

These women were frequently able to describe their medical problems and their treatment in great detail; husbands often deferred to their wives for details. When Peter was asked to recount events in his and Kim's medical history, he referred to a list of procedures and dates that Kim had written down to prepare him for the interview.

It is important to reiterate here that these women (and their husbands) were overwhelmingly middle class in terms of both income and education. It, is of course, quite possible (even likely) that living lives of privilege, responsibility, and perceived efficacy has socialized these women into the role of active strategists. It would be of interest to see if women with less income and education manage their infertility treatment differently.

CONCLUSION

I have explored some of the ways in which the biological, personal, and social drama of infertility is played out in the bodies of women. In the discourse of medicine, women's bodies are often seen in terms of mechanical metaphors—as flawed machines, in need of medical intervention. While infertile women make use of mechanical metaphors, they tend to mix their metaphors, to see their bodies not only as flawed machines but also as integral parts of self and as property over which they have the right to exert some control. Infertile women do not respond passively to medical definitions of themselves but rather act as independent agents who work the system to achieve the outcomes they desire.

Proponents and opponents of reproductive technologies differ with regard to their perception of the dynamics of the rise of the new techniques and of the role of infertile women in that process. Supporters often argue that the development of reproductive technology is propelled by demand from infertile couples and that because so many couples desperately want a child, it is proper to do anything reasonable to satisfy that wish. Opponents argue that individuals, especially women, are pressured into making use of the new reproductive technologies and are therefore more properly described as being exploited by these technologies than as taking advantage of them.

It is clear that infertility brings with it a certain sense of demoralization for the infertile women in this study. The experience of infertility is an experience of the failure of body and self, and the experience of infertility treatment is an experience of frustration, loss of control, and mortification. But these women do not present themselves as passive victims content to be treated as objects. Rather they appear as active strategists and negotiators who have learned to work the system in such a way as to maximize the control they do have. While they are certainly not in control of the situation, neither are they totally helpless. By acquiring knowledge about infertility and about their bodies, they appear to have found one means for taking back control over their lives that they feel has been stripped from them by infertility. Thus the data from this study suggest a different way to look at infertile women: as strategists doing the best they can in the context of a system in which they lack substantive power.

NOTES

This is a revised version of a paper originally presented in March 1994 at the annual meeting of the Eastern Sociological Society in Baltimore, Maryland. I wish to thank Lynn Davidman, Rosanna Hertz, Marcia Inhorn, Judith Lasker, and Frank van Balen for support, encouragement, and help with earlier drafts.

1. It should be pointed out here that Martin takes pains to point out that her list is not necessarily exhaustive. It is also interesting to note the similarity between Martin's range of responses to medicalization and Merton's (1949) typology of responses to cultural strains. Van Balen and Trimbos-Kemper (1994) have applied a modified version of Merton's typology to responses of infertile couples.

2. Thomas A. Leitko, Karen L. Porter, and the author conducted interviews during 1985 and 1986. Couples were located using the snowball sampling technique. Initial contacts were made through the local chapter of RESOLVE, an infertility support organization. No more than two referrals were accepted from any one respondent, and respondents were encouraged to help locate people who were not involved in RESOLVE. Of the twenty-two couples interviewed, twelve reported that at least one member of the couple was active in RESOLVE.

All interviews were tape recorded. Interviewers advised respondents that their voices were being recorded and assured them that the contents of the interview would be kept confidential. Interviewers were guided by a list of questions but were free to vary the order and the wording, based on their judgments about how the interview was progressing. Interviews lasted an average of an hour and a quarter. Subjects covered included the decision to bear children, treatment history, reactions to treatment, decisions regarding adoption and reproductive technologies, couple reaction to infertility, changes in lifestyle and social relationships, effects of infertility and infertility decision making on career, and effects of infertility on values, attitudes, and worldview. Interviewers were careful to be sensitive and responsive to respondents' comments rather than judgmental.

Findings from this research have been published in book form (Greil, 1991a). The present chapter represents a reanalysis of the data with a special focus on infertile women's use of body metaphors. Although there have been technological changes in the treatment of infertility, they do not appear to have had a significant impact on the issues addressed here.

3. The mean estimate of family income given by men was $48,000; by women, $38,000. Of the women, fifteen had completed college, as had sixteen of the men; eight women and six men had gone on to attain advanced degrees; the remainder were high school graduates. All of the husbands and thirteen of the wives were engaged in full-time employment outside the home at the time of the interview.

Eighteen of the husbands and ten of the wives worked in professional or managerial positions. All couples were white.

4. While the couples in this sample are white and above average in terms of income and education, infertility is actually more common among blacks and those with lower incomes (Chandra & Mosher, 1994; Hirsch & Mosher, 1987; Kalmuss, 1987; Mosher, 1982).

5. Furthermore, many of these respondents are active in RESOLVE, a self-help organization, and may be different in some significant ways from those who do not join self-help groups. Even those who are not RESOLVE members are seekers of treatment and are likely to differ in significant ways from infertile couples who have not sought treatment.

6. Eleven couples had adopted children by the time of the interview. One wife had had a successful pregnancy and four wives (including two who had already adopted at least one child) were aware of being pregnant at the time of the interview. Three of the twenty-two couples had biological children before their involvement with infertility and would therefore be classified as cases of secondary infertility.

7. This and all other names used in this chapter are pseudonyms.

8. Several studies have shown that it is possible to experience oneself as being "in control" even when one has been cast in a passive role. Sargent and Stark (1989) found that new mothers in their sample saw no contradiction between receiving epidural anesthesia and feeling in control, because they interpreted control in terms of alertness and being in control of oneself. Likewise, many of the mothers interviewed by Davis-Floyd (1992) were able to feel in control during their hospital births because they could control how they responded to hospital routines.

REFERENCES

Arluke, A. (1980). Judging drugs: Patients' conception of therapeutic efficacy in the treatment of arthritis. *Human Organization, 39*, 84–87.

Barker-Benfield, B. (1976). *The horrors of the half-known life: Male attitudes toward women and sexuality in nineteenth-century America.* New York: Harper & Row.

Becker, G. (1990). *Healing the infertile family.* Berkeley: University of California Press.

Becker, G. (1994). Metaphors in disrupted lives: Infertility and cultural constructions of continuity. *Medical Anthropology Quarterly, 8*, 383–410.

Becker, G. (1997). *Disrupted lives: How people create meaning in a chaotic world.* Berkeley: University of California Press.

Browner, C. H., & Press, N. (1996). The production of authoritative knowledge in American prenatal care. *Medical Anthropology Quarterly, 10*, 141–156.

Chandra, A., & Mosher, W. D. (1994). The demography of infertility and the use of medical care for infertility. *Infertility and Reproductive Medicine Clinics of North America, 5*, 283–296.

Chrisman, N., & Kleinman, A. (1983). Popular health care, social networks and cultural meanings: The orientation of medical anthropology. In D. Mechanic (Ed.), *Handbook of health, health care, and health professions* (pp. 569–590). New York: Free Press.

Clarke, A. (1988). The industrialization of human reproduction, c. 1890–1990. Plenary address of annual conference of the University of California Systemwide Council of Women's Programs. Davis, April 9.

Conrad, P. (1985). The meaning of medications: Another look at compliance. *Social Science & Medicine, 20,* 29–37.

Conrad, P. (1987). The experience of illness: New and recent directions. *Research in the Sociology of Health Care, 6,* 1–31.

Conrad, P., & Schneider, J. (1980). *Deviance and medicalization: From badness to sickness.* St. Louis: Mosby.

Davis-Floyd, R. E. (1992). *Birth as an American rite of passage.* Berkeley: University of California Press.

Ehrenreich, B., & English, D. (1979). *For her own good: 150 years of the experts' advice to women.* Garden City, NY: Anchor.

Feldman-Savelsberg, P. (1999). *Plundered kitchens and empty wombs: Threatened reproduction and identity in the Cameroon Grassfields.* Ann Arbor: University of Michigan Press.

Fisher, S. (1986). *In the patient's best interest: Women and the politics of medical decisions.* New Brunswick, NJ: Rutgers.

Fisher, S., & Todd, A. D. (1983). *The social organization of doctor-patient communication.* Washington, DC: Center for Applied Linguistics.

Goffman, E. (1961). *Asylums.* Garden City, NY: Doubleday.

Goffman, E. (1963). *Stigma: Notes on the management of spoiled identity.* Englewood Cliffs, NJ: Prentice-Hall.

Greil, A. L. (1991a). *Not yet pregnant: Infertile couples in contemporary America.* New Brunswick, NJ: Rutgers University Press.

Greil, A. L. (1991b). A secret stigma: The analogy between infertility and chronic illness and disability. In G. Albrecht & J. Levy (Eds.), *Advances in medical sociology,* vol. 2 (pp. 17–38). Greenwich, CT: JAI Press.

Handwerker, L. (1995). The hen that can't lay an egg (*Bu xia dan de mu ji*): Conceptions of female infertility in modern China. In J. Terry & J. Urla (Eds.), *Deviant bodies: Critical perspectives on difference in science and popular culture* (pp. 358–379). Bloomington: Indiana University Press.

Hayes-Bautista, D. E. (1976). Modifying the treatment: Patient compliance, patient control and medical care. *Social Science & Medicine, 10,* 233–238.

Hirsch, M. B., & Mosher, W. D. (1987). Characteristics of infertile women in the United States and their use of fertility services. *Fertility and Sterility, 47,* 618–625.

Inhorn, M. C. (1994). *Quest for conception: Gender, infertility, and Egyptian medical traditions.* Philadelphia: University of Pennsylvania Press.

Inhorn, M. C. (1996). *Infertility and patriarchy: The cultural politics of gender and family in Egypt.* Philadelphia: University of Pennsylvania Press.

Kahn, R. P. (1995). *Bearing meaning: The language of birth.* Urbana: University of Illinois Press.

Kalmuss, D. S. (1987). The use of infertility services among fertility-impaired couples. *Demography, 24,* 575–585.

Katz, J. (1984). *The silent world of doctor and patient.* New York. Free Press.

Martin, E. (1987). *The woman in the body: A cultural analysis of reproduction.* Boston: Beacon Press.

Martin, E. (1988). The fetus as intruder. In R. Davis-Floyd & J. Dumit (Eds.), *Cyborg babies: From techno-sex to techno-tots* (pp. 125–142). New York: Routledge.

Martin, E. (1994). *Flexible bodies: Tracking immunity in American culture from the days of polio to the age of AIDS.* Boston: Beacon Press.

McGuire, M. B. (1988). *Ritual healing in suburban America.* New Brunswick, NJ: Rutgers University Press.

Merton, R. K. (1949). *Social theory and social structure.* Glencoe, IL: Free Press.

Miall, C. E. (1985). Perceptions of informal sanctioning and the stigma of involuntary childlessness. *Deviant Behavior, 6,* 383–403.

Miall, C. E. (1986). The stigma of involuntary childlessness. *Social Problems, 33,* 268–282.

Mishler, E. (1984). *The discourse of medicine.* Norwood, NJ: Ablex.

Mizrahi, T. (1986). *Getting rid of patients: Contradictions in the socialization of physicians.* New Brunswick, NJ: Rutgers University Press.

Mosher, W. D. (1982). Infertility among U.S. couples, 1965–1976. *Family Planning Perspectives, 14,* 22–27.

Ong, A. (1995). Making the biopolitical subject: Cambodian immigrants, refugee medicine and cultural citizenship in California. *Social Science & Medicine, 40,* 1243–1257.

Osherson, S. D. & AmaraSingham, L. R. (1981). The machine metaphor in medicine. In G. Mishler, L. R. AmaraSingham, S. D. Osherson, S. T. Hauser, N. E. Waxler, & F. Liem (Eds.), *Social contexts of health, illness, and patient care* (pp. 125–142). Cambridge: Cambridge University Press.

Roth, J. (1972). Staff and client control strategies in urban hospital emergency services. *Urban Life and Culture, 1,* 39–60.

Rothman, B. K. (1989). *Recreating motherhood: Ideology and technology in a patriarchal society.* New York: W. W. Norton.

Sandelowski, M. J. (1990). Failures of volition: Female agency and infertility in historical perspective. *Signs, 15,* 475–498.

Sandelowski, M. J. (1993). *With child in mind: Studies of the personal encounter with infertility.* Philadelphia: University of Pennsylvania Press.

Sargent, C., & Stark, N. (1989). Childbirth education and childbirth models: Parental perspectives on control, anesthesia, and technological intervention in the birth process. *Medical Anthropology Quarterly, 3,* 36–51.

Scambler, G. (1984). Perceiving and coping with a stigmatizing condition. In R. Fitzpatrick, J. Hinton, S. Newman, C. Scambler, & J. Thompson (Eds.), *The experience of illness* (pp. 203–226). New York: Tavistock.

Scully, D. (1980). *Men who control women's health.* Boston: Houghton Mifflin.

Sennett, R., & Cobb, J. (1972). *The hidden injuries of class.* New York: Vintage.

Stimson, G., & Webb, B. (1975). *Going to see the doctor: Consultation process in general medical practice.* London: Routledge & Kegan Paul.

Synott, A. (1992). Tomb, temple, machine and self: The social construction of the body. *British Journal of Sociology, 43,* 80–100.

Synott, A. (1993). *The body social: Symbolism, self, and society.* London: Routledge.

van Balen, F., & Trimbos-Kemper, T. (1994). Factors influencing the well-being of long-term infertile couples. *Journal of Psychosomatic Obstetrics and Gynecology, 15,* 157–164.

Waitzkin, H. (1991). *The politics of medical encounters.* New Haven, CT: Yale University Press.

West, C. (1984). *Routine complications: Troubles with talk between doctors and patients.* Bloomington: Indiana University Press.

Young, K. (1997). *Presence in the flesh: The body in medicine.* Cambridge, MA: Harvard University Press.

SIX

Deciding Whether to Tell Children about Donor Insemination

An Unresolved Question in the United States

Gay Becker

As many as one in eight married couples in the United States experience difficulty conceiving a child, leading more than one million women a year to seek infertility treatment (SART, 1998). Although inadequacies associated with sperm are causal or contributory to almost half of all infertility, there has been little if any effective treatment for male infertility until the 1990s. As a result, the artificial insemination of women with the sperm of donors who are usually anonymous has been widely practiced in many countries for almost half a century. It is estimated that as many as thirty thousand children a year have been conceived in this manner in the United States alone (Shenfield & Steele, 1997), resulting in the birth of as many as one million offspring since the 1950s.

When male infertility is discovered and couples subsequently decide to use donor sperm to conceive a pregnancy, issues of biological continuity and stigma arise that affect the decision-making process about disclosure. Great significance is attached to genetic, or blood, relationships in the United States (Duster, 1990; Nelkin & Lindee, 1995; Schneider, 1980), where public approval for donor insemination (DI) is lower than for adoption or for other reproductive technologies that do not have third-party involvement (Klock, 1993). Moreover, there is apparently more stigma attached to male than to female infertility. The experience of stigma is defined as a negative sense of social difference from others that is so far outside the socially defined norm that it discredits and devalues the individual (Goffman, 1963).

It has been found that men who have been identified as having an infertility factor experience greater stigma than men who do not and that the stigma attached to male infertility is much greater than that attached to female infertility (Nachtigall, Becker, & Wozny, 1992). Other research has shown that higher guilt and blame levels are found among men who are themselves the infertile partner, when compared with men with infertile partners (van Balen & Trimbos-Kemper, 1994). Furthermore, there is less openness about infertility status in the case of male infertility (van Balen, Trimbos-Kemper, & Verdurmen, 1996).

Based on research with couples who used donor insemination in Great Britain, Snowden, Mitchell, and Snowden (1983) suggested that the underlying impetus for nondisclosure is protection of the infertile husband's feelings, as it avoids the risk of having the husband's potency, virility, or masculinity come under suspicion. They also observed that infertility is often ascribed to women, regardless of its actual source, to protect men from the stigma of infertility. The stigma attached to male infertility thus reflects cultural attitudes about masculinity and male sexuality.

Sexuality, conceptualized as part of gender (Butler, 1993; Grosz,1994; Ortner, 1996), is a moral domain (Foucault, 1986), and, as Howell (1997) notes, certain kinds of behavior are singled out for moral debates more than others, sexuality being one such arena. In a study of Great Britain's Warnock Report, Haimes (1993) found that assumptions about gender were embedded in the report itself and affirmed in committee members' interviews: semen donation was associated with "deviant" sexuality, while egg donation was associated with altruism. These characterizations symbolize deep-seated gender assumptions about what is natural—assumptions that became embedded in policy and lived out in practice. Following Douglas's (1966) observations about women's bodies as the site of symbolic transgressions of social boundaries, it can be argued that the use of male donors to achieve a pregnancy in a woman's body is a transgression of cultural rules about how children should be conceived. This practice challenges patriarchal concepts of what is natural for women and men and indicates the perceived threat to common understandings of the family, including sexuality within marriage, that the use of third parties engenders. Such societal views about women's bodies and "appropriate" male and female sexuality are, therefore, central to decisions parents make about disclosure.

Parents who use DI may view the decision not to disclose as one that protects them from the negative reactions of society, family, and friends, and it protects the child from being looked upon as different from others (Nachtigall, 1993). Although parents who decide not to disclose to their children often cite the principle of confidentiality (expressed as the social right to privacy, personal autonomy, and freedom from unwanted intrusion) as their justification, their comments frequently appear to anticipate the negative judgments of others and suggest that they are wary of subjecting themselves and their children to public scrutiny and judgment (Nachtigall, Becker, Szkupinski Quiroga, Pitcher, & Tschann, 1998). However, some have argued that the secrecy surrounding donor insemination may undermine family relationships and that children conceived by gamete donation may feel confused about their identity (Daniels & Taylor, 1993; Snowden, Mitchell, & Snowden, 1983). Children may also feel deceived by their parents if they eventually discover the facts about their conception (Golombok, Cook, Bish, & Murray, 1995).[1] The range of concerns women and men express about disclosure after the birth of a child and the stances they take once they have made a decision have yet to be fully addressed.

The decision about whether to disclose the use of a donor has become a critical focus of policy makers, health professionals, advocates, and parents. There has been a worldwide focus on whether disclosure decisions should be regulated at the national level, despite an inadequate research base from which to promulgate policy. In the United States, it is important to differentiate between national and state laws and policies that are put forward by special interest groups. For example, the American Society for Reproductive Medicine, the medical society of reproductive endocrinology, has a policy that only frozen sperm should be used in donor insemination. But such a policy should not be interpreted as mandatory law. On the other hand, among western European countries, the anonymity of donors is mandated in France, Denmark, Israel, Norway, Belgium, and Spain, while Sweden has a law mandating the availability of disclosure information to children on reaching the age of eighteen (Adair & Purdie, 1996; Daniels & Lalos, 1995; Freeman, 1996; Landau, 1998; Shenfield, 1994; Shenfield & Steele, 1997; Weil, Cornet, Sibony, Mandelbaum, & Salat-Baroux, 1994). In the Netherlands and in New Zealand, parents are urged to disclose to their children (Adair & Purdie, 1996; Brewaeys, Golombok, Naaktgeboren, de Bruyn, & van Hall, 1997); in Great Britain, donor offspring have the right to access their donors' genetic information when they reach eighteen, but not their donors' identity. And in Australia, a heated debate is currently under way about whether to mandate disclosure (Daniels & Taylor, 1993; Walker & Broderick, 1999). The voices of parents who have created their families through donor insemination are seldom heard in these debates. With limited information about how families manage these dilemmas, moral stances have prevailed in the literature and in the advice given to parents (Shenfield & Steele, 1997). Furthermore, flaws in much of the research carried out on disclosure decisions to date leave major questions unresolved (Broderick & Walker, 1995).

TWO STUDIES AND THEIR METHODOLOGIES

In research we conducted in the United States on donor insemination and family functioning (Nachtigall, Tschann, Szkupinski Quiroga, Pitcher, & Becker, 1997; Nachtigall et al., 1998), disclosure decisions about donor insemination were found to be the primary ongoing concern of parents who had used this method to create a family. This chapter draws on data from two related studies. In the first study, respondents were recruited from a single private practice in a predominantly urban five-county geographic area in the western United States. Four kinds of data were collected: (1) basic medical information about couples from reviewing their medical charts; (2) psychological scales measuring marital and parental satisfaction, stigma, and disclosure; (3) written answers to open-ended questions on a questionnaire; and (4) in-depth interviews with twenty couples who conceived a child through DI. Questionnaires were mailed to couples who agreed to participate, with an individual questionnaire for each partner. Couples were instructed to complete the questionnaire individually. Coded numbers were assigned to protect the anonymity of respondents. A number-coded, postage-paid envelope with individual inner envelopes was provided for the return of the completed questionnaires. Of a total of 184 couples who were successfully contacted, 102 women and 85 men completed and returned a questionnaire.

The second study was a general examination of the experience of infertility of 134 couples and 9 women who were interviewed without their partners, which took place in the same geographic area and drew on respondents recruited from physicians' private practices, clinics, adoption services, and a self-help group (Becker, 2000; Becker & Nachtigall, 1994). Twenty-one of the couples used donor insemination to conceive a child. These couples were interviewed two to three times over a three-year period. The disclosure decision was one of the most prominent themes to emerge from the open-ended interviews. The findings from the open-ended responses in the disclosure study's questionnaire were supported by the in-depth interviews from both studies, in which partners initially were interviewed together. Those participating in the general infertility study were subsequently interviewed alone as well.

This chapter draws primarily on the in-depth interviews to elucidate the complex issues with which parents grapple. I address heterosexual couples' decision-making process about disclosure after they have conceived a child through DI.[2] My purpose is threefold: (1) to describe the types of disclosure issues that continue to arise after the birth of a child; (2) to demonstrate that decisions about disclosure shape the way in which issues pertaining to the use of a donor are subsequently perceived; and (3) to examine the role of gender in this process.

MALE INFERTILITY AND THE DECISION TO USE DONOR INSEMINATION

Men in this study reported that they were shocked and distressed to learn of their infertility. Men who had no premonition that they might be infertile were more distraught than those who had some prior inkling of a problem, for example, because of a previous illness or surgery that had suggested their fertility might be compromised. Acceptance of the diagnosis of male infertility was a gradual process, and many men described how coming to terms with their infertility took years, not simply weeks or months.[3] The decision to use donor insemination was a complex one for men, because it meant that their infertility might become public knowledge. Jerry, although he has made a decision to disclose, is nevertheless reluctant to tell others about using a donor. Soon to become a father, he said:

> I will admit that part of it is my own stuff. Part of it is not wanting our child to find out too early or not wanting everybody in the world to know. But at the same time part of it is my own stuff around my ego, and, you know, feelings of inadequacy, of feeling like I couldn't father a child. I needed somebody else's sperm. It is still a little bit there.

David, a nondiscloser whose eldest child was eight, was philosophical in retrospect: "You are dealt your hand in life, and you do the best you can. It was hard enough, frankly, my being sterile, or impotent. Anyway, that was really hard." When David uses the word *impotent,* we see how he confuses sterility, a physiological problem, with potency, which refers to sexual function. Asked what his reaction was when he first learned about his infertility, he said:

> Bummer! But I always had some feeling in the back of my mind somehow that everything wasn't there. I have no vas deferens. So I have semen but no sperm. I have always wanted children since I was seven years old. I was always looking forward to having children. But then, I just got past it and decided, how do we have children?

TAKING A STANCE ON DISCLOSURE DECISIONS

In the questionnaire phase of the study, responses about disclosure were divided into three overall categories, based on the structured question: "I have told or plan to tell our child." Answers to this question were grouped by disclosure status: disclosers, nondisclosers, and undecideds. Fifty-four percent of the sample were nondisclosers, 30 percent were disclosers, and 16 percent were undecided. In only 1 of 65 couples did the partners report opposite disclosure intentions (1.5%); but in 8 couples one partner was undecided whereas the other was a nondiscloser; and in 5 couples one partner was undecided whereas the other was a discloser (Nachtigall et al., 1998). Analysis of the data from the interview portion of the study revealed that these categories continued to be extremely salient, thereby facilitating the analysis of ways in which women and men developed a stance on disclosure.

"Honesty" versus "Confidentiality"

The words that people chose to talk about disclosure issues reflected the stances they took on disclosure, as well as their current plans about disclosing. The major determinant in their decision about whether to tell children about the use of a donor was whether women and men viewed the disclosure issue as one of "honesty" (disclosers) versus "confidentiality" (nondisclosers). Yet even straightforward statements about disclosure or nondisclosure were often interwoven with parents' concerns about the possible repercussions of their decision and its effect on their child and family.

The majority of comments about confidentiality were by nondisclosers. Such statements included concerns that disclosure would interfere with the father-child relationship and that who raises the child is more important than the knowledge disclosure would bring. For example, many nondisclosers' comments about their disclosure stance recognized or anticipated the negative judgments of others, as well as unknown but potentially deleterious effects on their child. They frequently voiced or implied the concern that their use of donor insemination was information that could be viewed as prejudicial or socially unacceptable; therefore, they believed that their decision needed to be controlled and protected against unauthorized dissemination. Some respondents invoked their right to privacy or personal autonomy, while others saw the decision as freeing them from unwanted intrusion. Some implied protection of the family from stigma,[4] and many saw nondisclosure as the best means of shielding their children from possible harm. For example, Verna, a nondiscloser, said, "I don't think it is fair. I feel very strongly about not telling her. I don't think it is fair to Mitch [her husband]. He is absolutely the father. And that is the way it is. I don't think that it is fair to put any doubt in anybody's mind." Mitch added,

> I have been there at Verna's side. I was there when she was born, I coached Verna through it. I have been through the whole pregnancy thing together, and there is just that one biological aspect to it that is missing. And I would hate to think that after being a very devoted, hardworking father that something like that came out and that she would feel like, number one, she may feel slighted that I am not totally her father, and number two, if she would start acting different toward me because I wasn't the biological father, I would feel really sad. . . . It is certainly none of anybody else's business.

In contrast, statements about honesty were made primarily by women and men who planned to disclose. The word *secrecy* was used in a negative sense by disclosers, while the predominant sentiment expressed in nondisclosers' responses was fearfulness about the child's response should he or she inadvertently learn of the use of donor insemination. Statements about honesty included the conviction that secrets are dangerous, that openness is essential for family well-being, and that nondisclosure is lying. Disclosers worried about not being honest and were concerned about the morally right thing to do. Leslie, a discloser whose husband was originally undecided but who has agreed to disclose, commented:

> Before we actually took on this choice I talked to Jerry a lot about it, and the only way that I would do it would be to be open with the child about it. Because I didn't want to enter into any agreement about keeping that kind of secret because I think it can be really damaging.

Disclosers commented more on the ethical underpinnings of their decision, often citing honesty as a held value in and of itself and not as a justification, and some voiced the opinion that it was the child's right to know his or her biological origins and cited their respect for the child's future autonomy. Disclosers disavowed "secrecy" in the negative psychological sense of something kept hidden or unexplained or because they would feel uncomfortable not telling the truth, while others believed or feared that discovery was inevitable and were therefore concerned with adverse consequences. Trina, a discloser, viewed it this way:

> I think it is her birthright to know. I wish that it could be more open, that if she chose to meet her biological father that the curiosity would be just to see the person and that would be a possibility, even though I know it really is not. I wish that it was. So, to me, it is like your secrets make things a bigger deal of it; that is the conclusion that I have come to on my own. The more we try to pretend that everything is fine, the crazier-making it makes it. And I don't want her to live in that kind of atmosphere. So we have made that a goal within our own family not to keep secrets.

Concerns for the Child

Regardless of their disclosure decision, more than half of the parents voiced concerns on behalf of their children, most frequently about their children's future psychological well-being or healthy development of identity and self-esteem. Some nondisclosers said this uncertainty reinforced their decision. Jerry, although he feels vulnerable about disclosing, has decided to disclose:

> The thing came up about medical reasons, if he needed a donor or something. Or the high school biology class where he finds out that his blood couldn't possibly be from our combination. Something like that, and he is eighteen or twenty and then he finds out that I am not his father, then it would really be hard. So we thought that we would start telling him younger, when he is old enough to understand. And tell him in a real loving way that we really wanted him and wanted him so bad but we needed help in order

to have him. But also I do have this fear that, at some point, when he is in his rebellious stage, it will be like, Well, you are not my father, I don't like you anyway, or, I hate you, you are not my father, anyway. I felt like that about my father—and he was my father!

Some parents were concerned with the adequacy of genetic information in addressing medical problems that their children might face in the future, while others addressed potential difficulties in explaining the significance of the husband's medical history. Nelson, a discloser, commented:

> I think she should know because the whole genetic thing is exploding so fast that I think she is entitled to know. If there comes a time when it would be an advantage to know about the donor's genetic makeup, then I think that she should be able to know.

Others commented on the physical appearance of their offspring, especially dissimilarities between the child and parents and siblings. David, a nondiscloser, said, "Maybe some day our kids will think about it and maybe they will look at each other and they will look totally different, and they may say, 'Why do we look so different?' " Kathy, his wife, interjected, "But we have so many people who say that one is just like me and the other one is just like David. They say that pretty much all of the time. And I say, 'Yes, you are right.' "

Concerns about Parenthood

Men and women had many concerns about parenthood and the relationship of the child to the parents, especially to the father. A majority of parents commented on their concerns as parents, focusing on the meaning of parenthood and reflecting Snowden, Mitchell, and Snowden's (1983) observation that parents emphasize the social reality of the situation and minimize the genetic reality. All the parents were concerned with establishing the social father as the "real" father. These responses reflected men's and women's philosophies about parenthood. Regardless of their disclosure stance, both men and women emphasized the importance of a spiritual and emotional connection associated with being a father and the unimportance of biology. Curtis, a nondiscloser, said:

> Whoever brings up the child is the parent regardless of where the sperm came from. A child should belong in their family. Socialization is almost everything. These children are from your [wife's] body. We had them together. I was there for all three births. There is no difference. There is no difference whatsoever.

Although men and women diminished the importance to parenthood of the method of conception, some expressed lingering concerns about the role of biology. Jerry, a discloser, said:

I would prefer that he was mine, but he may be getting better genes, I don't know. I know that it is not going to be a big issue for me. There is a little bit of that, though. I can't deny that. There is a little bit of that ego stuff, but I really do look at him as my son, and our son, and that is the way that it is going to be. But it is just that when it comes to telling other people, it is not something that I am real out there with.

Men and women frequently stated their belief in the preeminence of the social parenting role and often reiterated the desire to establish the social father as the real father. Yet disclosing parents often expressed trepidation about the effects of disclosure on the father-child relationship that ranged in intensity from relatively mild to more profound. Jerry's wife, Leslie, commented, "I would hope that nobody would do this, but I have to admit that I have some fears that maybe someone else would somehow diminish Jerry's role as the father of this child because he wasn't biologically connected." David, a nondiscloser, shared the same concerns:

I don't want my kids to stop loving me because they think that there is someone else and then go on this bizarre trek trying to find their roots. I think it would make a difference. They are not old enough, they are not adults yet. I don't know what kind of father I am going to be necessarily, you know. I haven't done this before and I don't really want them to find an excuse to, not to not love me, but to go against me. That might be there anyway. So that worries me. Obviously, that is why we are not telling them, because I think their knowing is going to make a difference.

Parents' Ongoing Concerns for the Child

Although it would appear that the majority of parents had a clear-cut stance toward disclosure of one kind or another, their additional statements belied that apparent certainty. They repeatedly addressed concerns about possible repercussions from disclosure and nondisclosure decisions. Women and men, regardless of their stance, were concerned about what to convey to children and how to convey it. David, a nondiscloser, said:

It would be interesting to know how other people felt if they decided to tell their children because that would be a better alternative, I think, than the kids finding out fifteen or thirty years from now that we have been telling a lie for that long. That also might not be a problem, they might just think that it is pretty strange, but can understand why you didn't say anything, and that makes sense. I am going about my business and it would be no big deal. Or they could go the other way and just freak out and say, "How could you do this to me?" and "You didn't tell me the truth." That is what worries me and weighs on my mind—if they were to find out—what would happen.

Some parents expressed concern about how they would go about explaining donor insemination to a young child but worried that if they waited until the child was old enough to understand the actual procedure, psychological damage might already have been done. Other parents reported creating their own story to explain the child's conception so as to make it more acceptable or manageable or to deemphasize certain aspects of it. Trina, a discloser, practiced how she would go about telling her small child:

> You learn about sperm and egg and how babies are made. Sometimes they come together inside the mommy, sometimes outside the mommy, sometimes the sperm comes from the daddy, you know, and sometimes it takes two daddies. And one is your daddy, and one is a biological daddy.

Parents who planned to disclose were concerned that their children not learn of their biological origins from others. For example, Leslie said:

> In the beginning, of course, all my close friends knew anyway. And I went back to all of our close friends who have children already, of an age where they could hear, overhear their parents. Anybody that had a kid that was two and a half on up, I went to them and said, "I really don't want you talking about this." Because when our child is three, that kid will be six and could say something that could be really hurtful to our child. That was my concern. And they said they would be very careful.

Parents were also concerned about issues related to biological roots and used words such as "lineage," "heritage," and "history" in their discussions. Jerry, a discloser, said:

> I think it is fine if he wanted to look for his biological father. I wouldn't stop him, couldn't stop him. And I would want the same thing if I were in his position. But, again, my fears are more around him rejecting me. But that could happen anyway. Like a boy, he has to move apart from his father and it is a real normal thing. And I understand that. On an intellectual level. But on an emotional level I just don't want any additional rejection because he feels like I wasn't there for him or I wasn't biologically connected to him. But I accepted that when we accepted this method. And I know that it can happen and it probably will on some level.

Women and men, regardless of their approach, were concerned, above all, with helping their children to establish a strong, positive identity. Parents expressed the wish to have their child avoid identity confusion or possible hurt or uncertainty about themselves. Nelson, a discloser, said: "I would hate for her to have her friends tease her. Kids are brutal enough anyway. I don't know the answer. I just know I hope we do it right so that it works out all right for her."

Both disclosers and nondisclosers reported concern about what people would think of them and their children and addressed a range of specific concerns such as social acceptability and negative judgments. For example, one nondisclosing parent said, "I fear our child would be rejected for being only half-tied to the family." Some parents wished to avoid any uncertainty about the description and quality of their family relationship, while others worried about possible disruption or strain that the knowledge of DI would bring to the extended family. Trina, a discloser, concluded, "Individually you have to be clear on your values and what you as a family stand for and what is your mode of operating. And us being true to us. But what is right for us is not going to be right for another family."

Thus it would appear that the overriding concern of couples undertaking donor insemination is the desire to be a "normal" family. Their concerns reflect this imperative. From the vantage point of one nondisclosing parent, the ultimate question is how to normalize the use of donor insemination:

> I hope that in the years to come that there will be some more openness and some celebrity will come out and say that they are a DI child or that they had a DI child. You need something like that. We would like to be considered a normal family.

CONCLUSION: NEGOTIATING THE COMPLEXITY OF DISCLOSURE DECISIONS

Concern with having made the right decision is an underlying theme of the findings in this study. This research indicates that disclosure issues are not necessarily resolved at the birth of a child. Rather, women and men have ongoing concerns about disclosure, and these concerns change over time. There is no straightforward answer to disclosure decisions because the questions of who is the "real" father and how children will respond if they learn of a third party's involvement are of perennial concern to parents.

The stances that parents take reflect their efforts to achieve a sense of normalcy within the family and for their children. People strive to be normal, however they define normalcy, and those personal definitions are interactive with cultural notions of what constitutes normalcy (Becker, 1997). This desire for normalcy drives disclosure decisions, for example, when nondisclosers cite their fear of the child's reaction as a reason for nondisclosure or when disclosing parents state that they do not want secrets within the family. Thus women and men apparently develop specific philosophies not only about disclosure but also about parenthood and their role as parents in acting in the best interest of the child. While most parents develop strong ideas of what they believe is best for the child and the family unit, underlying worries persist. The statements of men and women reflect their concerns that they are treading uncharted ground and are ultimately uncertain about the wisdom of their actions. Their frequently expressed fears about having made the correct decisions for them as a family, about the child's well-being, and about the actions of others, as well as their wish to know more about disclosure, belies the certainty with which they portray their beliefs.

The ways in which men and women characterize their approaches to disclosure and nondisclosure are striking and suggest that stance on disclosure may affect the nature of family interactions. For example, in the quantitative part of this study, it was found that nondisclosing fathers who scored higher on stigma also reported less parental warmth and less parental fostering of independence (Nachtigall et al., 1997). The stance taken toward the overall issue of whether to disclose may therefore pervade family life, with far-reaching implications for the family constellation as a whole. Conversely, this finding also raises the question of how the lack of a stance on whether to disclose may affect family life and interpersonal relations. Indecision and uncertainty about such an issue may affect family functioning as well; but how uncertainty is expressed and what its effect on the family may be remain unknown.

Parents' concerns about disclosure also reveal ongoing worries about the emphasis U.S. society places on biology. Those men and women who elect to use a donor to create a family are reworking cultural meanings of parenthood. In their efforts to normalize the use of a donor to conceive a child, the women and men in this study were unanimous in their belief in the social father—that is, that the man who raises the child is the "real" father. This privileging of social parenthood over biological parenthood is *the* critical factor in parents' decisions to use donor insemination.

Recently in the United States and elsewhere, there has been a trend toward increased openness to the use of donor insemination (Shenfield & Steele, 1997). The introduction of donor egg technology in the United States and the propensity of many couples using this technology to do so openly has likely contributed to the increased receptivity. Nevertheless, the changes to date are small, and donor insemination, unlike donor egg technology, continues to be shrouded in secrecy to a great extent.

Public arguments for or against disclosure do not acknowledge the complexity of either the decision itself or the extent of parents' concerns. Nor do those arguments acknowledge the underlying root issue: that is, that cultural ideas about what is natural for men are as deeply ingrained as are cultural notions about what is natural for women. The use of a donor flies in the face of gender ideologies about sexuality. Men's discomfort about their infertility becoming a public matter reflects moral discourses about men, biology, and sexuality, in which men who use the sperm of another man to conceive a child are viewed as deviant.

Ultimately, the global controversy that continues to revolve around the use of donor insemination and its disclosure attests to how gender ideologies may propel policies of the state and constrain parental decision mak ing. The recent tendency to regulate donor insemination may create an ongoing dilemma, namely, that nation-states' efforts to control reproductive technologies by framing moral discourses on the use of donors may not only hamper individual agency, but may place further constraints on the potential to change far-reaching gender ideologies. Thus, until there are significant changes in attitudes about social fatherhood, it is likely that families created through donor insemination will continue to experience ongoing tensions associated with the disclosure process.

NOTES

The research "Donor Insemination and Family Functioning" was supported by grants from the Academic Senate of the University of California, San Francisco, and the California-Pacific Medical Center, San Francisco, Robert D. Nachtigall, Principal Investigator; Gay Becker and Jeanne M. Tschann, Co-Investigators. The research "Gender and the Disruption of Life Course Structure," RO1 AGO8973, was supported by a grant from the National Institute on Aging, National Institutes of Health, Gay Becker, Principal Investigator; Robert D. Nachtigall, Co-Investigator. Many thanks to the women and men who participated in this research.

1. Golombok and her colleagues (1995) found that parents in England feared the disclosure of donor insemination, and none in that study had disclosed to the child. But keeping the method of conception secret did not appear to have any negative impact on family relationships.

2. Single women and lesbian couples were not included in this study. See Tober (2000).

3. Based on the general research study on infertility that included a large number of men who declined to consider DI after learning of their infertility, it appears that men who opt to undertake DI may resolve their feelings about infertility more quickly than men who do not choose this option. See Becker (2000).

4. Parents who have used DI to conceive a child and have disclosed this to others have been found to experience lower "stigma scores" than parents who did not disclose (Nachtigall et al., 1997).

REFERENCES

Adair, V. A., & Purdie, A. (1998). Donor insemination programmes with personal donors: Issues of secrecy. *Human Reproduction, 11,* 2558–2563.

Becker, G. (1997). *Disrupted lives: How people create meaning in a chaotic world.* Berkeley: University of California Press.

Becker, G. (2000). *The elusive embryo: How women and men approach the new reproductive technologies.* Berkeley: University of California Press.

Becker, G., & Nachtigall, R. D. (1994). "Born to be a mother": The cultural construction of risk in infertility treatment. *Social Science & Medicine, 39,* 507–518.

Brewaeys, A., Golombok, S., Naaktgeboren, N., de Bruyn, J. K., & van Hall, E. V. (1997). Donor insemination: Dutch parents' opinions about confidentiality and donor anonymity and the emotional adjustment of their children. *Human Reproduction, 12,* 1591–1597.

Broderick, P., & Walker, I. (1995). Information access and donated gametes: How much do we know about who wants to know what? *Human Reproduction, 10,* 3338–3341.

Butler, J. (1993). *Bodies that matter: On the discursive limits of "sex."* New York: Routledge.

Daniels, K., & Lalos, O. (1995). The Swedish insemination act and the availability of donors. *Human Reproduction, 10,* 1871–1874.

Daniels, K. R., & Taylor, K. (1993). Secrecy and openness in donor insemination. *Politics Life Sciences, 12,* 155–164.

Douglas, M. (1966). *Purity and danger: An analysis of concepts of pollution and taboo.* London: Routledge..

Duster, T. (1990). *Backdoor to eugenics.* New York: Routledge.

Foucault, M. (1986). *The history of sexuality, volume 2: The use of pleasure.* New York: Vintage Books.

Freeman, M. (1996). The new birthright: Identity and the child of the reproductive revolution. *International Journal of Children's Rights, 4,* 273–297.

Goffman, E. (1963). *Stigma: Notes on the management of spoiled identity.* Englewood Cliffs, NJ: Prentice-Hall.

Golombok, S., Cook, R., Bish, A., & Murray, C. (1995). Families created by the new reproductive technologies: Quality of parenting and social and emotional development of the children. *Child Development, 66,* 285–298.

Grosz, E. (1994). *Volatile bodies: Toward a corporeal feminism.* Bloomington: Indiana University Press.

Haimes, E. (1993). Issues of gender in gamete donation. *Social Science & Medicine, 36,* 85–93.

Howell, S. (1997). Introduction. In S. Howell (Ed.), *The ethnography of moralities* (pp. 1–22). London: Routledge.

Klock, S. C. (1993). Psychological aspects of donor insemination. *Infertility Reproduction Clinics of North America, 4,* 455–469.

Landau, R. (1998). The management of genetic origins: Secrecy and openness in donor assisted conception in Israel and elsewhere. *Human Reproduction, 13,* 3268–3273.

Nachtigall, R. D. (1993). Secrecy: An unresolved issue in the practice of donor insemination. *American Journal of Obstetrics and Gynecology, 168,* 1846–1853.

Nachtigall, R. D., Becker, G., Szkupinski Quiroga, S., Pitcher, L., & Tschann, J. M. (1998). The disclosure decision: Concerns and issues of parents of children conceived through donor insemination. *American Journal of Obstetrics and Gynecology, 178,* 1165–1170.

Nachtigall, R. D., Becker, G., & Wozny, M. (1992). Effects of gender-specific diagnosis on men's and women's response to infertility. *Fertility and Sterility, 57,* 113–121.

Nachtigall, R. D., Tschann, J. M., Szkupinski Quiroga, S., Pitcher, L., & Becker, G.

(1997). Stigma, disclosure, and family functioning among parents of children conceived through donor insemination. *Fertility and Sterility, 68,* 83–89.

Nelkin, D., & Lindee, S. (1995). *The DNA mystique: The gene as a cultural icon.* New York: Freeman.

Ortner, S. (1996). *Making gender.* Boston: Beacon Press.

SART. (1998). Assisted reproductive technology in the United States and Canada: 1995 results generated from the American Society for Reproductive Medicine/ Society for Assisted Reproductive Technology Registry. *Fertility and Sterility, 69,* 389–398.

Schneider, D. (1980). *American kinship: A cultural account.* Englewood Cliffs, NJ: Prentice-Hall.

Shenfield, F. (1994). Filiation in assisted reproduction: Potential conflicts and legal implications. *Human Reproduction, 9,* 1348–1354.

Shenfield, F., & Steele, S. J. (1997). What are the effects of anonymity and secrecy on the welfare of the child in gamete donation? *Human Reproduction, 12,* 392–395.

Snowden, R., Mitchell, G. D., & Snowden, E. M. (1983). *Artificial reproduction: A social investigation.* London: George Allen and Unwin.

Tober, D. (2000). Romancing the sperm: Sexuality, technology, and alternative American families. Ph.D. dissertation, University of California, Berkeley/San Francisco.

van Balen, F., & Trimbos-Kemper, T. C. M. (1994). Factors influencing the well-being of long-term infertile couples. *Journal of Psychosomatic Obstetrics and Gynecology, 15,* 157–164.

van Balen, F., Trimbos-Kemper, T. C. M., & Verdurmen, J. (1996). Perception of diagnosis and openness of patients about infertility. *Patient Education and Counseling, 28,* 247–252.

Walker, I., & Broderick, P. (1999). The psychology of assisted reproduction, or psychology assisting its reproduction? *Australian Psychologist, 34,* 38–44.

Weil, E., Cornet, D., Sibony, C., Mandelbaum, J., & Salat-Baroux, J. (1994). Psychological aspects in anonymous and non-anonymous oocyte donation. *Human Reproduction, 9,* 1344–1347.

SEVEN

Conceiving the Happy Family

Infertility and Marital Politics in Northern Vietnam

Melissa J. Pashigian

Infertility in northern Vietnam is a serious issue because it threatens to hinder the development of ties that are believed to bind the conjugal unit, to link that unit to the previous generation, and to connect the living to the dead. Childlessness in a married couple challenges the very purpose of marriage in northern Vietnam, where the birth of children is intended to build the nuclear family unit, to fulfill extended-family expectations for filial piety, and to ensure the happiness and security that come with assuming well-established and well-recognized reproductive and gender roles. In this chapter I argue that to understand why women in Vietnam pursue often lengthy and arduous treatments for infertility, it is critical to make sense of how reproduction informs Vietnam-specific conjugal and generational relationships and the potential consequences for the marital relationship when children are not forthcoming. Also important to understanding the experience of infertility are women's expectations of how having children will change their daily lives and the affective content of their marriages. Indeed, a woman's efforts to find a solution to infertility are to a large degree shaped by her desire to form a special bond with her husband and his family. Preoccupation with infertility, especially by childless married women who are having difficulty conceiving, often involves fears regarding the consequences for married life that are tied to issues of ancestor worship, descent, and familial expectations. Beyond the family, childbearing and motherhood are celebrated in public culture in northern Vietnam through state media promotion of family planning. The presence of these public national images also shapes the experience of infertility by depicting an idealized version of the Vietnamese family; normative family values that valorize motherhood contrast sharply with the image of the childless couple.

In contemporary Vietnam, most women marry at some point during their lives. Approximately 88 percent of women ages twenty-five to forty-nine have ever been married (VNICDS, 1995). Just as it is not socially acceptable for Vietnamese women to remain single voluntarily (Belanger & Khuat, 1999), it is also not socially acceptable for married women of reproductive age to remain childless voluntarily. In the 1994 Viet Nam Intercensal Demographic Survey, no recently married women (married less than five years) indicated that they did not wish to have any children at all (VNICDS, 1995). Most women said they preferred two children, which is not surprising as the national family planning program promotes having no more than "one or two" children.

Northern Vietnam has had a population control agenda since 1961 (Decision 216-CP) (Uy Ban Quoc Gia Dan So va Ke Hoach Hoa Gia Dinh, 1996). After reunification in 1975, the Vietnamese government expanded its population planning efforts to include southern Vietnam. The family planning program was poorly funded during this period, and into the 1980s the intrauterine device (IUD) was promoted to the exclusion of other methods, including condoms and sterilization (Banister, 1993). Abortions were also available. In the late 1980s the formalization of the national family planning program and the introduction of a one-or-two-child policy followed in the wake of the Doi Moi (Renovation) economic reform policy of 1986, which initiated the shift from a centrally planned economy to a market economy in an effort to bring prosperity to Vietnam. An influx of foreign aid, some of which was earmarked for population control, has made sufficient resources available to widely communicate and enforce a family planning policy in the 1990s and beyond. Family planning efforts are focused on stabilizing a population with tremendous growth potential: more than 55 percent of Vietnam's population is under the age of twenty-five (VNICDS, 1997). But despite the national emphasis on reducing population growth aimed to benefit the nation, for women in northern Vietnam, not having any children is perhaps, on a personal level, cause for greater concern than having too many children. Although it should seem obvious in the analysis of reproduction that infertility is inextricably linked to fertility (Inhorn, 1994), this dialectical relationship is often overlooked, especially in the greater politics of population and family planning.

Reproduction thus serves as a site through which social life and the production and replication of culture can be examined. Reproduction provides a means for exposing contestations of social, political, and moral ideology, as well as cultural transformations. In the process of examining reproduction, multiple arenas of difference, involving generation, ethnicity, race, nationality, class, and gender, are revealed (Browner & Sargent, 1996; Ginsburg & Rapp, 1995). For the purposes of this chapter, gender and generation are particularly salient, and an exploration of infertility reveals the cultural framework on which childbearing is based in northern Vietnam.

This chapter offers an analysis of some of the reasons why northern Vietnamese women who have difficulty reproducing pursue lengthy searches for specialized fertility treatments (although I do not explicitly discuss the treatments themselves here), and it addresses the consequences for women when their searches fail.[1] The discussion follows two veins: the first concerns how womanhood and motherhood are conflated in a public culture that forms the larger context in which infertile women exist in northern Vietnam; and the second focuses on the cultural reasons for having children and the potential marital consequences of difficult reproduction and childlessness. How a woman experiences infertility is shaped by numerous conditions that influence and mitigate the circumstances of her marital and extended-family relationships. In other words, infertility in northern Vietnam is much more than simply having or not having a child. Women's efforts to have a child are, in fact, attempts to engage in normative identity formation and to establish links to others.

THE FIELDWORK AND STUDY POPULATION

This chapter is based on ethnographic research conducted over fourteen months in 1995 and 1997 on the social construction of infertility in urban northern Vietnam. During my fieldwork, I interviewed two groups of married women: thirty-nine women who were pursuing treatment for infertility (or had pursued treatment in the past) and a comparison group of ten women with at least one living child who had not experienced infertility. The latter were included in the study as a comparison group to determine how their reproductive and family experiences differed from those of women who were seeking treatment for infertility. In addition, I interviewed husbands of key informants, except in cases in which the wife was pursuing treatment secretly. Questionnaires, ethnographic interviews, and reproductive and life histories were used to collect information. Interviews took place at a major state maternity hospital in Hanoi that offered infertility services, at a state maternity clinic in Hanoi, and in women's homes in and around the city.

The women in this study came from central Hanoi, the outskirts of the city, and villages in adjacent rural provinces. They ranged in age from 21 to 55 (women who were pursuing infertility treatments ranged in age from 21 to 44, with a mean age of 32). Most of the women had at least a junior high school education (not unusual for Vietnam) and came from lower- and middle-class backgrounds. (Class distinctions, less apparent under a centralized economy, have become more readily apparent again in the past ten years with the rise of a middle class). All of the women were employed in addition to being responsible for their households. They worked as laborers in rice fields, market vendors, small shop proprietors (in their own homes or elsewhere), teachers, and government workers.

Of the thirty-nine women who had difficulty reproducing, twenty (51%) had never been pregnant, and nineteen (49%) had been pregnant previously. Of those who had been pregnant in the past, eight (42%) were childless, having aborted or miscarried at least one previous pregnancy; nine (47%) had one living child but were having difficulty bearing a second child; and before the start of research, two women in this group (11%) successfully had children after seeking medical assistance.

It is impossible to know how many of these women were not the main cause of the infertility. Women are usually the ones who seek treatment, and many husbands are never tested for infertility. Therefore, referring to this entire group of women with the highly medicalized term "infertile" might be misleading. Rather, in the Vietnamese lexicon, the term *vo sinh* (literally, "without birth") describes the problems that the women in this study faced. In a hospital consultation, when the gynecologist asks, "What is your medical problem?" the patient frequently responds, "I am without birth [vo sinh]." This indigenous term does not distinguish between those who cannot conceive, those who conceive but miscarry, and so on. Instead, it refers to the outcome, whether a birth is achieved or not, which is ultimately what matters the most within the social and family structure in northern Vietnam.

FAMILY PLANNING POLICY AND CONSTRUCTIONS OF MOTHERHOOD

The multifaceted identity of women in northern Vietnam comprises mother, wife, and worker. Women are known as the pillars of the family, industrious workers who support not only their families but the nation as well. Thus, besides any desire to have children for personal reasons such as love and affection, there exists an entirely separate public adulation of motherhood with which women contend as they shape their identities as married women. The emphasis on motherhood reflects its importance culturally and politically. The state-constructed image of women, which reflects current interpretations of the country's history, is that of strength, control, and contribution to building and protecting the nation through industriousness and control over fertility. The most obvious public emphasis on woman as mother, not surprisingly, is found in the national family planning program.

Population policy and planning in Vietnam have been implemented to stem overpopulation and to prevent future population explosions, which, it is feared, will cause social, economic, and environmental instability. The goal is to reduce the population growth rate to replacement level by the year 2015. The official discourse is family size reduction in the quest to reduce the number of births to no more than two children per family through the promotion of contraceptives and birth spacing of three to five years.

The nationally constructed image of women as mothers is omnipresent, particularly on national family planning campaign billboards adorning the streets. These billboards depict what is referred to as the "happy family," which is composed of wife, husband, and no more than two children in compliance with legislated family size limits.[2] A common slogan on the billboards reads, "Have only one or two children in order to raise them well." The idealized family is depicted as relatively prosperous and nicely dressed. The implication is that they are prosperous because they have no more than two children. These billboards, along with family planning brochures and motivational materials used by family planning cadres, also contain depictions of the "crowded" family, which is poor, whose members wear tattered clothing, and whose numerous crying children drain the family's resources. Messages state directly or imply that by having no more than two children, a couple cannot only be well-off but can also enjoy the happiness and harmony that a small family ensures (cf. Gammeltoft, 1999).

But the messages have a dual meaning. They also imply that happiness comes with having *at least* one child. Embedded in the family planning messages is the assumption that married couples will have at least one child, that fertility and procreative ability are accessible to all. The family planning campaign primarily targets women, as do the penalties for "breaking the plan" (these include fines and temporary job termination). However, the messages apply only to those women who can reproduce; there is no social space for someone who cannot. It is ironic and somewhat contradictory that a message designed to reduce the fertility rate in effect also endorses childbearing.[3]

The emphasis on motherhood by government entities is not limited to family planning programming but is also present in some motivational campaigns to build the nation. On painted placards that line the streets of Hanoi women are depicted as workers and citizens, contributors to the transformation of Vietnam into a competitor in the world market. In these national campaigns, motherhood is reified as a means to a stable society and a prosperous country as Vietnam makes the transition from a centralized economy to a market economy.[4] Women are believed to be instrumental in keeping the population in check and producing upstanding, moral children, brought up with "traditional Vietnamese values." The official image of the contemporary "national" woman—the woman-mother-worker—is perhaps best conveyed in the enormous gilded statue that greets visitors in the vestibule on the first floor of the Vietnam Women's Museum in Hanoi. The statue depicts a larger-than-life woman standing erect, holding a child on her left shoulder, facing into the wind, her short hair blowing back. Her face and posture exude confidence and strength. Her stylized *ao dai* (long tunic-style dress) is also flowing in the wind around her body, her right hand rigidly poised at her side suppressing waves that represent difficulty and strife. The statue, titled "Vietnamese Mother," is displayed in a circular room. Rising a single story above the statue is a lattice of gilded metal and a constellation of fluorescent lightbulbs that forms a dome symbolizing a woman's breast. The image conveys the idea that Vietnamese womanhood encompasses strength against adversity, capability, self-possession, and motherhood.

The cultural salience of motherhood in Hanoi validates a way of life in which childless women are unable to participate. Childless women are surrounded by images that promote women as mothers. Media depictions do not glamorize everyday life but for the most part reflect it. For example, a television interview with a celebrity singer, who could easily pass as one's next-door neighbor, took place in her modest living room, her husband sitting nearby, her two young children sitting on her lap. The setting was intended to show her as much in her role as mother, fulfilling her maternal duties as she sat for the interview, as in her dual (if not secondary) role as an artist.

Thus motherhood is prominent in national public life as one of the most important roles for women, despite the fact that most women are also active in the labor force. More than 90 percent of Vietnamese women participate in the labor force (Desai, 1995; State Planning Committee, 1994). Nonetheless, care for the family is still highly vested in women. In the national representation of women, work, womanhood, and motherhood, childless married women of reproductive age are not discernible. Yet the average individual readily acknowledges the difficulties that childless women face. Many married women in their reproductive years, even if not infertile themselves, can cite someone they know personally or someone they have heard of (in their neighborhood, or among friends of relatives) who is experiencing or has experienced infertility. Although family planning may be the national preoccupation, in terms of the politics of everyday life, to the average person deficient fertility is equally if not more salient than what the state considers high fertility.

EXPECTATIONS OF MARRIAGE AND REASONS TO HAVE CHILDREN

An important aspect of having children in Vietnam is the establishment of harmonious relationships with the living, as well as ritualized respect for the dead. Childless women expect that the birth of children will create a closer relationship with their husbands, increase the chances of having

harmonious relationships with their in-laws, and, in the case of a son, contribute to the husband's filial piety by producing a descendant who continues the lineage and maintains ancestor worship after the death of his parents. It is widely held by both men and women, regardless of their fertility
status, that the purpose of marriage is to have children and that few couples
can attain a special and coveted form of marital sentiment with each other
without the birth of children. This strongly held view continues despite the
fact that there has been a move toward so-called companionate, or "love,"
marriages in contemporary Vietnam.

Unlike its neighbor China, where historically the extended-family system
has been prevalent, the nuclear family has been the main social unit in
Vietnam for many centuries (Whitmore, 1984). A nuclear family is composed of a couple and their children. Therefore, while the union of a
couple in marriage is regarded as the initial step in family formation, until
a couple has children (including through adoption) "building a family"
(xay dung gia dinh) is viewed as incomplete.[5] It is not socially acceptable for
a married woman to choose not to have a child. To do so would be an
affront to her husband's filial piety, in particular, his obligation to his parents to produce descendants, and a potential threat to the stability of her
marriage.

In the northern Vietnamese context, giving birth and raising children
are believed to create a special bond between husband and wife, a bond
that will help the conjugal relationship flow more smoothly. A child links
the emotions of husband and wife. The reason most widely cited by women
in this study for wanting to have children has to do with the establishment
of *tinh cam* with their husbands. *Tinh cam* refers to emotion, sensibility,
feeling, and sentiment that arises within oneself and can be shared mutually.[6] Establishing tinh cam with one's husband is important regardless of
whether a marriage is companionate or arranged. Tinh cam is different
from and can exist independently of love *(tinh yeu)*. It is a feeling that when
established, is believed to bind a couple together. Women and men, regardless of their fertility status, universally expressed the belief that without
having at least one child, it is extremely difficult for a husband and wife to
feel tinh cam for one another, and therefore it is difficult for them to find
happiness together.

Thus, while "happy family" is the term used by the national family planning program to signify a small and therefore prosperous family, happiness
in the family is more broadly interpreted locally to mean harmonious social
relations among family members. The presence of marital tinh cam is
closely related to the presence of harmony and an absence of family conflict
and strife (cf. Rydstrom, 1998). Childless women in particular said they
long for the "cheerfulness" that they expected the introduction of children
would bring to a home and for the happiness that they associated with

establishing a family. Children are thought to create a boisterous house-hold, and happiness is expected to follow as relations between wife and husband and wife and in-laws become closer. Children create a new focal point, refocusing attention from the woman to her child.

Family happiness and harmonious relationships are particularly signifi-cant to a recently married woman because she is now a new member of her husband's family. She must not only establish a relationship with her hus-band but also with his parents, especially if they live in the same household. The roles of each household member are often highly affected by gener-ation and by affinity. Having children fulfills the desires, expectations, and obligations of oneself and others, whether these desires, expectations, and obligations include (in varying degrees of importance) the continuation of ancestor worship, the continuation of the lineage, or the creation of tinh cam. While a childless woman of reproductive age who is attempting to conceive may focus on the tinh cam she wishes to develop with her husband by having a child, having a child may at the same time also fulfill concurrent expectations of parents-in-law for whom, for example, filial piety may be of utmost importance. The expectations of others and the obligation to the patriline may not seriously encroach on the lives of a given married couple, but the birth of a child may mute or make moot the so-called needs of other relatives, thereby creating family harmony. In general, women with-out children hope that having a child will cement their relationship with their husbands and endear them to their in-laws by meeting their expec-tations of building a family.

Harmony is symbolized by a family in which extended family members relate amicably, filial piety is observed, and ancestors are appropriately wor-shiped such that they look out for their descendants on earth. On a func-tional level, ancestor worship and continuing the patriline are invoked as traditional reasons to have children, particularly sons. Worshiping the cult of the ancestors and family descent are two cultural practices that influence the perceived need to bear children in this context. Ancestor worship is widely practiced in this region, and family altars can be seen in most homes. At these altars, children make offerings to the spirits of deceased parents and other relatives to ensure that the souls of the ancestors are taken care of and are not abandoned to wander aimlessly in the spirit world, or wreak havoc on the living for being neglected. Food is offered, and paper money and paper clothing are burned to provide necessities for deceased relatives in the spirit world.

Only a son can continue a kin group's practice of ancestor worship, as daughters are considered to be members of their husbands' families once they marry (Mai, 1991). The primary responsibility for maintaining the family altar is traditionally passed through the paternal line from eldest son to eldest son. If an infertile woman is married to an eldest son, the pressure to bear a child, particularly a boy, can be more intense than if she is married to a younger son. Yet much depends on the family's adherence to Confucian-influenced patriliny, which emphasizes the importance of the eldest son.

The perceived necessity to bear a son varies among women pursuing treatment for infertility. But among the women in this study, there was general agreement that if a woman's firstborn is a son, she will not need to worry about securing her position in the family if no additional children are forthcoming. Some women experiencing secondary infertility following the birth of a daughter came to the hospital for treatment hoping to have a boy. They often explained that their husbands were the eldest sons in their families, and they wanted to have a boy in addition to a daughter. These women expressed less concern about marital stability and their family relationships, because if they were ultimately unable to conceive a second child, they had at least already produced one. Haughton and Haughton (1995) have shown that among ever-married women with at least one living child, son preference is strongly valued in Vietnam, but it does not highly influence fertility behavior.

A number of patrilineal practices that valorize males have been deemed "feudal" by some well-educated urban women. Cuc, a highly educated health care worker who lived in Hanoi and had not experienced infertility, explained that son preference was a vestige of an old belief system to which she said she did not subscribe.[7] She and her husband were perfectly happy with their daughter and had no plans to have another child. But she added that her family situation also lent itself to her progressive perspective, as her husband was not the eldest son and she therefore did not have to worry about having a son. Cuc's reflection on her own family situation reveals a kind of complicit resistance to established social values, but it is resistance within the safety of socially circumscribed boundaries. Her personal situation affords her the ability to disagree with tradition but does not compel her to flagrantly resist that which she contests.

The reality of family formation does not always lend itself to the ideal practice of ritual and support of patrilineal descent. With regard to the importance of sons, there are cases of tradition tempered to fit personal needs. For the eldest son, having a boy serves the dual purpose of continuing ancestor worship and also ensuring patrilineal descent. Tuyet, whose husband is an eldest son, endured three miscarriages and a difficult pregnancy before she finally gave birth to her daughter at age thirty-nine. Unlikely to bear another child, let alone a son, because of her age and reproductive history, this family took exception to the patrilineal transfer of the altar from eldest son to eldest son. Adapting tradition to fit the needs of their family lineage, the altar was passed to the husband's younger brother who already had a son who could ensure both continuity in ancestor worship and continuation of the bloodline. The exception made in this family relieved the pressure Tuyet felt to produce an heir for her husband's family. The adjustment this family made to how ancestor worship would proceed in the next generation reflects the flexibility of culture, not in complete deviation from a traditional practice, but, in this case, to the end of adhering to established norms.

Although it is agreed that women who have a son first are secured in their family, most childless women said they would be satisfied with either a daughter or a son as long as they could have just one child. When faced with the prospect of having no children, a child of either sex can help to bring the marital relationship closer together, a high priority for women. In such cases, preferences of in-laws and complicating factors of ancestor worship and descent, although not always entirely separable from the conjugal relationship, are somewhat peripheral when producing even a single child, regardless of sex, is at stake. In addition, reasons for having children, especially sons, commonly cited in academic literature—for example, old age security and additional family labor (Cain, 1984)—may still be factors for some, but they were rarely cited by women in this study who were having difficulty reproducing. Old age security may be inconsequential when the need to guarantee marital stability in the short term is more pressing. One woman explained that without a child and the associated tinh cam, a marriage and family relationships could become disordered, threatening family harmony and potentially leading, in worst-case scenarios, to divorce, separation, polygyny, or adultery by the husband.

CONSEQUENCES OF INFERTILITY

Indeed, the marital consequences for women that arise as a result of childlessness and reproductive difficulties in northern Vietnam are many and varied. Women, especially in the early years of marriage, feel a sense of urgency to resolve their reproductive difficulties in order to demonstrate their fertility quickly so that their relationships with their husbands will not deteriorate. Some of the childless women in this study expressed concern about the stability of their marriages, as well as their husbands' feelings about their childlessness. Women talk in general about men taking second wives, but polygyny, which was made illegal in Vietnam in 1959 (Luat Hon Nhan va Gia Dinh, 1998), is an especially sensitive issue for childless women who feel insecure about their marriages and living situations. The primary concern is that during the period in which a couple is unsuccessful in their attempts to conceive a child, the husband may seek a second wife to increase the chances of having offspring. In some cases, this is done openly. In other cases, a second household is set up clandestinely.

Although the majority of infertile couples are strongly committed to one another, polygyny is nevertheless a concern in some marriages. One woman, Trang, who was particularly forthcoming about her personal life recollected the attempts her husband made to take a second wife. She described that after thirteen years of marriage and nine years of trying to conceive a baby, her husband, Minh, under pressure from his mother to start a relationship outside his marriage in order to have a child, began a relationship with a woman in his mother's village. This woman became pregnant and one year into the relationship gave birth to a baby girl. Minh asked Trang if he could bring this woman and her baby to live with them so that they could raise the child together, although there was some doubt about whether he was the baby's biological father. Furious, Trang forbid him to see this woman and refused to let her and the baby move into their house. Pointing out that the practice of taking a second wife was illegal, she told him to give her a divorce. Instead he remained in his marriage but continues to bring clothing and money to this woman and the child. He refused a paternity test requested by Trang and continues to claim the child as his own. In this case, Trang blamed Minh's behavior on the encouragement by his mother and the promiscuity of the single woman with whom he was involved but considered him to be a good husband.

Men with second wives are even portrayed sympathetically at times. In a telling letter to an advice column printed in a widely circulated national women's newspaper, one woman from the south who had been married thirty years wrote about her experience. In the letter the woman explained that early in her marriage she had a hysterectomy for health reasons. Both she and her husband were extremely dejected that they would not be able to have children. Her husband eventually brought her a child to raise. She said it made her very happy to take care of a child and her husband also seemed to cheer up with a child's presence in their home. But, unfortunately, the child became ill and died. Eventually she told her husband that they should separate so that he could have a family with someone else. He did not want to. The letter goes on to describe how ultimately he began a relationship with another woman and they had a child. He was very open with his wife about the new relationship. She was hurt but at the same was time happy for him and periodically visited them once he moved to be with his new family. Her question to the advice columnist was whether she should continue her relationship with her husband as is, no longer that of "husband and wife," or whether she should divorce him (*Bao Phu Nu Viet Nam*, February 23, 1995). This woman's concern was that if she remarried, she would have "nothing": she would no longer have her current husband, she would not have a child, and she would not have emotive sentiment with the new husband. The advice columnist lauded the husband for continuing to support his wife and not divorcing her so that she would not have to fend for herself, and she suggested that the husband might return to her some day since they had spent many years together already. The implication was that the first wife was better off in her current situation than if she were divorced.

That men can be both despised and lauded for polygyny reflects a practice that, when used to increase the chances of progeny, is at times culturally understood and treated with empathy but also criticized and disdained. Whether polygyny is more common among infertile couples than those who do not experience childlessness is an open question. Despite the threat of polygyny, many of the infertile couples in this study were committed to each other, and either one or both partners pursued treatment to have a child.

Divorce and permanent separation are additional risks associated with childlessness. Childless women fear losing their husbands and their support networks. Divorce, which had been shunned, is becoming increasingly more common in Vietnam. When women are divorced, their options are to try to live without any family and support themselves (difficult but possible), to return to live with their parents or a sibling's family, or to remarry. If it is common knowledge that a woman cannot reproduce, her chances of remarriage can be diminished, particularly in villages in the countryside where anonymity and privacy are rare. One childless woman who came to the hospital from a distant rural village was clearly devastated by a recent turn of events in which her husband had abandoned her for a new wife. She had elected to move in with her parents who lived in a nearby village and was not communicating with her husband's family. She came to the hospital for the last treatment she could afford in the hope of being cured so that she could reconcile with her husband.

Although divorce or separation can significantly alter the stability of a woman's living situation, a woman's life is not completely destroyed, especially if she has natal relatives to whom she can return. In addition, because it is permissible and common for women to work outside the home in Vietnam, women can reestablish their income-generating power with some effort even if they change locales. Finally, there is also a legacy of Vietnamese women who never married during the 1970s and 1980s because of war and migration (Goodkind, 1997). Some cohorts of women were past the acceptable marriage age by the end of the Vietnam–U.S. war, and for younger cohorts of women who came of age at the end of the war and after, there were fewer men available to marry because of wartime casualties. That these women have successfully survived without marriage has set a new precedent.

Paradoxically, some women ask for a divorce themselves in order to free their husbands to marry again, in the chance that he may conceive with another woman. Several women stated they felt guilty, believing that *they* were preventing their husbands from having a child, and they had asked their husbands for a divorce. (In each of these cases, the husbands declined.) One woman asked her husband if she could find him a second wife, a situation she found preferable to divorce. Divorce, as a threat, is also a tool for women, not all of whom cower in the face of marital dissolution. As in the case of Trang and Minh, she wielded the threat of divorce in an attempt to prevent her husband from taking a second wife. In other words, women who are childless are not always powerless in their marriages, perhaps attributable in part to the historical legacy of powerful women and earlier attempts at gender egalitarianism under communism.

Changes in marital status are among the severest social consequences of infertility for women, but there are notable complications in common daily interactions. Most childless women in this study did not feel they suffered overt ostracism; however, their childless state was sometimes used against them. A woman who worked as a fruit seller in the market explained, "Sometimes people who don't like me [in the marketplace] put me down because they want to be superior to me. They tell me I will never have a child." The women in the market were not targeting her for her lack of children per se, she said, but her childlessness was used as fodder. In-laws who are unsympathetic might also blame a daughter-in-law for not bearing a child, rebuking her for not wanting a child badly enough.

In addition to such insults, expressions of sympathy mark difference as well. Well-intentioned "preoccupation" with a couple's conception can create uncomfortable social pressure. Yet there is also marked sympathy for couples who are childless. Men and women who have no experience with infertility in their own lives sympathetically describe the lives of women who cannot bear children as *kho* (miserable), referring to the difficulties women have in bonding with their in-laws and husband, the threat of marital dissolution, and the general disappointment they must experience in a quiet, small household. While family and friends may be preoccupied with a couple's conception difficulties, most women who participated in this study said they thought that their friends and family on both sides wanted only what was best for them and thus hoped for children for them. Friends and relatives sometimes suggested the names and addresses of doctors and traditional healers or offered "medicines" to relieve the problem. Questions from acquaintances, such as "Do you have any news yet?" are common in conversation with married women of reproductive age. Although such questions are banal, they may seem prying or pressuring to women who are having difficulty reproducing.

The infertile women who participated in this study consistently described their current family life without children as sad *(buon)*. Without children in their future, they expected life to continue to be sad. Sadness meant, among other things, that without a child everyday life would be filled primarily with work. Exhausted after hours of labor, a short television break for those who can afford a set might be the only leisure activity of the day before going to sleep. A common perception is that husbands and wives tire of one another unless there is a child to distract them.

Some couples who did not have children said that they did not frequently visit or receive visits from others. Sunday, typically the one day off per week, is reserved for visiting friends and relatives, especially with children in tow, or going for a motorbike ride in and around town. Some childless couples did not consider themselves entitled to the same social prerogatives as those with children. For instance, Hang and her husband, Hong, had been married for ten years. They were pursuing infertility treatments because they had not yet produced any children. Hang explained, "We would buy a motorbike if we had a child, to take the child out. When we have a child we will buy one. With a child we can go out happily. Without children there is only me and my husband, tired of one another." While this isolation may be involuntary (i.e., being included less frequently in activities that involve children), to some extent it is self-imposed.

In northern Vietnam, women who experience secondary infertility in the years after their first child's birth and elect to pursue treatment find themselves in a liminal state: they pass as mothers, but at the same time they personally experience infertility and attempt to achieve the idealized but elusive two-child family. Physiologically, these women may be experiencing infertility, but socially this may be imperceptible, as they are mothers of one child in a society where "one or two" children are acceptable. Because they are able to access social networks by virtue of being mothers, they are buffered from some of the social consequences of infertility experienced by childless women. Despite the cultural presence of patrilineal descent traditions, having proved fertility with a daughter was often sufficient. Indeed, there were some women experiencing secondary infertility who, along with their husbands, hoped to have a second daughter.

Most women with a child who pursued treatment for secondary infertility were more relaxed about the success of the treatment process than were childless women. For these women, part of the motivation for having a second child was to provide companionship for their first child now that, having assumed the role of mother, they were more secure in their marriage. One woman who had been pursuing treatment for six months decided she would try for one more month and then give up. She said that if she did not have another child, things would still be satisfactory in her family.

Similarly, most childless women whose husbands had children from a previous marriage said they did not feel spousal pressure to reproduce. For the most part, these women were encouraged to pursue fertility treatments for their own happiness, not for their husbands' fulfillment. In cases in which the husband's children lived with them, a woman might be told by her husband that it was not crucial to have children of their own as she had his children to raise. But this was not a fully satisfactory option from the perspective of these women, as they wished to have a child with their husbands in order to "bind" the two of them together and build tinh cam.

Although each of the categories of women described above falls under the rubric *vo sinh,* how and when the absence of birth occurs, combined with particulars of family structure and interpersonal relationships, shapes the effect of reproductive difficulties on their lives. Nevertheless, to stave off the potential consequences of childlessness, virtually all of the women in this study felt compelled to seek treatment for their reproductive difficulties, even if that meant intermittent treatment over the years as funds were available and when they could afford time away from work.

CONCLUSION

Childbearing for women in contemporary northern Vietnam is closely associated with establishing ties of sentiment with one's husband and closer bonds with his family. Childbearing engages generational issues by linking the worlds of the living and the deceased through ancestor worship and descent. When childbearing fulfills each of these needs, people expect that happiness and family harmony will be achieved.

Infertility is extremely salient in contemporary Vietnam and is well recognized, even by those who do not experience infertility, as provoking serious social consequences for a woman because she is not afforded the conventional means by which to integrate herself into her marital family. Thus a woman's experience of infertility is tied to the gender politics of marriage in Vietnam. Some women's experiences are mitigated by specific family circumstances, such as the timing of the onset of infertility or the presence of children from a husband's previous marriage and the degree to which a family rigidly adheres to traditional practices, as in the case of ancestor worship and descent. But if adherence to tradition and cultural practices in a given family are not flexible enough, the consequence may be marital dissolution. Thus, in many ways, the consequences of not having any children in Vietnam are viewed as more difficult than having too many children.

Vietnam is currently undergoing profound social and economic change and women's roles are being influenced by often contradictory modern and traditional cultural practices. As social change continues to take place, the experience of infertility and the flexibility with which people adapt cultural ritual to their personal situations are likely to change. Although women who experience infertility cannot integrate themselves in their husband's family in conventional ways, they are not simply victims of circumstance. As shown in this chapter, they are also social actors who will continue to work to negotiate their position in their marriages, albeit some more successfully than others.

NOTES

The research on which this chapter is based was generously supported by a dissertation grant from the Wenner-Gren Foundation for Anthropological Research and the University of California, Los Angeles. The University of California Office of the President provided dissertation writing support. I owe special thanks to Marcia Inhorn and Frank van Balen for their detailed readings, insightful comments, and editorial vision for this chapter. The chapter has also benefited from comments at earlier stages by Carole Browner, Nancy Levine, Gina Masequesmay, and Cynthia Strathmann, to whom I am grateful.

1. In this chapter I limit my comments to northern Vietnam. While there may be some commonalities in the social experience of infertility in northern and southern Vietnam, cultural and treatment differences do exist.

2. Exceptions to family size legislation are made for ethnic minority groups, couples in which one or both partners were married previously, and couples with two disabled children.

3 To its credit, a clause buried in the text of the family planning policy states that women who are unable to bear a child may be given assistance in bearing a child if they so desire, further complicating the contradictory nature of fertility regulation (see Banister, 1993). Unfortunately, the financial and technical assistance necessary to assist a desiring couple as stipulated by the clause is limited.

4. Market reforms and an influx of commercial goods have forced significant social changes during the 1990s. Economic and social reforms have been heavily controlled by the government to prevent social unrest as class differences widen.

5. In some cultures adoption can be an alternative to biological reproduction for infertile couples. However, in Vietnam this option is not popular (see Inhorn [1996] for discussion of the unpopularity of adoption in Egypt). There are numerous folk beliefs and cultural taboos regarding adoption. Not knowing the family of an adopted child is a large impediment to adoption. There is concern about whether the child's biological ancestors (alive or deceased) led decent lives or committed immoral acts. If the child comes from inauspicious stock, then it is possible for one's family to be beset by negative events through these ancestors. Furthermore, the child may have inherited a tendency toward negative behavior and may therefore reflect poorly on the adoptive family. There is additional concern that the adopted child will leave the adoptive family to seek her or his birth mother. Finally, because the adopted child is not biologically related to the social parents, there is concern that adopted boys in particular will not have a vested interest in the family and will not pray to the adoptive family's ancestors after the adoptive parents are deceased.

6. I would like to thank Keith W. Taylor for discussions about the meaning of *tinh cam.*

7. All names of respondents are pseudonyms.

REFERENCES

Banister, J. (1993). *Vietnam population dynamics and prospects.* Berkeley: University of California Institute of East Asian Studies.

Belanger, D., & Khuat, T. H. (1999). Too late to marry: Failure, fate or fortune? Women's paths to unmarried life in two rural villages of North Vietnam. Paper presented at the annual meeting of the Association for Asian Studies, Boston, MA.

Browner, C. H., & Sargent, C. F. (1996). Anthropology and studies of human reproduction. In C. F. Sargent & T. M. Johnson (Eds.), *Medical anthropology: Contemporary theory and method* (pp. 219–234). Westport, CT: Praeger.

Cain, M. (1984). *Women's status and fertility in developing countries: Son preference and economic security.* World Bank Staff Working Papers No. 682. Washington, DC: World Bank.

Desai, J. (1995). *Vietnam through the lens of gender: An empirical analysis using household survey data.* Hanoi: United Nations Development Program.

Gammeltoft, T. (1999). *Women's bodies, women's worries: Health and family planning in a Vietnamese rural community.* Surrey: Curzon Press.

Ginsburg, F. D., & Rapp, R. (1995). Introduction: Conceiving the new world order. In F. D. Ginsburg & R. Rapp (Eds.), *Conceiving the new world order: The global politics of reproduction* (pp. 1–17). Berkeley: University of California Press.

Goodkind, D. (1997). The Vietnamese double marriage squeeze. *International Migration Review, 31,* 108–127.

Haughton, J., & Haughton, D. (1995). Son preference in Vietnam. *Studies in Family Planning, 26,* 325–337.

Inhorn, M. C. (1994). *Quest for conception: Gender, infertility, and Egyptian medical traditions.* Philadelphia: University of Pennsylvania Press.

Inhorn, M. C. (1996). *Infertility and patriarchy: The cultural politics of gender and family life in Egypt.* Philadelphia: University of Pennsylvania Press.

Luat hon nhan va gia dinh va nhung van ban huong dan thi hanh (Law of marriage and family). (1998). Hanoi: NXB Chinh Tri Quoc Gia.

Mai, H. B. (1991). A distinctive feature of the meaning of reproduction in Confucian family tradition in the Red River Delta. In R. Liljestrom & Tuong Lai (Eds.), *Sociological studies on the Vietnamese family* (pp. 49–56). Hanoi: Social Sciences Publishing House.

NCPFP (National Committee for Population and Family Planning) (1993). *Population and family planning strategy to the year 2000.* Hanoi: NCPFP.

NCPFP (National Committee for Population and Family Planning). (1996). *Population and family planning program in Vietnam.* Hanoi: NCPFP.

Rydstrom, H. (1998). *Embodying morality: Girls' socialization in a North Vietnamese commune.* Linkoping, Sweden: Department of Child Studies, Linkoping University.

Socialist Republic of Vietnam. (1995). *Vietnam government country report on social development.* Hanoi.

State Planning Committee–General Statistical Office. (1994). *Vietnam living standards survey 1992–1993.* Hanoi.

Uy Ban Quoc Gia Dan So va Ke Hoach Gia Dinh. (1996). *Ky yeu chinh sach dan so va ke hoach hoa gia dinh Viet Nam* (Summary of Vietnam's population and family planning policy). VIE/93/P07. Hanoi: Nha Xuat Ban Thong Ke.

Viet Nam Intercensal Demographic Survey 1994. (1995). *Major findings.* Hanoi: Statistical Publishing House.

Viet Nam Intercensal Demographic Survey 1994. (1997). *Population structure and household composition.* Hanoi: Statistical Publishing House.

Vu, M. L. (1991). The gender division of labour in rural families in the Red River Delta. In R. Liljestrom & Tuong Lai (Eds.), *Sociological studies of the Vietnamese family* (pp. 149–163). Hanoi: Social Sciences Publishing House.

Vu, Q, N. (1994). Family planning programme in Vietnam. *Vietnam Social Sciences, 1(39),* 3–20.

Whitmore, J. K. (1984). Social organization of Confucian thought in Vietnam. *Journal of Asian Studies, 15,* 296–306.

EIGHT

Positioning Gender Identity in Narratives of Infertility

South Indian Women's Lives in Context

Catherine Kohler Riessman

How, in a context such as India where strong pronatalist attitudes mandate motherhood, do women construct gender identities when they cannot be mothers? Making babies is how women are expected to form adult identities the world over, and in non-Western "developing" societies the gendered consequences of infertility can be grave (Inhorn, 1994; Unisa, 1999). Psychological theories consider maternity the central milestone in adult female development (Ireland, 1993). Yet women find ways to compose lives that accommodate, and sometimes resist, dominant definitions. How is this identity work done as women move into and beyond the childbearing years?

Recent work on adult identity development questions formulations about identity as singular and continuous (Mishler, 1999). Building on these ideas and drawing on a social constructionist perspective, I show how identities are constituted in and through spoken discourse. In symbolic exchanges—conversations being the most basic—individuals interpret their pasts to communicate how they want to be known. By talking, listening, and questioning, human actors generate definitions of their situations that are in turn taken for granted as "real" (Bamberg, 1997; Harre & van Langenhove, 1999). Gender identity in particular is accomplished interactionally, continually renegotiated in linguistic exchange and social performance (Davies, 1989; Cerulo, 1997; Kessler & McKenna, 1978). Narratives developed during research interviews provide a window into the process. When we tell stories about events in our lives, we perform our preferred identities (Langellier, 2001).

I examine the personal narratives of three South Indian women who are in their forties and fifties, selected from a larger corpus of interviews with married childless women completed during fieldwork in Kerala in 1993–1994. Interviews, conducted by me and my research assistant, Liza George, were tape recorded and subsequently transcribed and translated where necessary (seven interviews were in English, the rest in Malayalam).[1] We encouraged women to give extended accounts of their situations, including the reactions of husbands, family members, and neighbors. We did not interview husbands, so their perceptions of infertility are not included except as wives represent them. (For a full description of method, see Riessman [2000a, 2000b].) The three women chosen for analysis here are among the oldest in my sample and probably past childbearing age. Constructing gender identities and meaningful lives without biological children is a salient issue for them.

Study of personal narrative is a form of case-centered research, often described as narrative analysis (Riessman, 1993, 2002). Investigators from several theoretical perspectives have adapted the methods to study issues of health and illness (Bell, 2000, 1999; Frank, 1995; Langellier, 2001; Mattingly, 1998; Mattingly & Garro, 2000). I use the approach pioneered by Mishler (1986a, 1986b, 1991, 1999), which includes the following distinctive features: presentation of and reliance on detailed transcripts of interview excerpts; attention to the structural features of discourse; analysis of the co-production of narratives through the dialogic exchange between interviewer and participant; and a comparative approach to interpreting similarities and differences among participants' life stories. I compare narratives the women develop to explain infertility, and analyze positioning in relation to identity claims. "The act of positioning . . . refers to the assignment of fluid 'parts' or 'roles' to speakers in the discursive construction of personal stories" (Harre & van Langenhove, 1999, p. 7). I analyze how narrative structure, positioning, and performance work together in women's constructions of their identities as childless women.

Several levels of positioning are my analytic points of entry into the "personal stories." First, they developed in an immediate discursive context, an evolving interview with a listener-questioner. At this level, women position themselves in a dialogic process. They perform their preferred identities for a particular audience—my research assistant and me in this case. We are also located in social spaces and bring views about infertility to the conversations, positioning the women. Second, the narratives are positioned in a broader cultural discourse about women's proper place in modern India, a "developing" nation that is developing new spaces (besides home and field) for women to labor. I show how attention to the shifting cultural context and the proximate interview context assists interpretation. Third, the women position themselves in relation to physicians (and medical technology) and vis-à-vis powerful family members in their stories. Taken together, the angle of vision of positioning in narrative provides a lens through which to explore how middle-aged women construct positive identities when infertility treatment has failed.

I now turn to the case studies, beginning with a brief description of each woman and the contexts of conversation. Detailed transcriptions of excerpts of interviews are included so that readers can examine the narratives in dialogic exchange.

THE NARRATIVES

"I think that it must be because I am so old"

Asha, who has never been pregnant, is a forty-two-year-old Hindu woman. She completed secondary school and is employed as a government clerk. Typical of women in Kerala, she has benefited from the state's educational policies: girls attend school as often as boys, and, because of similar levels of education, secure government jobs are occupied by both women and men, in contrast to other states in India.[2] Asha and her husband, from a "backward" (Dalit) caste, receive some food and housing assistance from the government. On the day we met her, she was making her second visit to the infertility clinic of a government hospital. She had previously gone for biomedical treatment for infertility in another hospital, as her narrative describes. Biomedicine is widely available in Kerala, and the hospital to which she came this time is the tertiary care center for a large district. We learn Asha had come reluctantly in the excerpt (below), but she was not reluctant to be interviewed; we spent nearly an hour talking together in a private room while she was waiting to be seen by the doctor. Liza, my twenty-six-year-old research assistant, told Asha we wanted to understand "the experience of being childless from women's points of view." The open-ended interview was in Malayalam, translated periodically for me, and Asha said she felt "comforted" by it. Although our questions focused mostly on issues of infertility and societal response, Asha directed the interview to other topics of importance to her. During the first few minutes, for example, when asked about the composition of her household and other demographic "facts," Asha's extended responses hint at complexities in gender relations: her husband is twelve years her junior and will become unemployed shortly ("we will be managing on my income alone"). The meaning of these issues only became clear later. At this point, Liza asked her about not having children.

> L: What do you think is the reason why you do not have children?
>
> A: I think that it must be because I am so old.
> That is my opinion.
> Other than that, no other problem.
> There is this [name] hospital in Alleppey
> there— I had gone there for treatment.

Then the doctor said that— after doing a scan
the way through which the sperm goes
there is some block.
And so they did a D&C.
When the results came—when we gave money to the lab
they said they did not see any problem.
After that they said I must take five pills.
I took them.
Then that also did not work.
Then they said that I must have an injection.
I had one.
They said I must come again after that.
After I had the first injection
I was disappointed when it did not work
I had hoped that it would be all right after the first injection.
When that did not happen
then I was very much disheartened.
Then when they said to come again—
then I didn't go after that. . . .

[describes how a neighbor persuaded her to go to the infertility clinic]

If God is going to give, let him.[3]

Asha's explanation for infertility takes a classic narrative form: she em-
plots a sequence of events related to medical treatment, which she locates
in time and place, and she provides evaluation or commentary on their
meanings. Typical of "fully formed" (Labov, 1982) narratives, hers is tightly
structured and uninterrupted by the listener. Asha was forty years old at
the time of the events, had been married two years, and could not get
pregnant. We do not know, at this point in the conversation, why she married so late; the average age at which women in Kerala marry is twenty-two
(Gulati, Ramalingam, & Gulati, 1996).

In terms of how Asha positions herself, she answers our question directly
and offers her present understanding of "the reason" for infertility ("it must
be because I am so old"), which contrasts with the technical diagnosis offered by a physician she consulted in the past ("there is some block"). It is
her location in the life course, she says, not some internal flaw, that is
responsible for the infertility. The narrator is agent, the real expert, wise
and realistic about the meaning of age for fertility; she positions the physicians as "they"—the other—who depend on medical technology (a scan,
a D&C, pills and injections). As the knowing subject, Asha deflects blame;
age is not something she is responsible for. Her positioning aligns the listener with the narrator in a moral stance: the "I" knows better than the
"other."

Asha carefully names every procedure and reports how she followed the prescribed regime, perhaps because of the setting of the interview and her expectations about us. She positions herself for the medical context, so that she will be viewed as a "good historian" and a "compliant patient." But biomedicine failed her. It also failed to make room for emotions: no one relates to her disappointment in the narrative performance. Asha became "disheartened" when treatment did not work, and she did not return to the hospital.

In a lengthy episode (not included here) Asha performs a conversation with a neighbor in her village, who got pregnant after treatment at the infertility clinic where our interview took place. "She told me if I came here [to clinic] it will be all right." Asha said to the neighbor, "I will still have this problem of my age." The neighbor responded by saying she had seen "people who are forty-five years" in the waiting room of the clinic. Asha then agreed, very reluctantly, to try the clinic as "a last resort." As she reasoned, "there will be no need to be disappointed" because she will have tried everything.

Asha concludes the narrative with a coda that looks to religion rather than science ("If God is going to give [children], let him"). Like the first line of the narrative or abstract ("I think it must be because I am so old"), the coda acknowledges that health involves more than narrow technical problems in the body that doctors can fix. A theodicy frames the account of infertility—beginning and ending it—suggesting resistance to the biomedical model and secular beliefs about health (Greil, 1991).

There are several puzzlements in Asha's sparse narrative. Because the interview was translated from Malayalam, close examination of word choice is not appropriate, but other narrative strategies can be examined, for example, the characters she introduces in the performance and the way she positions herself in relation to them. Absences are striking: there is no mention of husband or family; only once does she use a plural pronoun ("when we gave money to the lab"). She does not say that her husband accompanied her for treatment or if he was examined by doctors—customary in Indian infertility clinics. In contrast to the richly peopled stories about infertility told by other South Indian women, there are few characters in Asha's: anonymous doctors ("they"), a neighbor, and Asha herself. We get the impression of an isolated, singular "self," negotiating infertility treatment on her own—a picture that is at odds with the typical family-centered fertility search I observed in fieldwork (Riessman, 2000b) and with Indian views of familial identity (Roland, 1988).

Information from later in the interview contextualizes Asha's performance in the excerpt and informs understanding of the process of her adult identity formation. Her life story is in some ways typical of the life course of women from the rural areas of Kerala, although in key respects it is unique. She relates that her natal family was large and very poor, and when marriage proposals came, her parents could not raise the dowry. Asha also says she was not interested in marriage ("married life, I did not want it from childhood on, I was one of those who did not like it"). Both of her parents died when she was a young woman, and she received a small inheritance when the property was divided among the siblings. She bought a little gold, took out a loan, got a job, won some money in the lottery, and eventually accumulated enough to buy a small piece of land with a thatched hut ("all of it I bought by myself"). Such autonomous actions contrast with stereotypes about women in India, but Asha's actions are not atypical in Kerala. Government policies are fostering women's power and economic independence as part of rural development efforts, including micro credit schemes and enterprises, in addition to affirmative action policies for historically disadvantaged castes (Gulati et al., 1996; Jeffrey, 1993). Without parents, however, arranging a marriage was difficult. In response to a question I asked about "her change of heart about marriage," Asha educated me: "If you want to get ahead in the future you must have a husband . . . when we become old there must be somebody to look after us." Like Indian women generally, she was constrained by gender ideology; Asha needed a husband to move forward and receive social recognition—to "get ahead"—and to have children—necessary in a country without social welfare programs for the aged. Instrumental views about having children to ensure parental caretaking are common in India (Jeffery, Jeffery, & Lyon, 1989; Uberoi, 1993).

At thirty-eight Asha went to a marriage broker to fix a marriage—an unusual move that was necessary because her brothers had left the region. The arranged intercaste marriage (Asha married "down") concealed a significant age discrepancy—Asha was twelve years older than her husband—which she discovered later. Because of her education and the context of women's employment in South India, she has secure earning capacity as a government clerk, while her husband faces unemployment. He wants children, however, and she fears she will be on her own again ("If we do not have children, the marital relationship will break up"). Like other rural women (Riessman, 2000b), Asha's in-laws blame her for the fertility problems and pressure her to get treatment. Constructing a positive gender identity without children is extremely problematic for Asha because of ideologies about compulsory marriage and motherhood.

In this context, the narrative excerpt above makes sense: "as a last resort" Asha decides to begin infertility treatment again, at age forty-two, even as she wisely knows she is "too old." The absence of family and husband in the excerpt masks their role in the decision. The husband's absence raises other questions, however. Given the complexities of their gender relations—she is significantly older and the primary wage earner—and the precarious status of their marriage, we might ask: Is Asha repositioning herself as a single woman? One might be tempted to read her story as one of victimization—a South Indian woman who faces divorce because of infertility—but her narrative performance as a competent "solo self" suggests a more complex reality. There is a consistency to her identity before marriage and the one she puts forward as the marriage is ending.

"I think I was overworking"

My interview with Sunita took place in a different context than the one with Asha, and her life circumstances are also dissimilar. Sunita is a forty-six-year-old Hindu woman from a Brahmin subcaste. She works as a university professor and has a Ph.D. Her husband owns an established business. Married for twenty-two years, they had planned to have "at least two children." I interviewed Sunita alone, in her home, in English; she was totally fluent, even using a Western argot. She was obviously familiar with the conventions of Western research interviewing and succinctly answered my beginning demographic questions, until I asked one ("And have you ever been pregnant?") that immediately prompted a lengthy narrative about a sequence of events that led to a miscarriage twenty years previously—the only time she had been pregnant. The context of the miscarriage was crucial to Sunita's understanding of infertility: she elaborated the circumstances several times during our long interview.[4]

C: And have you ever been pregnant?

S: Yeah I think it was the second or third year of marriage   1
that I was pregnant
then in the third month I started spotting.
I think I was overworking.

And uh since it was a choice marriage, I had a lot of–   2
We were trying to get my in-laws
to be more amenable to the whole situation.
In-laws were against the marriage.

And uh so I used to work the whole day,   3
then go to their place to cook in the evening for a family of seven.
Then uh pack the food for two of us and bring it home [laughs] . . .

[interaction about living separately and traveling between two households]

I think uh that uh was overdoing it.

And then I carried some of the food stuff you know,   4
the grains and things, the monthly stuff, groceries,
from that place,
because my mother-in-law insisted that I carry it *that* day.

And the next day I started spotting   5
and I was so frightened because uh, you know,
I didn't know really what to do.

So I rang up my doctor and told her   6
and she said, "You just lie down, and come in, you're okay,
but only thing I think you need to rest."
You know, "don't move around" and things like that. . . .

[tells of miscarriage]

So uh it *was* quite traumatic at that point.

But the doctor—in fact I was very thin.   7
I weighed under one hundred pounds.
So the doctor said, "Look you have to put on weight
before you uh decide to get pregnant again . . ."

And after that I stopped going every day to my in-laws   8
because my husband said, "This is ridiculous, I mean you know."

Sunita, unlike Asha, positions her infertility in a web of family obligations that result in "overworking." She was twenty-six years old at the time of the miscarriage, several years into a "choice"—not arranged—marriage, and her in-laws were not "amenable to the whole situation." Sunita attempts to be the good daughter-in-law: going "to their place to cook in the evening for a family of seven," after she has worked "the whole day" at a job, and before she returned home with food prepared for her husband. (Double shifts are typical for employed South Indian women, although the triple shift Sunita reports is unusual—a consequence of the couple's decision to live apart from the joint family and also have her perform the cooking duties expected of a new daughter-in-law.) In the context of heavy physical demands made by her mother-in-law, a miscarriage occurs, which Sunita attributes to "overworking."

Sunita structures the narrative in ways that ensure her attribution will be heard by the listener-reader. In the dialogic process she places her audience—me—in a dual position: a sympathetic woman listener, who understands about the heavy demands of combining career and family, but also an outsider who may not understand the additional demands placed on Indian women. She invites me into an Indian narrative world in stanzas 2 and 3, by providing orientation about choice marriage, family hierarchy, and the obligations of brides to in-laws. Understanding that I am being educated, I ask questions. In lines deleted from the transcript, I ask, "You were living separately from your in-laws?"; she responds by clarifying that she and her husband were "living some distance away." They chose not to become part of a joint family, yet she performed cooking responsibilities as the newest bride, as if she had become part of the joint family. The audience positions Sunita as the dutiful daughter-in-law and enters into her point of view.

With cultural context and an alliance between teller and audience established, Sunita commences the narrative plot in earnest in stanza 4. Time shifts from the general to the particular (*"that"* day). She positions key characters in her drama: a demanding mother-in-law ("she insisted that I carry it"), an attentive personal physician ("she said 'You just lie down . . . ' "), and a concerned husband (after the miscarriage, he says going to cook every day for the in-laws is "ridiculous"). Sunita's positionings offer clues about her preferred identity; she represents herself as an Indian woman who observes tradition and authority relations, deferring to mother-in-law and husband.

Sunita and Asha position characters in their performances in distinctive ways. Both are first-person accounts and consequently privilege the "I." But Sunita's voice exists in the context of meaningful relationships—with a mother-in-law, husband, and personal physician. The physician, for example, is given a spoken role ("You just lie down . . .") and a gender ("she"), in contrast to Asha's anonymous physicians ("they"). In Sunita's account, the physician is represented as a supportive advocate concerned with the lifeworld of her patient ("I think you need to rest . . . you have to put on weight"), not simply the gynecological expert who relies on one medical technology after another as in Asha's representation. Attending to emotions connected to the events also varies: there is no mention of physician response when Asha refers to "disappointment" when treatment failed; when Sunita "was so frightened" when she began spotting, her physician offers reassurance ("you're okay"). These differences probably reflect the contrasting class positions and related medical experiences of the two women: Sunita had a personal physician she "rang up," and Asha got treatment at a local hospital clinic, where she probably saw a different doctor every visit. Asha positions herself economically throughout her "solo" life story: she explicitly mentions paying for treatment and her belief that a child would provide security in old age. Sunita's relational life story takes class privilege for granted: she never mentions money explicitly and appears to want a child for "completeness," instead of economic security.

Sunita returns to the miscarriage and the role her physician played much later in the interview. We had been talking for more than an hour, and I was asking about the reaction of others to her childlessness, including "your husband's family." She responded by saying she thinks her mother-in-law has "always felt guilt . . . she has always felt she has been the cause of that miscarriage." When I asked, "Because of the traveling and bringing all the food?" Sunita agreed and immediately returned to the storyworld to elaborate the earlier narrative. New information emerges: when her doctor learned of the heavy physical work Sunita had done at her mother-in-law's insistence and of her mother-in-law's statement ("I've had five children, I've done the same work as you, I've carried things such as these"), the physician expressed anger: "Don't you do such stupid things." Sunita interpreted the physician's statement as a clear message to take care of herself, not her mother-in-law. As Sunita performs the role of the woman physician, she appears to identify with her young patient, who is caught in a web of obligations and authority relations typical in Indian families, with which the physician must have been familiar. A new daughter-in-law is expected to provide household services in her mother-in-law's home, until the time she achieves full status as a woman, that is, has a child. Sunita positions her physician as an ally against inequality—ironically, in the case, between a mother- and daughter-in-law, both women, but separated by age and status in a hierarchical family system. Sunita's representation suggests she was empowered by the medical relationship. The physician's authority enabled her to break away from traditions of generational deference. Together with her husband, the physician enabled her to say no.

Yet there is something missing from the narrative: there is no explicit reference to blame. In accounting for infertility, Sunita never expresses anger or holds her mother-in-law responsible, nor does she fault herself for "overworking." Can such thoughts and emotions even be imagined in the South Indian context? The issue of blame must remain implicit. My interpretation here is supported by material from elsewhere in the interview and also from a letter Sunita wrote to me. (I had sent her a draft of a book chapter [Riessman, 1997], which drew heavily from our interview conversation, and asked for her reactions to my interpretation of her narrative account.)

Sunita performed a conversation with her mother-in-law as our interview was drawing to a close. To elaborate why her mother-in-law might feel "guilty," Sunita related a conversation the two women had on a long train ride as they returned from the funeral of a close family member; Sunita had repositioned herself as a valued daughter-in-law in the twenty years that had passed since the miscarriage. She reconstructs their conversation: Her mother-in-law said, "I've never had the courage to ask you. . . . You *had* conceived so why couldn't you conceive again? . . . It shouldn't have happened that way." Sunita says to me, "I tried to tell her 'I don't blame you.' " In the brief exchange, Sunita refers to the conversational rules the two women observed: they went "round and round," she says, circling the question of blame. Still positioning herself as a traditional Indian woman and dutiful daughter-in-law, Sunita follows her mother-in-law's lead about how to conduct herself ("since she went round and round I also had to go round and round"), just as twenty years earlier she had followed her mother-in-law's instructions, leading (she implies) to miscarriage . Elsewhere (Riessman, 1997), I interpret the exchange by arguing that generational tensions cannot be addressed openly in contemporary India. Political issues about women's proper place in modern Indian families remain private, cast as interpersonal conflicts between women. Because the available discourse is interpersonal, the two women go "round and round" about blame and forgiveness.

Sunita's letter in response to my draft manuscript ignored my political interpretation and concurred with my interpersonal one. Here is precisely what she wrote:

> Till you interviewed me I had not reflected very deeply about the events in my life. On reflection I think that your interpretations about the blame-forgiveness is quite right, though I had not consciously perceived it in that way before. My ability to deal with my not having children was because I know there was nothing medically wrong with me or my husband. Moreover, my husband's acceptance of me as a complete woman facilitated my own acceptance of myself as a complete person. This has enabled me to enjoy all the children in my life.

Sunita puts forward several identities in the letter. First, it is typed on university letterhead, which brings her professional self into our exchange. Second, she emphasizes that there is nothing "wrong" with her medically. Like Asha, she claims an identity without medical fault and consequent blame. Unlike Asha, however, Sunita can claim a secure identity as a wife, even without progeny. She says her husband's acceptance of her as a "complete woman" has enabled her to accept herself as a "complete person." Her word choice here is puzzling: it could suggest some continuing uncertainty about gender identity in the absence of motherhood, or it could be read as a statement about the superiority of "personhood" over motherhood and womanhood. Finally, she refers to enjoying "all the children in my life." Here, Sunita is recalling a continuing theme in our interview—the many nonbiological children with whom she has important relationships (the children of servants and colleagues and nieces and nephews). Sunita chooses to locate herself in a "complete" life—how she wants to be known.

I now turn to a third, and final, interview, which contrasts with the first two in identity construction processes.

"You are perfectly- [normal], no defect at all"

Gita, who had two miscarriages, is a fifty-five-year-old Hindu woman from a lower caste (Ezhava, historically composed of agricultural and industrial workers). She completed a law degree and practices family law in a municipality. Her high educational attainment is not unusual in Kerala, where women have the highest levels of education (and literacy) in all of India (Gulati et al., 1996). Gita's husband, now retired, is also professionally educated. They invited us into their home, after Gita had been asked by an intermediary if she was willing to be interviewed for a research project on childless women. She readily consented. She greeted me at the door in fluent English, so I conducted the interview (my research assistant was also present, as was Gita's husband for the first half hour of the long interview).

The topic of my research—infertility and its consequences for women—was not particularly salient for Gita. I did not realize this at the time, but it became clear when working later with the transcript. Early in the interview she gave many hints about her preferred identity that I missed: when asked demographic questions about educational attainment, for example, she responded with a lengthy account that included the name of each school she had attended, from primary school through postgraduate school, and the history of her career since. When I asked how long she had been married and the number of children they had expected ("one boy, one girl"), she began a story about the first miscarriage but quickly switched topics: it was a "late marriage" (at thirty-five), because she had "not wanted to marry." In a lengthy "aside" (my formulation at the time), Gita said that "so many proposals" came because of her professional status as a "lady lawyer," but she refused them. She told me she was "active in politics, you know, the liberation struggle movement," referring to the time when the Communist Party came to power. She vividly performed a conversation with her mother that occurred after her brothers married and her father died: "I am old," her mother said, "very old, I cannot safeguard you, so get married." A year passed before Gita agreed, and then she asked the family to "fix [her] marriage." She had decided she "wanted a companion." Gita brought out photograph albums of the wedding celebration, naming the judges in the pictures and "all the lady lawyers—all in good positions."

At this point in the trajectory of the interview, I requested that we "go back" to the pregnancy and miscarriage, my interest; that is, I positioned Gita as an infertile woman. Looking back, I am embarrassed at the abruptness, and also at my formulation at the time of the "digressions."

> C: Now I am going to go back and ask some specific questions. Were you ever pregnant?
>
> G: Pregnant means— You see it was three years [after the marriage].
> Then I approached [name of doctor]
> then she said it is not a viable—[pregnancy]. . . .
>
> So she asked me to undergo this operation, this D&C.
> And she wanted to examine him also.
>
> Then the second time in 1974- in 75,
> next time—four months. . . .
>
> Then she wanted [me] to take bed rest
> advised me to take bed rest.
>
> Because I already told you
> it was during that period that [name] the socialist leader

led the gigantic procession against Mrs. Indira Gandhi
the prime minister of India, in Delhi.

And I was a political leader [names place and party]
I had to participate in that.

So I went by train to Delhi
but returned by plane.
After the return I was in [name] Nursing Home
For sixteen days bleeding.

And so he was very angry.
He said, "Do not go for any social work
do not be active," this and that.
But afterwards I never became—[pregnant]. . . .

Then my in-laws, they are in [city]
they thought I had some defect, really speaking.
So they brought me to a gynecologist,
one [name], one specialist.

She took three hours to examine me
and she said, "You are perfectly- no defect at all."
Even though I was forty or forty-one then.
"So I have to examine your husband."

Then I told her, "You just ask his sister,"
she was- his sister was with me in [city].
So I asked her to ask her to bring him in.
He will not come.

Then we went to the house.
So then I said, "Dr. [name] wants to see you."
Then he said, "No, no, I will not go to a lady doctor."
Then she said she would not examine him
they had to examine the—what is it?—the sperm in the laboratory.
But he did not allow that.

Positioning is a vivid point of entry into the narrative and our interaction generally. Gita clearly performs her preferred gender identity—"lady lawyer" and "political leader"—and minimizes the importance of motherhood, over the objections of husband, in-laws, and interviewer. Like the family (but for different reasons), I attempt to position Gita in a world of fertility. In the opening lines she briefly obliges, mentioning two pregnancies—the outcomes of which I have to clarify (deleted from the transcript). She quickly changes topics to what "I already told you"—the primacy of her political world. The two worlds are linked by a miscarriage. Ignoring her doctor's advice "to take bed rest" during the second pregnancy, she "had to" participate in a major demonstration against Indira Gandhi, who was seeking reelection. Traveling from Kerala to New Delhi to participate in the protest probably involved a three-day train trip in 1975. Despite her return by plane and a sixteen-day nursing home stay for "bleeding," we infer that Gita lost the pregnancy (a fact I confirm with a question a few lines later).

Gita shifts topics to the response of various family members. Her husband was "very angry" and ordered her not to "be active." Her in-laws "brought" her for infertility treatment to a specialist in a major South Indian city. In both instances, she positions herself as the object of others' displeasure, without responsibility herself. Yet readers might question this attribution: she had ignored her physician's advice, and she was "forty or forty-one" years old when evaluated subsequently by the specialist who, Gita says, found "no defect." As with Asha's infertility, age may have been a factor. Gita had conceived twice but could not sustain pregnancies—also suggesting a possible "defect." Instead, she locates responsibility in her husband, who refused to be examined by a "lady doctor" and will not allow his sperm to be tested. Gita returns several times in the interview to his refusal to be tested.[5] By these actions, she can enact the gender identity of a "perfectly" normal woman, with "no defect at all."[6]

Gita's narrative contrasts with both Asha's and Sunita's in its multitude of characters. The performance is richly peopled—with political figures, "lady" lawyers and doctors, concerned in-laws, a helpful sister-in-law, and an involved husband. Gita's positioning of characters puts forward a relational identity, complete without motherhood. Later in the interview, she supports my interpretation here. Resisting (once again) my positioning of her in the world of biological fertility, she says explicitly: "Because I do not have [children], I have no disappointments, because mine is a big family." She continues with a listing of many brothers, their children, and certain nieces who "come here every evening . . . to take their meals." Here she explicitly challenges bipolar notions of parental status—either you have children or you don't. She performs a gender identity that challenges the normative script for women in India. She is constructing a life that explicitly resists the master narrative: biological motherhood is supposed to be the central axis of gender identity.

CONCLUSION: RETHINKING IDENTITY

Throughout the world, adult identity for women is normatively organized around the milestone of motherhood, and the norm is particularly strong in India. To be sure, there are currents of change in the motherhood mandate with economic liberalization, which is influencing ideas about marriage and reconfiguring family forms. Nevertheless, arranged marriage continues to be the dominant form and pronatalism remains, even if diversity is possible in the timing of marriage and childbearing, especially among India's growing middle class. While "delay" may be tolerated, women are ultimately expected to marry and reproduce (Riessman, 2000b).

Married women who cannot bear children must construct gender identities based on other principles than motherhood. Three case studies suggest diverse possibilities for women as they age in South India. I examined the identity work women did in interviews to communicate how they wanted to be known—positively, not as victims, but as agents of lives that had accommodated infertility. The stories women developed were my focus, because narratives are a particularly significant genre for representing identity and its multiple guises in different discursive contexts (Mishler, 1999). Social positioning in the stories—how narrators chose to position audience, characters, and themselves—was my point of entry, because "fluid positionings, not fixed roles, are used by people to cope with the situation they find themselves in" (Harre & van Langenhove 1999, p. 17).

However difficult events may have been in the past, all three women performed positive identities in the present that transcended stigma and victimization. Significantly, none of the women blamed themselves for infertility in their interpretive accounts: fault lay with age (Asha), a husband's refusal to be tested (Gita), and, implicitly, a mother-in-law's demands for heavy housework (Sunita). Whatever the "truth" may be, each woman had constructed an explanation that left her without blame and responsibility. The women's age is hugely significant also: all were beyond the typical childbearing years and consequently could look back on their reproductive lives. As all narrators do, they recast the past in light of present concerns and values. All three had developed subjectivities apart from motherhood. Social location is also significant: the women were employed, although they differed considerably in social class (and caste) origins. Elsewhere (Riessman, 2000a, 2000b), I analyze age and social class as important mediators of women's experiences of the stigma of infertility. The case studies here represent women who are economically comfortable (Gita and Sunita) or occupationally secure (Asha, Gita, and Sunita)—certainly not representative of Indian women in general or women in Kerala, even with their relative advantage in literacy and status. My point is not to generalize from cases to populations but to extend boundaries theoretically about possibilities for identity construction among childless women as they age, even in contexts such as India where pronatalism strongly shapes constructs of female status and identity. In Kerala, possibilities for "modern" women are considerable, given the political-economic context and women's historic access to education. Schooling enlarges interpretive capacities, self-concept, and women's bargaining power in marriage, and it encourages social participation.

The case studies reveal diversity and a plurality of identities that develop over time, even in the same woman. Kristeva expresses it well: female identity is "subject in progress," "always becoming" (cited in Ireland, 1993, p. 108). The case studies provide yet another challenge to psychological theories of adult identity that emphasize a universal trajectory (Erikson, 1959) and to some feminist theorizing that essentializes women's development. As Mishler (1999, p. 111) states, a "notion of identity as socially distributed or as existing only within a matrix of changing relationships is not easy to grasp, particularly since it runs counter to traditional deeply entrenched views of identity as coterminous with and 'belonging' to the individual person."

My analysis raises questions for social research on infertility and identity construction processes. Previous work emphasizes infertility as a disruption in the expected life course (Becker, 1994). But this is true only "if we think of identity formation as a progressive development from childhood to adulthood, and of personal narratives as functioning primarily to provide a sense of continuity by reframing and smoothing over the impact of discontinuities and disruptive events" (Mishler, 1999, p. 61, citing Cohler, 1982). The narratives of the women I interviewed certainly emphasized bodily disruption—miscarriages—but the case studies do not suggest identities organized on the basis of metaphors of disruption.

Previous research has examined young couples in the midst of (often desperate) fertility searches, where discontinuities in the expected life course may be particularly difficult. Not much is known about the interpretive accounts of women past childbearing age who are involuntarily childless. The case studies here present some beginning insights about pathways of adult identity when motherhood cannot be the central axis of self-definition. They begin to suggest that South Indian women might find other ways of interpreting infertility and constructing identities more easily than U.S. women professionals (see chap. 5, this volume)—an intriguing possibility that challenges cultural stereotypes. Pathways of gender identity are always influenced by cultural context, in Western countries and developing ones alike. Despite constraints, however, women do not simply follow cultural plots in storying their lives. Encountering infertility, they interpret it and compose lives that adapt to, resist, and sometimes reach beyond the master narrative of motherhood. Infertility is positioned differently in older women's lives, compared to younger ones. Thus, in closing, I would suggest that future research, in both Western and non-Western settings, needs to examine further the contrasting meanings of infertility over the life course.

NOTES

For research assistance, I thank Liza George, Celine Suny, and Leela Gulati; A. K. Chacko, Kaveri Gopalakrishnan, and P. K. Shamala, my physician sponsors; and Chandran and James, my village sponsors. For critiques of earlier versions, I thank

Elliot Mishler, Wendy Luttrell, Marcia Inhorn, Frank van Balen, an anonymous reviewer, and the Narrative Study Group. Deepest thanks go to the women who taught me about childlessness during fieldwork. The Indo-U.S. Subcommission on Education and Culture, Council for the International Exchange of Scholars, provided financial support for fieldwork.

1. Malayalam is a member of the Drividian family of languages spoken in South India. My representation of the translated interviews has benefited from conversations with Liza while in India and with India specialists since my return to the United States. (See Riessman [2000a] for a fuller discussion of translation and interpretation issues.)

2. Kerala, located along the extreme southwestern coast of India, is an exceptional state on a variety of indicators: a 75 percent literacy rate for women (vs. 39 percent for India), a life expectancy at birth of 73 years for women (vs. 57 years), and a sex ratio of 1,036 females per 1,000 males (vs. 929). The "effective" female literacy rate in Kerala, which excludes 0- to 6-year-olds, approaches 86 percent (Gulati, Ramalingam, & Gulati 1996). There is debate about the precise causes of the state's advantaged position (*New York Review of Books*, 1991). On the political economy, special ecology, and unique history of Kerala, see Jeffrey (1993); Nag (1988).

3. Deleted from this and subsequent transcripts are brief exchanges in which I ask for clarification. These are denoted by ellipses (. . .).

4. I have represented the structure of the narrative thematically in stanzas (a series of lines that are about the same topic, adapted from Gee [1991]).

5. The actual responsibility for infertility in this and the other cases is unclear. Kerala's infertility clinics require both spouses to be tested, and about a third of the time the problem lies in the husband's sperm. Male responsibility for infertility is acknowledged in the region. Elsewhere (2000b) I have described women's management of male responsibility: they do not disclose it in order to deflect stigma but instead absorb the "fault" themselves.

6. For a detailed structural analysis of Gita's narrative, see Riessman (2002).

REFERENCES

Bamberg, M. G. W. (1997). Positioning between structure and performance. *Journal of Narrative and Life History, 7(1–4)*, 335–342.

Becker, G. (1994). Metaphors in disrupted lives: Infertility and cultural constructions of continuity. *Medical Anthropology Quarterly, 8*, 383–410.

Bell, S. E. (1999). Narratives and lives: Women's health politics and the diagnosis of cancer for DES daughters. *Narrative Inquiry 9(2)*, 1–43.

Bell, S. E. (2000). Experiencing illness in/and narrative. In C. Bird, P. Conrad, A. Fremont and S. Levine (Eds.), *Handbook of medical sociology,* 5th ed. (pp. 184–199). New York: Prentice-Hall.

Cerulo, K. A. (1997). Identity construction: New issues, new directions. *Annual Review of Sociology, 23*, 385–409.

Davies, B. (1989). *Frogs and snails and feminist tales: Preschool children and gender.* Sydney: Allen & Unwin.

Erikson, E. H. (1959). *Identity and the life cycle: Selected papers. Psychological Issues 1 (1)*, 1–171.

Frank, A. W. (1995). *The wounded storyteller: Body, illness, and ethics.* Chicago: University of Chicago Press.

Gee, J. P. (1991). A linguistic approach to narrative. *Journal of Narrative and Life History, 1(1)*, 15–39.

Greil, A. L. (1991). *Not yet pregnant: Infertile couples in contemporary America.* New Brunswick, NJ: Rutgers University Press.

Gulati, L., Ramalingam, & Gulati, I. S. (1996). *Gender profile: Kerala.* New Delhi: Royal Netherlands Embassy.

Harre, R., & van Langenhove, L. (Eds.). (1999). *Positioning theory.* Malden, MA: Blackwell.

Inhorn, M. C. (1994). *Quest for conception: Gender, infertility, and Egyptian medical traditions.* Philadelphia: University of Pennsylvania Press.

Ireland, M. S. (1993). *Reconceiving women: Separating motherhood from female identity.* New York: Guilford.

Jeffery, P., Jeffery, R., & Lyon, A. (1989). *Labour pains and labour power: Women and childbearing in India.* London: Zed.

Jeffrey, R. (1993). *Politics, women and well being: How Kerala became "a model."* Delhi: Oxford University Press.

Kessler, S. J., & McKenna, W. (1978). *Gender: An ethnomethodological approach.* Chicago: University of Chicago Press.

Labov, W. (1982). Speech actions and reactions in personal narrative. In D. Tannen (Ed.), *Analyzing discourse: Text and talk* (pp. 219–247). Washington, DC: Georgetown University Press.

Langellier, K. (2001). "You're marked": Breast cancer, tattoo and the narrative performance of identity. In J. Brockmeier and D. Carbaugh (Eds.), *Narrative and identity: Studies in autobiography, self and culture* (pp. 145–184). Amsterdam: John Benjamins.

Mattingly, C. (1998). *Healing dramas and clinical plots: The narrative structure of experience.* New York: Cambridge University Press.

Mattingly, C., & Garro, L. C. (Eds.) (2000). *Narrative and the cultural construction of illness and healing.* Berkeley: University of California Press.

Mishler, E. G. (1986a). The analysis of interview-narratives. In T. R. Sarbin (Ed.), *Narrative psychology: The storied nature of human conduct* (pp. 233–255). New York: Praeger.

Mishler, E. G. (1986b). *Research interviewing: Context and narrative.* Cambridge, MA: Harvard University Press.

Mishler, E. G. (1991). Representing discourse: The rhetoric of transcription. *Journal of Narrative and Life History, 1(4)*, 255–280.

Mishler, E. G. (1999). *Storylines: Crafts artists' narratives of identity.* Cambridge, MA: Harvard University Press.

Nag, M. (1988). The Kerala formula. *World Health Forum, 9(2)*. Geneva: World Health Organization.

New York Review of Books. 1991. Letters: The Kerala difference. October 24.

Riessman, C. K. (1993). *Narrative analysis.* Qualitative Research Methods Series, No. 30. Newbury Park, CA: Sage.

Riessman, C. K. (1997). Telling, transcribing and analyzing: Methodological considerations for work with personal narratives in the social sciences. In L. C. Hyden & M. Hyden (Eds.), *The study of storytelling* (pp. 30–62). Stockholm: Lieber. [In Swedish]

Riessman, C. K. (2000a). "Even if we don't have children [we] can live": Stigma and infertility in South India. In C. Mattingly & L. C. Garro (Eds.), *Narrative and cultural construction of illness and healing* (pp. 128–152). Berkeley: University of California Press.

Riessman, C. K. (2000b). Stigma and everyday resistance practices: Childless women in South India. *Gender & Society, 14(1)*, 111–135.

Riessman, C. K. (2002). Analysis of personal narratives. In J. R. Gubrium & J. A. Holstein (Eds.), *Handbook of interviewing* (pp. 695–710). Thousand Oaks, CA: Sage.

Roland, A. (1988). *In search of self in India and Japan: Toward a cross-cultural psychology.* Princeton, NJ: Princeton University Press.

Uberoi, P. (Ed.). 1993. *Family, kinship and marriage in India.* New Delhi: Oxford University Press.

Unisa, S. (1999). Childlessness in Andhra Pradesh, India: Treatment-seeking and consequences. *Reproductive Health Matters, 7(13)*, 54–64.

NINE

Childlessness, Adoption, and *Milagros de Dios* in Costa Rica

Gwynne L. Jenkins

With Silvia Vargas Obando and José Badilla Navas

Costa Rica has been celebrated as an international success story in health development (Harrison, 1981). Among its many successes, Costa Rica has achieved one of the "earliest and fastest . . . fertility transitions in the developing world" (Rosero-Bixby & Casterline, 1994, p. 439). Declining birthrates, increasing acceptance of family planning, and diminishing "ideal" family size have been lauded by demographers and health specialists as part of the overall picture of health "modernization." For this tiny country of 3.3 million people, the creation of a health profile rivaling the "developed" world is a point of national pride.

As in other so-called developing nations, the experience of infertility has languished unattended within Costa Rica's contradictory sociocultural framework, which deeply values children and family life while practicing a health politic that emphasizes the limitation of childbearing. Little research has been generated specifically to define the extent and contours of infertility and childlessness in Costa Rica (Vaessen, 1984). Rather, knowledge of infertility in Costa Rica has been produced principally as a spin-off of research on fertility and women's health (e.g., CCSS, 1994; Melendez, 1995; Oberle, Rosero-Bixby, & Whitaker, 1993). "Uncontrolled" births in "undesirable" circumstances that capture the attention of national health politicians and academic researchers—including adolescent pregnancy, unwed mothers, and female-headed households—are the subject of close scrutiny as threats to what is considered the traditional family in Costa Rica.

Adoption receives considerably more discussion than childlessness. The principal objects of concern, however, are controversial adoptions by foreigners who allegedly snatch up Costa Rican children through payoffs to cut the bureaucratic red tape slowing down legal adoptions among nationals (e.g., Solano, 1998). There has been little attention to the national adoptive triad (Terrell & Modell, 1994): the women who give up their children, the adoptive families, and the adopted children. The characteristics and social experiences of the Costa Rican birth mothers and the Costa Rican families seeking to adopt are nearly unknown (except for Rojas Chávez & Martínez Cabezas [1982]), and the experiences of adopted children in Costa Rica are totally unexplored.

FIELDWORK: FROM INATTENDANCE TO INTEGRATION

When I began my fieldwork in 1990, it was the study of pregnancy and birth rather than infertility and childlessness that drew my attention. For sixteen months I lived in Buenos Aires, one of the poorest and most rural townships in Costa Rica, where I interviewed midwives, laypersons, both men and women, and health care providers about the transition from home to hospital birth. Ironically, I lived with a childless couple, Silvia and José, during most of this research. It was Silvia who taught me Spanish, making ample use of the patience she undoubtedly acquired as a grade school teacher. José sometimes participated in the lessons and brought us pineapple to refresh our spirits—a product of the plantation where he worked as a solderer. Our relationship was ideal for my work. Silvia was the daughter of a midwife and a well-liked member of a respected family. She knew everyone, and everyone knew her. She and José excelled at interpreting that which befuddled me and intuitively understood the difficulties and peculiarities of my experience as a foreign researcher. They facilitated my work through countless acts of generosity, large and small.

I interpreted their childlessness as nonproblematic based on my own experiences. Silvia was about the same age as my eldest sister, who intentionally chose not to have children, and only a few years older than my middle sister, who delayed childbearing until her early thirties. From my perspective, Silvia and José were a young, vibrant couple with many years ahead of them before they needed to be concerned about childbearing. Silvia and José's calm demeanor and general silence about children reinforced this interpretation. In fact, I recall only one conversation with Silvia about their desire for children. It was 1990: I was twenty-one, Silvia twenty-seven. As we sat in a small restaurant, with wood-slat walls painted turquoise blue, we savored the chill of ice cream after the sweltering heat of a long bus ride. Silvia told me she and José had been asking God for children but had not conceived. I told her I was certain one day she would call me in the United States to tell me she is pregnant. The conversation turned to another subject.

The day I returned to Costa Rica in early 1997 to complete my fieldwork, I called Silvia and José from the capital to announce my arrival. On hearing my voice, Silvia launched into a story that so took me by surprise I thought

I was falling victim to my rusty Spanish: they were adopting a baby girl. The newborn's mother came to Silvia's sister just the night before, asking her if she knew someone who would adopt the two-day-old baby. Silvia was going to the regional capital with the mother and baby the next day to testify before the government and begin adoption proceedings. We both agreed that it was a miracle. "All that's missing is the basket," laughed Silvia, comparing the events to finding a baby on their front stoop with a note pinned to its diaper.

Silvia and José's story of childlessness and adoption is a story of pain, suffering, dedication, religious conviction, and elation. It is a story of risks and struggles with the high stakes of marital stability in the face of social intolerance. When I suggested publishing it in a volume on childlessness globally, they agreed to the idea for two very personal reasons. First, they felt that discussing their experience of childlessness and adoption was one way to testify to the will of God in their lives and the inestimable blessing they received when they adopted their daughter. Second, they hoped that sharing publicly—for the first time—the social stigmatization of unwanted childlessness, which they had suffered in silence, would contribute to better understanding of the experience and greater sensitivity to the plight of infertile couples.

As an anthropologist, my desire to undertake this work arose from a mixture of personal and professional objectives. Having lived with Silvia and José, I witnessed the joy and transformation in their lives engendered by the adoption of their daughter. Furthermore, I came to realize that despite having lived with them for many months and known them for many years, I never recognized how powerfully they felt their childlessness: it was a deeply hidden, highly guarded part of their lives, only hinted to me on rare occasions. Probing the meaning of childlessness became both a personal and a professional endeavor. Personally, it was a way to engage the people who had supported my fieldwork, although at times it was undoubtedly painful to them, to share in their lives, and to reciprocate their generosity by providing them with a means to tell their story. Professionally, it was the chance to move beyond studying the meaning of "reproduction" simply in terms of pregnancy and birth. As Inhorn (1994, p.23) points out, "Fertility and infertility exist in a dialectical relationship of contrast, such that understanding one leads to a much greater understanding of the other."

I felt—and Silvia and José agreed—that this should be a collaborative project. As a result, for the most part this chapter was written in the field. We taped discussions about their experience of childlessness and adoption. We read articles on adoption and infertility from Costa Rican sources and books that helped Silvia and José to cope with childlessness (e.g. Inhorn, 1994; Kleinman & Kleinman, 1995; López & Zúñiga, 1988; Love, 1988;

Terrell & Modell, 1994). We discussed biblical stories and passages that were meaningful to them. As I began to write their story and integrate their experience with the available research on childlessness and adoption in Costa Rica, Silvia and José reflected on my translation, adding information and suggesting changes. They played a significant role in this project, and they repeatedly declined anonymity. Of course, I alone am accountable for any shortcomings.

This is an experience-near account, as advocated by Kleinman and Kleinman (1995). The "ethnography of experience" they propose is a strategy to grapple with the complex and power-laden relationship of individual physical and emotional experience occurring within a local moral world. Kleinman and Kleiman pose suffering as a compelling window to the social universe. Although endured physically and psychically on a day-to-day basis by the individual, suffering is interpersonal and intersubjective. Suffering is created, exacerbated, and ameliorated by the social world and its power to define the issues having "overbearing practical relevance" to the individual. Ethnography of experience intends to locate and interpret "what is at stake for particular participants in particular situations[,] . . . [an] orientation [that] will lead the ethnographer to collective (both local and societal) and individual (both public and intimate) levels of analysis of experience-near interests" (1995, p. 98). "Nearness" is a strategy to resist caricatures and other ethnographic violence to human experience while maintaining the complexity, indeterminacy, and sublime nature of particular suffering.

When I began preparing for this work, this potent strategy came to mind immediately as a way to dignify Silvia and José's experiences and to help me address the uneasy tension of my dual role as friend and ethnographer. Indeed, the world of infertility and childlessness described by Silvia, in particular, was a shrouded world, filled with anguish and otherness born in silence. It was clearly an experience of suffering. What was at stake for the couple can be summed up in a single word: everything. Their experiences reflect the public and private nature of suffering engendered by childlessness, and the circumstances of their adoption indicate the parallel worlds of shame and humiliation layered on unacceptable motherhood, particularly as experienced by poor, single, adolescent mothers like the young woman who gave her newborn to Silvia and José. The intersection of these local moral worlds of birth and parenting resulted in the event that Silvia and José define as the greatest *milagro de Dios*—miracle of God—in their lives.

This is a highly individualistic account, yet it resonates with the social meaning of pregnancy and parenthood in Costa Rica, the influence of family and community on the experience of childlessness, and the importance of faith in God to reconcile difference, soothe suffering, and resolve the dilemma of childlessness. In my research on birth in the hinterlands of Costa Rica, I was repeatedly reminded of the fervent Christianity that helped women and men to make sense of life's triumphs and tragedies, especially on the issue of pregnancy and birth. Older women who lived their adult lives in a nearly constant state of pregnancy considered child-bearing a castigation from God. Many confided in hushed tones that they had prayed to God to stop punishing them and end their childbearing. The midwives who attended women in some of the worst and most dangerous circumstances believed it was the power of God that moved their hands and guided their decisions. Families believed that mothers and children lived and died according to God's will, and fervent prayer helped them through the uncertainty of childbirth. Nothing happened, good or bad, but for the will of God. It should not be surprising, then, that the currency of faith and prayer that is critical in childbearing would likewise play a central role in childlessness. It is the key discourse through which Silvia and José made sense of their years of childlessness and subsequent adoption. It is the tie that binds this ethnography.

PLANS MADE AND PLANS UNDONE

After their wedding in 1982, Silvia and José moved into a small rented home in Buenos Aires, the town where Silvia grew up. Buenos Aires was the municipal seat and the hub of a region dramatically expanding with immigrants poaching virgin farmland and seeking employment at the pine-apple plantation. But Buenos Aires was still small enough to create the sense that everyone knew each other. It was an example of the often-repeated saying, *pueblo chiquito, infierno grande,* or small town, big hell. The eyes of the community follow the individual's actions, criticizing and commenting on the conduct of personal lives. After dating for two years, for example, people in the community had already begun to ask Silvia and José when they would marry. Silvia was still in high school, though, and determined to finish her education first, so their courtship continued another three years. Their wedding portrait shows them standing side by side, their expressions resolute and serious. Silvia was nineteen, and José was twenty-seven.

When I asked them about their plans as newlyweds, they spoke with one voice: their first goal was for Silvia to complete her college education and become established as a teacher while José established himself as a solderer at the pineapple plantation. Their second goal was to build a home on the piece of land Silvia inherited from her mother. Their third goal was to have children after Silvia received her college degree. During a premarital counseling retreat sponsored by the town's Catholic church, they decided to have only the children they could care for adequately and imagined that three would be an ideal number.

Parenthood is a critical component of gender identity and self-esteem in the Costa Rican context. Melendez (1995) found that both men and women desire childbearing so as to experience parenthood and as a mechanism to solidify their conjugal relationships. Fatherhood, however, was not as central to men's adult identities as motherhood was to women; indeed, women of all ages consider motherhood a quintessential component of their adult identity (cf. Low, 1978). Melendez (1995, p. 191) hypothesizes that infertility is devastating to both women and men but that "in the case of a man the reason is related more to his fear that he could not attract or hold on to a mate unless he could father children, rather than infertility undermining his self-identity." For both men and women, the absence of children may be a threat to the stability of the conjugal relationship. But for women, gender role expectations, vulnerability, and public reputation are more keenly implicated in parenthood. The morality of childbearing and the high stakes of pregnancy are shouldered principally by women as they negotiate adult identity and conjugal stability.

Silvia and José's early decision that she should finish her education illustrates that they had a broader view of their roles, identities, and strategies for marital cohesion. Silvia, José, and I discussed Melendez's (1995) conclusions about parenthood and the fulfillment of adult gender identity. Silvia agreed that motherhood was central to many women's feelings of "wholeness." For her, however, motherhood was not the defining essence of womanhood. Rather, she felt that there are many other facets of life that make a person whole: attaining intellectual and economic goals, having a fulfilling marital relationship, and, most important, knowing how to respect oneself and others. Parenthood was important to both Silvia and José, but so were education, economic stability, and marital harmony. Based on my observations of a number of households, their relationship is one of rare equality and mutual respect. But their broad conceptualization of their adult roles was not necessarily shared or understood by their community.

Silvia finished college and qualified as a grade school teacher in late 1986, and she began working as a teacher in a local school in early 1987. After four years of delaying conception, Silvia and José decided to *pedir un bebé*—to ask for a baby. Much like the social pressure to marry that they experienced, they had begun to receive overt questions from the larger community about children. Questions such as "Why are you passing so much time without children?" and "Can't you have children?" were initially explained away by Silvia's wish to complete her education. But when Silvia did not become pregnant in their first year of trying, the couple themselves began to wonder. They decided to make the most of this unforeseen window of opportunity for as long as it lasted, and over the next two years Silvia traveled every other week to a university in the north of the country to finish an advanced degree in teaching.

Both Silvia and José agreed that she felt more acutely the social pressure to bear children. At a personal level, she defined her experience as an accumulating feeling of "emptiness" when it became apparent that they would not conceive. The experience of childlessness was one of difference and abnormality. Her role as a teacher was one lens through which she assessed childbearing and motherhood in the context of her community:

> Working with children, you begin to think and to analyze how it could be that within a single classroom, you're teaching twenty-five or thirty kids and all of them come from a home in which their mother knew what it was to give birth, as a normal part of her life. Maybe they were women with many children, who didn't value them, didn't value them as a blessing from God, women that were simply fulfilling their function because that's the way it is. One begins to see, and to question why. Why me? Why am I different? You're in that room with all these children, without knowing what it is to feel such happiness when you see this child after giving birth, what a wonderful emotion it must be to feel. And to know that I didn't have this right. Now, I say it normally. But in that moment, you feel that your chest will tear out. The pain is indescribable.

Innumerable small reminders of childlessness surfaced daily: when her female friends discussed their children, when she helped her students prepare Mother's Day presents, and when she was assigned to teach sexual education to older children. Silvia withheld the depth of her pain from everyone—even José—rather than burden them with her frustrations and anxieties.

Silvia and José did not feel pressure from their families over their initial decision to delay childbearing, nor did they feel pressure or guilt from their families about their subsequent inability to conceive. However, the small town increasingly became a big hell, primarily for Silvia. People who were little more than casual acquaintances took the liberty of overtly asking why they were childless. José had his share of questions, but Silvia was more consistently subjected to scrutiny as children and parenthood were more overtly defined as women's arenas. Silvia recounted one event illustrative of the public scrutiny of childlessness. She was walking past a crowded bus stop when a woman she hardly knew asked her why they did not have children. Silvia kept walking, forcing herself not to turn around or acknowledge the question. The indiscretion of the question in this highly public setting, from someone she hardly knew, showed the hardness and cruelty of people who had never experienced childlessness. Although the public discussion of infertility was more directly aimed at Silvia as a woman, the blame for infertility was not. For both Silvia and José, the question that most acutely demonstrated the inability of the larger community to understand the feelings of abnormality and difference felt by infertile couples was, *¿Cuál de los dos no sirve?*—Which of the two of you doesn't work?

INTERVENTION AND CRISIS

Silvia and José were not alone in their difficulty conceiving. Yet infertility in Costa Rica is only documented as a brief addendum to research reports. One survey of married women's reproductive health found that 8.1 percent of women reported having difficulty conceiving at some point in their lives, 5.4 percent had sought medical advice for the inability to conceive, and 3.2 percent had been diagnosed with infertility. The estimated prevalence of infertility among married women between twenty-five and forty-four years of age based on that survey was 2.2 percent, although this limited sample probably underestimates infertility rates (Oberle et al., 1993; cf. CCSS, 1994; Vaessen, 1984).

Male infertility has been the subject of greater public anxiety in Costa Rica than has female infertility. It came to the forefront of national consciousness as a result of a massive lawsuit against Dow Chemical and other transnational corporations, filed by twenty-five thousand banana workers (including six thousand Costa Ricans) left sterile after exposure to agrochemicals (Villalobos, 1997). Fear of male sterilization as well as fear of the unknown effects of agrochemicals on human reproduction are keenly felt in Buenos Aires. As the site of the largest pineapple plantation in the world, local anxiety emerged in my everyday interactions with locals ranging from physicians and ambulance drivers to waitresses and housewives. It could be heard in gossip about plantation workers taken off the job after routine medical testing revealed them to be at risk for sterility, for example, and in the multitude of jokes and folklore about the consumption of chemical-laden pineapples causing "hormonal" changes and wildly affecting sexuality and fertility.

After nine years of marriage, Silvia, now twenty-eight, decided to seek help. The tension, conflicts, and fears that surrounded this decision were palpable as Silvia and José described to me this difficult interval in their lives. José did not believe that any earthly intervention would give them a child, because both childlessness and childbearing were the will of God and God alone. Silvia decided her own course of action and began taking a homeopathic therapy used successfully by a friend. The effects of the therapy proved disastrous both physically and emotionally. Within days of starting the therapy Silvia developed heavy and continuous uterine bleeding, and within two weeks she was hospitalized for blood loss so severe that the doctors were uncertain she would live. After recovering physically, however, the emotional stakes of childlessness rose as Silvia and José's individual needs came into overt conflict.

This traumatic experience compelled Silvia to consult a physician about their continuing childlessness. The physician diagnosed uterine growths that can cause increased miscarriages but explained that the cause of the couple's infertility could be identified only through extensive fertility evaluations. He recommended testing José before subjecting Silvia to grueling examinations. When Silvia explained that José would certainly refuse testing, she received a shocking response: the physician quipped that she was growing old and if she really wanted a child, she should leave her husband and set off in search of conception. For Silvia, there was no choice: she wanted a child but not at that price.

Silvia defines this moment as the beginning of a period of crisis in their married life. The first five years of childlessness were hard to understand, but the couple remained hopeful, thinking that it took many couples five years to conceive. But the second five years began with Silvia nearly losing her life to a fertility therapy, followed by the realization that they might never conceive unless they sought medical intervention. They were entrenched in a crisis of desires. José was certain that if God wanted to give them a child, this would occur the "natural" way, without medical assistance.

For four years after her visit to the physician, Silvia repeatedly asked José to submit to medical evaluation, and he repeatedly refused. In retrospect, José acknowledged he did not experience childlessness with the acute feelings of emptiness that Silvia experienced. The small, day-to-day reminders of childlessness were small wounds that refused to heal and brought Silvia to tears when in the privacy of her home. It was this pain—the pain that continuing infertility was causing his wife—that finally compelled José to agree to testing at some point in the future. However, that point never arrived: José repeatedly committed to testing, then put off the exams for a later date. For José, the tests represented a refutation of the belief that only God could make it possible to have a child. If God wanted them to have a child, he reasoned, God would deliver that child to them. Silvia, however, was not willing to give up on the idea of earthly interventions.

I returned to Costa Rica on a regular basis between 1994 and 1997, when Silvia and José were entrenched in this crisis. I lived in their household but often left for many days at a time to pursue my research in the hinterlands or in the capital, returning to rest, transcribe my interviews, and enter my field notes into my computer. At times I felt an edginess in the household and accepted their occasional silences and withdrawal as a basic need for privacy. Otherwise, their crisis was completely hidden from me.

RESIGNATION TO CHILDLESSNESS

Silvia finally decided that the only way to survive emotionally and maintain her marriage was to stop asking José to go to the doctor and seek resignation to the will of God. She prayed to God that He would grant her tranquillity and peace—that she would not suffer sadness and feelings of difference or abnormality but rather be able to participate in the discourse of parenthood and feel "normal." Silvia had seen the emotional decay that other women in the community had suffered as a result of the accumulated pain of childlessness. In rural Costa Rica, the appropriate reaction to both physical and emotional pain is to withhold its public expression. Emotional privacy and individual stoicism in both men and women are valued as a sacrifice of one's self in order to protect the comfort of others. For some childless women, the price of maintaining this facade of indifference was increasing hatred of women who were pregnant, hatred of children, and loss of marital stability in the wake of failed reproductive interventions. Silvia understood that she needed to achieve tranquillity and resign herself (as had her husband) to the will of God in order to achieve a sense of normalcy and avoid succumbing to destructive feelings.

It was after Silvia began to feel that God had granted her tranquillity that the couple first considered adoption. After suffering physical abuse, one of Silvia's students and her sister were removed from their home by the government and placed in a group home run by nuns. Silvia and José brought the girls home to stay with them for Christmas in 1996. The day they returned the girls to the group home, Silvia and José had a conversation that they feel portended the will of God in their lives.

On this day one of the nuns sat down to discuss adoption with them. Silvia had already expressed her desire to adopt one of the girls, even though José continued in his belief that if God wanted them to have a child, the child would come to them. They wondered aloud if adding a child to their household, after years of living "alone" as a couple, would jeopardize their marriage. Contrary to the dominant model for couples in Costa Rica, they had created marital stability in the absence of children by developing an expanded definition of their adult identities, based on the pursuit of goals such as higher education and careers. Would one or the other become jealous of the attention and emotions directed toward a new baby? Could they strike a new balance as a working couple in the face of the commitment required by parenting? In essence, could they change the patterns developed over fourteen years of marriage without destroying the marital shelter they created in the face of public and private suffering?

The nun suggested that they pray over it. Many times, she told them, one receives messages and signs from God but chooses to ignore them. They must be careful not to "close the door" on God. In recounting this eventful day, Silvia and José remembered that as they sat in front of their house after speaking with the nun, a shooting star flashed through the sky from east to west. Thinking back, José imagined that he and Silvia were wishing for the same thing at that moment because—although they did not know it at the time—this was also the night a young single mother gave birth to her second child in the local health clinic less than half a kilometer from their home.

In Costa Rica, the shifting countenance of childbearing and family structures has been the subject of intense debate. Single mothers and female-headed households, along with teen mothers, divorces, and consensual unions, are considered by many to be national scandals and part of the overall disintegration of the traditional family (Low, 1978; Melendez, 1995; Reuben, 1997). The young woman who gave birth the night Silvia and José saw the shooting star is representative of this phenomenon. Her child was one of the 18 percent of all children born annually to adolescent women, and she was among the 40 percent of adolescent mothers who are neither married nor in consensual unions (DGEC, 1994).

Until recently, out-of-wedlock pregnancies brought shame to the pregnant woman's family and would often result in her being forced out of the family home. Young women are willing to run the risk of jeopardizing their public reputation as "moral" women, however, as they seek to both solidify their relationship with their male partners and achieve adult female identity through motherhood (Melendez, 1995). Although unwed mothers are still subject to scorn and shame, they are increasingly tolerated in Costa Rican families. A single mother, for example, might stay in her parents' household along with her child or children, a family formation that I witnessed repeatedly in my research on birth in the hinterlands. However, the socioeconomic circumstances of her family may limit the number of children the family can support. Furthermore, a single mother's ability to participate in wage labor is increasingly compromised as she has more children. There is little that women can do to terminate an unwanted pregnancy; abortion is illegal except in cases of medical necessity, although illicit abortions are known to occur (Low & Newman, 1985). Married women may suffer similar consequences from pregnancy; women with "too many" children are criticized for their lack of "care" in avoiding pregnancy, such that some hide their pregnancies to delay public scrutiny.

Adoption is one solution to this dilemma. The patterns noted by Rojas Chávez and Martínez Cabezas (1982) more than fifteen years ago are implicated in the contemporary phenomenon of adoption in Costa Rica. When asked why they were giving up a child for adoption, the single most important reason women cited was that they could not afford to keep it. Single mothers constituted over 45 percent of all women who gave up their children for adoption in the late 1970s, and the majority of women (married and not married) who gave up a child for adoption already had one or more children (Rojas Chávez & Martínez Cabezas, 1982; see also López & Zúñiga, 1988).

FAITH, FULFILLMENT, AND REINTEGRATION

Two days after the shooting star fell, one of Silvia's sisters telephoned to say that a young woman had come to ask her if she knew someone who would adopt a baby. According to the young woman, it was her sister's baby and her sister was unable to keep it. José and Silvia agreed that Silvia should go to see the baby, as José preferred not to get involved until they knew more about the circumstances and the mother's decision to give the baby up. Silvia was immediately taken with the newborn, but because it was being given up by an aunt, not the mother, adoption would be impossible. Silvia and José had recently seen a case on the evening news in which a baby was stolen from its mother and given to a family for adoption, and they feared being drawn into similar circumstances.

Soon after Silvia left for home, the young woman confessed that she was in fact the baby's mother. She explained that she was a single mother living in her parents' household. This was her second child. She was working as a domestic to support herself and her first child, and neither she nor her impoverished family could afford another child. Her initial secrecy about her identity makes sense in this social context. Bearing a child as an unmarried woman brings with it the social stigma of having engaged in sexual intercourse before marriage. Giving up a child adds a second—and weightier—social stigma. Just as unwed mothers are accused of immorality, women who give up their children are criticized with the saying, *Ni los perros dejan sus hijos en la calle*—Not even dogs abandon their children in the street. In addition to private feelings of frustration and loss, women who give up their children for adoption bear the burden of public scrutiny and social stigma when they leave their community pregnant and return empty-handed (cf. Modell, 1986).

The young woman's personal search for parents for her newborn was a common strategy for establishing the adoptive triad. In the Costa Rican context and especially in rural areas like Buenos Aires, personalism and the small town ethos dominate. One Costa Rican social worker suggested to me that this strategy, known as direct adoption, is the most important means for biological mothers to locate safe homes for the children they cannot keep. But this strategy created a dilemma for all members of the adoptive triad. Because the birth mother lived locally, Silvia and José wondered what role she would take in the baby's life and feared further heartbreak should she change her mind and seek to regain custody of the child. They also feared that the gaze of the small town would be bent on discovering the identity of the birth mother and undermining their legitimacy as parents. In sympathy for the young woman's situation and hoping to diffuse some of these anxieties, Silvia and José offered to support her by letting her live in their household with both children, if she wanted to keep her baby. She did not.

José said repeatedly that if God wanted them to have a child, He would bring the child to them. The arrival of this newborn, practically at their doorstep, could only be interpreted as God's fulfillment of their deepest desire in response to their faith. This was the message from God, portended in the nun's advice, in the shooting star, in their reconciliation to the will of God. Silvia and José decided to begin the custody process the next day. That night the emotional barricade Silvia had built to protect herself from the torment of childlessness broke down:

> Afterward, that same night, we prayed to God and thanked Him for everything He has done. This day, we prayed and out came all the feelings that I'd held inside, hidden, in silence. Oh, my God! It was in that moment that I realized— although I'd had a few years of living resigned [to it]—all of this history came out. Everything that had happened, everything, so many nights of thinking, and unanswered questions, and discomforts. So many things, in this moment. Things came into my mind that even I didn't realize, they were from so deep inside of me. . . . Feelings of frustration, pain. Everything that had happened. So many small things that had happened. In that moment, I felt how deep the emptiness had been. I felt a happiness that was so great, so great! After we prayed, José said that he didn't know that I was able to keep such pain inside of me! But even I didn't realize how deep it was—it surprised even me. It's like you're born again, as another person—with a different mind.

Silvia and José felt an uncomfortable mixture of overwhelming joy in their new daughter and sympathy for the difficult choice the young woman had made. They felt that the birth mother did what she had to out of love for the baby and as part of a divine plan. For years they had prayed for a child to make their marriage complete, and God united their needs with the needs of the young woman and her baby in the best interests of each member of the adoptive triad. The next day Silvia and the young woman traveled to the regional capital to begin the lengthy process of legal adoption.

The number of children adopted each year in Costa Rica is difficult to estimate (PANI, 1997a, p. 11). Some direct adoptions are never made legal and go unreported, while others that take place behind the closed doors of lawyers' offices may not be counted because of an inadequate system of census taking. Still others languish for years unfinalized in legal limbo and create an overrepresentation of adoptions annually in national statistics. The available data suggest that in 1997, the year Silvia and José began the process of adopting their daughter, some 489 children were known to have been adopted by new families (of which about 20 percent were international adoptions), and another 461 children were known to be in various stages in the prolonged process (PANI, 1997b, p. 24; cf. Solano C., 1998).

The news that they decided to adopt the baby was received by family and friends with an intense public celebration (including social visits and gifts) that reintegrated them into the community as new parents. Silvia felt this transformation most profoundly at a singular moment: when she stepped off the bus from the regional capital with the baby in her arms, she imagined it was how other women must feel when making the journey from the hospital in the regional capital with their newborns. As a member of the household during this joyous time, I watched and joined in as friends came by and commented on the perfection of the baby and wondered aloud if she looked more like Silvia or José. Continuing this somatization, José commented one afternoon that I should have brought one of the midwives I studied to the house to give Silvia a *sobada,* a massage used to help women prepare for and recover from birth—in other words, to physically reintegrate them as mothers.

This complete surrender to the joy of parenthood helped them to adjust to their new identities, particularly as the gaze of the community was once more turned on them. They had to explain their new status as parents to the larger community—a process they have faced with a mixture of joy and stoicism. The adoption is no secret, but they keep the details (including the identity of the birth mother) to themselves. They learned to deal with a *pueblo chiquito* under worse circumstances. The public transition to parenthood has been less problematic for José than for Silvia. He has not suffered anxiety over identifying himself unequivocally as the father of his new daughter. Silvia initially feared being called a liar if she did not qualify her motherhood by explaining the adoption to those who asked, but she now feels it is unnecessary to discuss the adoption with casual acquaintances. She decided to resist the temptation to explain and allow herself the luxury of unmitigated motherhood. They have only once seen the birth mother since the adoption, when she stopped by the house briefly to show the baby to her sister. Silvia felt butterflies in her stomach, fearing the young woman's intentions. Silvia gathered her courage and asked the young woman if the baby still seemed like her own daughter. The young woman said no. Thus fulfillment is still accompanied by anxieties for Silvia and José. What is at stake, however, is more priceless than anything preceding it: their right to fully parent their daughter.

CONCLUSION

Childlessness and childbearing are key symbols in an ambiguous, contradictory local moral world. At stake in childbearing, for both men and women, are innumerable permutations of morality and immorality, joy and suffering, fulfillment and loss. Becoming a mother is key to the fulfillment of adult female identity, and procreation is the reification of the social bond between women and men. Yet the circumstances of childbearing may be subjected to painful inflections when viewed by the public "big hell" of small town Costa Rica, particularly for women. Some women are abandoned by their male partners when they become pregnant. Unwed mothers (especially adolescents) are left to bear the brunt of public disapproval while their male partners escape unscathed. Married women may be criticized as "careless" if they have too many children. In contrast, childless women are asked to publicly elaborate on "the problem" of their infertility. Childbearing is clearly a realm in which women unduly bear the literal and figurative burden of "too many" or "too few," "too late" or "too early," "moral" or "immoral." Childbearing's significance is complex, contradictory, changing, and seldom wholly good or bad. In the narrative of childbearing and childlessness, as in other narratives of human experience, "the human veracity . . . is its concentration of multiple divergent meanings" (Kleinman & Kleinman, 1995, p. 107).

Kleinman and Kleinman (1995, p. 98) suggest that human conditions such as suffering "offer a resistance in the flow of life to the elaboration of life plans." When they were first married, Silvia and José took childbearing for granted as a natural and unquestioned part of their lives. Fourteen years of struggling to cope with childlessness destroyed this notion and repeatedly turned the meaning of childbearing on its head. Childbearing was no longer a natural part of married life, nor was it determined by human will. Childbearing was a miracle, precious and divine, because it happened only according to God's will. Among those blessedly ignorant of the suffering and pain experienced by childless couples, this perspective was superseded by the contradictory Costa Rican context that emphasizes controlling the birthrate, eliminating undesirable births, and reproducing the so-called traditional nuclear family.

Throughout their story it was not only suffering and pain but also transcendence that was at stake in Silvia and Jose's daily experience. Seeking to transcend childlessness threw Silvia and José directly into conflict, as their individual needs, meanings, and modes of action conflated into an emotional crisis that put their marriage in jeopardy. Left with no other choice, Silvia decided to seek tranquillity through God in order to protect herself from the daily public reminders of childlessness. The adoption of their daughter resolved this crisis, however, through a divinely ordered series of events interpreted not only as fulfilling their prayers for a child and completing their marriage but also as relieving a young woman of the social burden of yet another fatherless child.

EPILOGUE

Each afternoon as I typed and edited this piece at the dining room table, Silvia sprawled out on a nearby sofa conversing with me about the shape it should take as it slowly evolved. José was at work, and Silvia would have been at work were she not on sick leave. The keys of my laptop clicked furiously whenever our conversation ebbed, and Silvia stroked and coddled her swollen belly in silence. Occasionally she called me over to feel some surge of movement. At age thirty-four (and approaching her fifteenth wedding anniversary), she was six months pregnant. For Silvia and José, the shocking realization that she was pregnant was only explicable as a continuation of the miraculous arrival of their adopted baby girl. From the moment their daughter entered their home, they felt their lives were complete and fulfilled. The seemingly impossible pregnancy was explained by them as proof of the divinity of childbearing and the will of God, not only to sustain them during their years of pain, but also to create a second miracle in their lives:

> It's like the doctor said, this [pregnancy] is the work of God that one has to recognize, because it doesn't happen when humans want it—but when God wants it. This is certain. You have to understand that many times, you cry and cry and pray to God. But it's that this is not the time that God wants. . . . [O]ne of my friends was talking to José and said that [this pregnancy] was a blessing from God, that it was the love of God that I was given the blessings of this pregnancy. José said that the truth is that the blessing isn't from this moment [and isn't new]. The blessing began when we adopted our daughter. From that moment, everything has been beautiful. The blessings began with her.

"People say," Silvia commented to me one afternoon, "'Oh, that always happens,' that people get pregnant the minute they adopt. What a pack of lies! There are many, many people who adopt and never get pregnant, and never will. People don't think about the things they say." I was one of those people. I had said it to them the night they called my husband and me in the United States to tell us the good news, in recognition of my auspicious comment in a small restaurant seven years before. What comfort I had taken in the idea that the body can be released from the chains of infertility if only allowed the chance. The words startled me, listening to them after days of hearing Silvia and José's story, and I understood the exasperation in her voice.

When Silvia and José decided to share their story for this volume, one of their primary motivations was to make public their lived experience of childlessness and adoption. In doing so, they purposefully went against the social rules that encourage private suffering—and did so to criticize those very rules and to describe their own framework for the miracles of their life. Silvia and José forthrightly acknowledged that many men and women in Buenos Aires experience childbearing as an unavoidable "fact" of life, a cross to be borne, or even a curse. Not everyone shared their passionate desire for childbearing, a common and "natural" desire painfully heightened by its denial. They acknowledged the injustice of the social rules that permitted public revelation of their infertility and cast them as abnormal. They chose to break the silence to raise consciousness. They hoped that it would encourage understanding among those who knowingly or unknowingly thrust daily reminders of childlessness before them and that other couples might be allowed the tranquillity they sought for themselves.

As I began the long trip back to the United States, I sat again on the sweltering bus to the regional capital, slowly reading *Cuando los niños no llegan* (Love, 1988), the Spanish version of *Childless Is Not Less* (Love, 1984). Silvia gave it to me so that I might better understand their story. She read much of it aloud to me the day before I left, commenting on the truth it told in each passage. It was an appropriate exchange, we agreed, because I gave them a copy of *Qué se puede esperar cuando está esperando* (Eisenberg, Murkoff, & Hathaway, 1998), the Spanish edition of *What to Expect When You're Expecting* (Eisenberg et al., 1994), to celebrate their pregnancy. As I read the book, its cover permanently curled and pages well thumbed, it occurred to me that I was twenty-eight years old: the same age Silvia was when she nearly died in the pursuit of children and she and her husband sank into a period of marital crisis. I too was married and childless, although by choice, as far as I knew. I wondered what the man sitting next to me was thinking, as he glanced awkwardly at me, a foreigner reading a Spanish book on childlessness. I shifted uncomfortably, and a fleeting thought shot through my mind, burning a path of shame: should I hide the cover?

Kleinman and Kleinman (1995, p. 99) remind us that in our work "[t]he task is to interpret patterns of meaning within situations understood in experience-near categories." "[Y]et," they add, "ethnographers also bring with them a liberating distance that comes from their own experience-near categories and their existential appreciation of shared human conditions." In my case, the act of doing ethnography highlighted the problems created by my own experience-near categories and by the unquestioned (and unrecognized) distance that I brought to childlessness. These traits were far from liberating, but they were instructive. It was only in the process of doing ethnography that it became possible to step into the vast, well-hidden emotional space of childlessness in Silvia and José's lives.

NOTE

I would like to thank Marcia Inhorn, Frank van Balen, and Judith Modell for their generosity and collegiality in helping to shape this piece. I am especially indebted to Pamela Sankar for her careful reading, penetrating insights, and open door. My heartfelt gratitude goes to Silvia and José, for the innumerable ways they continue to enrich my life. This piece is dedicated to Silvia and José's children, *con mucho cariño*.

REFERENCES

CCSS (Caja Costarricense de Seguro Social). (1994). *Fecundidad y formación de la familia: Encuesta nacional de salud reproductiva de 1993*. San José, Costa Rica: Caja Costarricense de Seguro Social, Departamento de Medicina Preventiva, Programa Salud Reproductiva.

DGEC (Dirección General de Estadística y Censos). (1994). *Estadisticas vitales: Población, nacimientos, defunciones, matrimonios*. San José, Costa Rica: Publicacions Dirección General de Estadística y Censos, Ministerio de Economía, Industria y Comercio.

Eisenberg, A., Murkoff, H. E., & Hathaway, S. E. (1994). *What to expect when you're expecting*. New York: Workman.

Eisenberg, A., Murkoff, H. E., & Hathaway, S. E. (1998). *Qué se puede esperar cuando se está esperando*. New York: Workman.

Harrison, P. (1981). Success story. *World Health, February–March*, 14–19.

Inhorn, M. C. (1994). *Quest for conception: Gender, infertility, and Egyptian medical traditions*. Philadelphia: University of Pennsylvania Press.

Kleinman, A., & Kleinman, J. (1995). Suffering and its professional transformation: Toward an ethnography of interpersonal experience. In A. Kleinman, *Writing at the margin: Discourse between anthropology and medicine* (pp. 95–119). Berkeley: University of California Press.

López, F., & Zúñiga, R. (1988). Adopciones en Costa Rica: La pobreza ampara el drama de la mujer marginada. *Universidad, 20(5)*, 12–13.

Love, V. (1984). *Childless is not less*. Minneapolis, MN: Bethany House.

Love, V. (1988). *Cuando los niños no llegan*. Caparra Terrace, Puerto Rico: Editorial Betania.

Low, S. M. (1978). Family formation in Costa Rica. In W. B. Miller & L. F. Newman (Eds.), *First child and family formation* (pp.128–144). Chapel Hill: Carolina Population Center, University of North Carolina.

Low, S. M., & Newman, B. C. (1985). Indigenous fertility regulating methods in Costa Rica. In L. F. Newman (Ed.), *Women's medicine: A cross-cultural study of indigenous fertility regulation* (pp. 147–160). New Brunswick, NJ: Rutgers University Press.

Melendez, D. A. (1995). The cultural context of adolescent childbearing in Costa Rica. Ph.D. dissertation, University of California, San Francisco.

Modell, J. (1986). In search: The purported biological basis of parenthood. *American Ethnologist, 13(4)*, 646–661.

Oberle, M. W., Rosero-Bixby, L., & Whitaker, P. (1993). A descriptive epidemiology of infertility in Costa Rica. In R. H. Gray, H. Léridon, & A. Spira (Eds.), *Biomedical and demographic determinants of reproduction* (pp. 126–131). Oxford: Clarendon Press.

PANI (Patronato Nacional de la Infancia). (1997a). *Cumplimiento de la convención sobre los derechos del niño: Informe de la República de Costa Rica.* San José, Costa Rica: Patronato Nacional de la Infancia.

PANI (Patronato Nacional de la Infancia). (1997b). *1997 resumen estadístico — Informe anual.* San José, Costa Rica: Patronato Nacional de la Infancia, Departamento de Informática.

Reuben, S. S. (1997). *Características familiares de los hogares costarricenses.* San José: Universidad de Costa Rica.

Rojas Chávez, C., & Martínez Cabezas, B. (1982). *En torno a la problematica de la adopción.* San José, Costa Rica: Patronato Nacional de la Infancia, Departamento de Investigaciones.

Rosero-Bixby, L., & Casterline, J. B. (1994). Interaction diffusion and fertility transition in Costa Rica. *Social Forces, 73(2)*, 435–462.

Solano C., M. (1998). Costa Rica, vitrina de adopciones. *La Nación Digital, January 18.*

Terrell, J., & Modell, J. (1994). Anthropology and adoption. *American Anthropologist, 96(1)*, 155–161.

Vaessen, M. (1984). *Childlessness and infecundity.* World Fertility Survey, Comparative Studies No. 31. Voorburg, the Netherlands: International Statistical Institute.

Villalobos, C. A. (1997). Proponen arreglo a esterilizados. *La Nación Digital, June 15.*

PART III

The Infertility Belt

TEN

Problematizing Fertility
"Scientific" Accounts and Chadian Women's Narratives

Lori Leonard

Large portions of Central Africa have long been characterized by unusually low fertility. Before the turn of the twentieth century, European explorers and colonial administrators noted the "fragility," even depopulation of some Central African societies, and historical demographers have since substantiated these claims (Caldwell & Caldwell, 1983; Headrick, 1990; Romaniuk, 1968). Despite recent increases in fertility in some Central African states, women in this region continue to bear fewer children than expected for a largely noncontracepting population and fewer children than other African women of similar social and economic circumstances (Cohen, 1993; Frank, 1983; Tambashe, 1992; United Nations, 1991).

Knowledge of Central Africa's fertility "problem" has been shaped primarily by demographic and epidemiological discourse on the distribution and causes of the phenomenon. More recently, ethnographic accounts of African women's experiences have appeared in the literature, adding emic[1] perspectives. I examine the ways in which these two broadly defined literatures problematize fertility and assess the extent to which the respective constructions diverge. I use empirical data from a study of fertility problems in southern Chad to illustrate areas of overlap and disjuncture. I begin, however, with a brief historical overview of work conducted from demographic, epidemiological, and ethnographic stances. The summaries that follow are by no means comprehensive; rather, they highlight only the most significant milestones in our understanding of what has become known as Central Africa's "infertility belt."

THE DEMOGRAPHY OF FERTILITY PROBLEMS IN CENTRAL AFRICA

Early demographic data on the fertility problems plaguing Central Africa were derived from the analysis of post–World War II sample surveys and censuses of varying quality. By piecing together, in a series of increasingly detailed maps and tables, fertility estimates for "tropical" Africa, demographers at Princeton University's Office of Population Research were among the first to document the existence of contiguous areas of curiously low fertility in the center of the continent (Brass et al., 1968; Coale, 1968; Coale & Lorimer, 1968; Page & Coale, 1972; van de Walle & Page, 1969). Included in this infertility belt were at least portions of the Democratic Republic of the Congo, the Central African Republic, the Sudan, Gabon, Cameroon, and Niger (Coale, 1968). Southern Chad, the geographic focus of this study, resisted classification until 1964, when the country's first partial census was conducted (Service de Coopération, 1966); previous "head counts" undertaken by colonial administrators resulted in data that were so scant, "irregular," and "unreliable" as to be virtually unusable (Headrick, 1990; Reyna & Bouquet, 1975). According to the census data, the average parity of southern Chadian women at the end of their reproductive years hovered around 5.0, with 12 percent of these women remaining childless (Service de Coopération, 1966). Estimated birth- and total fertility rates, while lower than average for the continent, were higher than those for other Central African women, leading demographers to conclude that the "belt" extended to, but stopped short of, southern Chad (Page & Coale, 1972; van de Walle & Page, 1969).

Among more recent sources of demographic data on African fertility are the World Fertility Survey (WFS) and the Demographic and Health Survey (DHS), two standardized, large-scale surveys of health and fertility conducted in selected countries, or regions of a country, with representative samples of the population. The WFS was carried out in nine sub-Saharan African nations between 1977 and 1982, the DHS in twenty-nine countries between 1986 and 1997. Although several of the Central African nations with historically low fertility (e.g., Gabon, the Democratic Republic of the Congo) are not represented in either survey, available data suggest that rates of childlessness and infertility have generally declined across the continent (Arnold & Blanc, 1990; Mammo & Morgan, 1986). Larsen (1995, 1996), for example, documented declines in childlessness of more than 60 percent between the administration of Tanzania's National Demographic Survey in 1973 and the DHS nearly two decades later and similar, though less dramatic, declines over roughly the same period in Cameroon and Nigeria.

THE EPIDEMIOLOGY OF FERTILITY PROBLEMS IN CENTRAL AFRICA

Early speculation about the causes of Central Africa's fertility problems was wide-ranging: poor hygiene, nutritional deficiencies, endemic disease, alcoholism, abortions, and even widespread apathy in the face of European demands for labor were hypothesized to play a role (Adadevoh, 1974; Caldwell & Caldwell, 1983; Retel-Laurentin, 1967; Romaniuk, 1968). A handful of in-depth investigations—notably those conducted by Retel-Laurentin in the Central African Republic (1967, 1978) and in Burkina Faso (1973) and by Romaniuk (1968, 1980) in the Democratic Republic of the Congo—narrowed the range of probable causes and focused attention on sexually transmitted diseases (STDs). Clinical evidence (scant and often based on cursory examinations carried out under field conditions), survey data, ecological correlations between sexual freedom or "promiscuity" and birthrates, and marked declines in infertility following the mass distribution of penicillin all provided support for this view (Allard, 1955; Central Statistical Office, 1975; Retel-Laurentin, 1973; Romaniuk, 1968, 1980).

From 1979 through 1984, in an effort to characterize global patterns of infertility using diagnoses derived from standardized protocols, the World Health Organization (WHO) sponsored a multicenter clinical investigation. Conducted in thirty-three medical centers in twenty-five countries, including four in sub-Saharan Africa, the study enrolled close to 8,500 couples, more than 5,800 of whom were eventually diagnosed. Compared with women evaluated in other centers, African women were more likely to report a history of an STD and of pregnancy complications, to suffer from bilateral tubal occlusion, and to be given a diagnosis suggestive of infection (Cates, Farley, & Rowe, 1985).

THE ETHNOGRAPHY OF FERTILITY PROBLEMS IN CENTRAL AFRICA

Local reflections on and interpretations of fertility problems, largely the products of ethnographic inquiries, have appeared in the literature much more recently (Boddy, 1989; Devisch, 1985; Ebin, 1982; Feldman-Savelsberg, 1994, 1999; Gerrits, 1997; Inhorn, 1994a, 1994b, 1996; Kielmann, 1998; Sangree, 1987; Sundby, 1997). Anthropologists working in different parts of the continent have described how women make sense of the inability to conceive or bear children, the range of treatments they seek when faced with reproductive failure as well as the patterns those searches take, and the lives and experiences of those for whom therapies are unsuccessful. These reports have underscored the human dimensions of reproductive failure and the centrality of childbearing to African women's identities and social welfare.

In its emphasis on emic experience, the ethnographic literature represents a departure from previous modes of studying fertility problems. This departure raises questions about the ways in which problems are defined and, in turn, the extent to which the multiple constructions speak to each other. How do fertility problems, as measured, mapped, and explained by demographers and epidemiologists, relate to the problems constructed by African women and their ethnographers? Do local narratives regarding problematic or inadequate fertility resemble or even closely mirror "scientific"[2] narratives grounded in biological models of reproduction? How do the biocentric constructions–those centered within the bodies, generally of women—of demographers and epidemiologists relate to the accounts of those actually experiencing the problems?

The aim of this chapter is to examine these questions using reports from women living in an urban center in southern Chad. Rather than use demographic or epidemiological criteria to diagnosis problems, women were asked for their self-assessments. From this perspective, problems occurred when individuals judged themselves to have had difficulty getting pregnant or having a child when getting pregnant or having a child was desired. However, before examining Chadian women's constructions of fertility problems, the following section examines, in a more general fashion, the ways in which the failure of African women to reproduce has been problematized.

PROBLEMATIZING FERTILITY

"Scientific" Constructions of Fertility Problems

The fertility problems of African women have been defined in a variety of ways in demographic, epidemiological, and clinical reports (see table 1). Among the constructs used are "childlessness," "infertility" (often subdivided into primary and secondary cases), "sterility," "infecundity," and "subfertility." Each of these measures provides an indication of the likelihood that women are physiologically incapable of reproducing; however, their use is conditioned in several important ways.

First, the fertility outcome on which the classification of African women as "fertile" or "infertile," "fecund" or "infecund," rests is based on a mechanistic model of "normal" physiological processes presumed to occur under "natural fertility" conditions (Bongaarts, 1978; Henry, 1961). Under such conditions, fertility outcomes are thought to be mediated by a small set of intermediate variables or proximate determinants, including, among others, factors such as contraceptive use and effectiveness, the prevalence of induced abortion, the duration of postpartum infecundability, and the frequency of intercourse (Bongaarts, 1982). While the way in which infertility or any other problem is defined may vary, sometimes greatly, from one investigation to another, within a given study strict rules pertain. In the context of the WFS, for example, women who had not given birth in the preceding five-year period were classified as "infecund" (with the proviso

TABLE 1 Conceptualizations of Fertility "Problems"

Measures Used	World Fertility Survey	Demographic and Health Survey	World Health Organization Multicenter Investigation
Childlessness	Women with no living children[a] Women who have never experienced a fertile pregnancy[b]		
Primary infertility	Women who have never experienced a pregnancy[c]	Women with no live births[d] Women who have never experienced a fertile pregnancy	Couples who have never been pregnant and have been trying, unsuccessfully, to achieve pregnancy for at least one year
Secondary infertility	Women who have experienced only one fertile pregnancy[e] Women infecund at different ages		Couples who have previously been pregnant at least once and have been trying, unsuccessfully, to achieve pregnancy for at least one year
Infecundity	Self-reported infecundity[f] Women responding affirmatively to the following question: "As far as you know, is it physically possible for you and your husband to have a child, supposing you wanted one?"[g] Behavioral infecundity Women with an open birth interval of five or more years who did not use contraception during that interval and were continuously married for the last five years		

TABLE 1 Conceptualizations of Fertility "Problems" (continued)

Measures Used	World Fertility Survey	Demographic and Health Survey	World Health Organization Multicenter Investigation
Aggregate infecundity	Women who either report themselves infecund or are classified as behaviorally infecund		

[a] In calculating both measures of childlessness, the base population was restricted to currently married women who had been married for at least five years.

[b] A "fertile pregnancy" was defined as either a pregnancy that resulted in a live birth or a current pregnancy.

[c] In calculating primary infertility, the base population was restricted to currently married women who had been married for at least five years.

[d] In calculating primary infertility, the base population was successively restricted to ever-married women, currently married women, women married five or more years, and women in their first union.

[e] In calculating secondary infertility, the base population was restricted to currently married women who had been married for at least five years.

[f] Asked of all currently married women who were not pregnant and not using a method of contraception.

[g] Variations of this question included the following: "Can you have more children?" "Do you think that you and your husband could have another child?" "Do you think that you can become pregnant (again)?"

that they met a number of behavioral and sociodemographic conditions). The use of biology to problematize fertility permits useful generalizations about the prevalence of problems and comparisons of the experiences of different groups according to a given standard but leaves no space for the particularistic experience of women who define problems differently–in this case, as something other than not having a child in the past five years.

Second, the chosen fertility outcome is applied only to specific segments of the population. In the example given above, only noncontracepting women married for the previous five years were eligible to be "infecund" and thus to have a fertility problem if problems are conceptualized as infecundity. While many, or even most, unmarried or contracepting women may view their failure to produce a child in the previous five years as unproblematic, some might disagree and indeed might be in the unmarried state precisely because of fertility problems.

Third, given the standardization of fertility outcomes and target populations, "infertility," "infecundity," "sterility," and other similar problems are static measures, held to be meaningful across time and place. Global comparisons of fertility problems, including cross-national, regional, and even continental comparisons, have been made on the basis of WFS, DHS, and WHO data (Arnold & Blanc, 1990; Cates et al., 1985; Vaessen, 1984). Similarly, survey data from numerous sources have been used to make comparisons of the prevalence of selected problems across time (Larsen, 1995, 1996; Mammo & Morgan, 1986; Sala-Diakanda & Lohlé-Tart, 1982). These types of analyses are useful in indicating the relative burden of fertility problems in different areas of the world; at the same time, however, they presume that fertility problems in Botswana are the same as those in Nigeria, Venezuela, and Bangladesh and that problems documented in the 1960s are the same as those documented in the 1990s.

Narrative Constructions of Fertility Problems

Ethnographic reports suggest that African women and men use a number of different models to interpret and explain fertility problems. Social, spiritual, and relational disruptions, in addition to physical ones, are cited as causes. In a study of healers' interpretations of "infertility" among the Aowin of Ghana, Ebin (1982) contrasts the explanations provided by spirit mediums, whose focus is on ascertaining which of the women's social relations need attention in order to appease the wrath of the gods, with those provided by herbalists, who attend instead to women's physical complaints. Among the twenty-five Aowin women in Ebin's study seeking treatment from a spirit medium, the diagnoses included, among others, disruptions in relations with neighbors, cowives, husbands, and matrilineal kin. Herbalists, by contrast, used knowledge gained in school and through appren-

ticeships and interactions with other herbalists to interpret and treat physical symptoms, entirely disregarding clients' personal relationships.

Few ethnographers have explicitly analyzed or reported the ways in
which their informants define problems. Many have focused on childlessness—one outcome apparently perceived to be problematic from both etic
and emic perspectives. Others have adopted scientific constructions of fertility problems or have studied women (generally to the exclusion of men)
seeking Western or indigenous treatment without systematically analyzing
or reporting the precise motivations for those visits. Clues are to be found,
however, in some ethnographic texts. Inhorn (1994b), for example, chron-
icles the long and so far unsuccessful "search for children" undertaken by
Hind, a twice-married, thirty-one-year-old "infertile" Egyptian woman.
Hind's fertility was first perceived as problematic by her in-laws, five months
after her first marriage at the age of twelve, and led to the intervention of
family members and Hind's participation in a ritual bath with a small, dead
baby. Hind's fertility was again judged problematic two months after her
second marriage, which occurred when she was sixteen, by her mother in-
law, who proclaimed "there is nothing" and pressured her to undergo a
number of painful, frightening, and ultimately unsuccessful therapies. In
another example, Gambian women and men interviewed by Sundby (1997)
reported that a marriage of seven years' duration should end in divorce if
no children are produced and cited the Qur'an for support. In his work
with the Tiriki of Kenya, Sangree (1987, 1992) provides perhaps the most
comprehensive account of a sub-Saharan African community's construction of fertility problems. The Tiriki expect group members to have six or
more children, at least two of whom are sons, and routinely sanction
women who bear less than three children.

> Those with at least two sons but less than a total of six children receive ex-
> pressions of mild condolence together with expressed hopes and assurances
> that it may not be too late to parent a few more children. For women who
> are approaching the end of their reproductive years without having borne a
> minimum of three children, and for older men with less than two sons, how-
> ever, the matter is much more serious; they are treated as though they were
> of questionable worth as human beings, or as if they were actually defective!
> . . . Tradition demands that a woman's husband's lineage provide her with
> food and shelter, including her own cooking hearth, until she dies, but only
> if she has borne her husband at least three children, regardless of their sex.
> . . . Older men, most of whom have at least some property with which to re-
> ward those who look after them in their old age, suffer primarily from mark-
> edly lowered respect from their peers, and probably experience concorrelate
> damaged self-esteem, if they have less than two living sons. For example, the
> epithet, "one-legged" may be used by his peers to address or refer to a man
> who has only one son alive who can be expected to mourn for him at his
> funeral, regardless of how many living daughters he may have fathered. And

a sonless man is reminded repeatedly as he gets older that he is becoming "very short!" (Sangree, 1987, pp. 213–214)

Thus, while the reproductive histories of those who figure in ethnographic accounts may concurrently earn them the label "infertile," "sterile," or "infecund," these histories may also reflect alternate reproductive ideals, such as the desire for sons or a family of a particular size or sex composition.

Ethnographic texts also affirm that problems are not exclusive to married women in multiyear partnerships. Hind's five-month period of barrenness following her first marriage, although not sufficient to qualify her for inclusion in a WHO-like clinical investigation or for classification as "infertile" in demographic studies, was sufficiently problematic from her family's perspective to warrant potentially iatrogenic intervention. Indeed, ethnographic texts reveal that problems are not even exclusive to women. Because they are more likely to be considered the source of problems and to take the initiative in seeking help, women are the usual focus of such inquiries; however, the above extracts from Sangree's work attest to the fact that men also suffer.

Finally, the examples of locally defined fertility problems provided in the preceding paragraphs, although limited in number, clearly suggest that the criteria used to make such assessments are context-specific. Empirical examples are scarce; yet, at least in theory, problems may be defined differently by different subgroups in a given population, and multiple definitions of problematic fertility may exist concurrently. Longitudinal studies are also lacking; however, it seems plausible to suggest that what constitutes a problem might take on different meanings over the life course of an individual and, on a community level, that conceptions of problematic fertility are likely to be revised over time as norms shift and cultural values change.

Having briefly outlined the ways in which African women's fertility has been problematized by demographers, epidemiologists, clinicians, and ethnographers, I turn now to an examination of the ways in which women living in an urban center in southern Chad assessed the adequacy of their own fertility. Their narratives were collected as part of a larger study of fertility problems that took place in 1993 and 1994.

CHAD, SARH, AND THE SARA

Chad is a vast, landlocked, and largely arid country, located near the center of the African continent. From 1889 until 1960 Chad was a French colony and for most of that period (from 1905 to 1958) formed part of French Equatorial Africa, a loosely governed federation that also included the present-day states of the Central African Republic, the Congo, and Gabon. In

Chad, colonial influence was largely confined to the south, which its administrators dubbed *le Tchad utile,* or useful Chad (Collelo, 1990).

Fort Archambault, renamed Sarh in 1972, was one of the first colonial outposts established in le Tchad utile. Currently, Sarh has 70,000 inhabitants, is the third largest urban center in the country, and serves as the capital of the Moyen-Chari, one of Chad's fourteen administrative regions, or *préfectures.* The Sara are the predominant ethnic group in Sarh and, with a population of nearly 1.7 million (Bureau Central du Recensement, 1995a), make up between one-fourth and one-third of the population of Chad. A conflation of a number of smaller ethnic subgroups, the Sara are patrilineal and patrilocal; members trace their lineage to the *gir ka,* or common ancestor. Marriages are strictly exogamous, and polygamy is commonly practiced.

The experience of colonialism, particularly the obligatory cultivation of cotton and the structural and organizational changes that accompanied its introduction, served to unite the multiple Sara subgroups that were formerly organized as much smaller clan- or lineage-based units (Collelo, 1990). The colonial period also brought the Sara increased access to educational opportunities and exposure to Western religious influences. Christian missionaries—American Baptists and, later, French Catholics—settled in southern Chad as early as the mid-1920s. According to the 1993 census, fully 85.2 percent of Sara are Christian: 51.9 percent of them Catholic and 33.3 percent Protestant. Animism remains the religion of 5.2 percent of all Sara; few (1.7 percent) have adopted Islam (Bureau Central du Recensement, 1995a). Protestant mission schools were opened in the Moyen-Chari by the end of the 1920s, and state-sponsored secondary schools were established two decades later. Access to Western education allowed the Sara to dominate the postindependence government, and this imbalance in turn fostered resentment among members of other groups and exacerbated ethnic tensions that eventually culminated in a protracted civil war.

Despite urbanization and increased access to education, Chad's economic development has been slow. In 1997 the World Bank ranked the Chadian economy, with an estimated GNP per capita of U.S. $180, as the world's sixth poorest (World Bank, 1997). The vast majority of Sara continue to subsist on small-scale agriculture, and the group's economy remains centered almost exclusively on agricultural production. Millet, sorghum, and peanuts are the most important staple crops, while cotton continues to provide the only cash revenue for most Sara families.

Until very recently, little data were available on the fertility of the Sara. Estimates of birth- and fertility rates were based on extrapolations and projections from partial censuses conducted in 1964 and again in 1968 (Service de Coopération, 1966). However, the country's first complete population census was completed in 1993, followed, in 1997, by a DHS. According to census data, the average total fertility rate of Sara women is 6.0, surpassing, slightly, the national average of 5.6 (Bureau Central du Recensement, 1995b). Among women fifty years of age and older, 11 percent of those living in the Moyen-Chari (proportions are not provided for ethnic groups) and 12 percent of those living in Chad had never given birth to a live child. Estimates from the DHS place the average total fertility rate higher—at 6.6 for the country (data for ethnic groups are not provided), making it among the highest on the continent (Ouagadjio et al., 1998). The DHS estimates of childlessness are substantially lower than those derived from census data: only 4.3 percent of women ages forty-five to forty-nine and only 2.5 percent of women ages thirty-five to forty-nine are childless.

METHODOLOGY

Fieldwork for this study was conducted over the ten-month period from October 1993 through July 1994 and employed both epidemiological and anthropological field methods (Dunn & Janes, 1986). Data presented in this chapter are those collected through semistructured household interviews with a sample of 170 women and from less structured, follow-up and supplementary conversations with 21 women with self-defined fertility problems.

Cluster sampling was used to select women to participate in the study. Block-by-block census maps and aggregate population figures for each of seventy-four census tracts in urban Sarh were obtained from the Bureau of the Census in N'Djaména; five of the seventy-four tracts were selected, with the probability of selection proportionate to the size of the tract. The author and a female research assistant who was Sara and lived in Sarh went door-to-door to document the number of eligible informants and to ask permission to conduct interviews. In selected tracts we interviewed, on alternate blocks, women who were of Sara ethnicity, aged fifteen or older, and currently residing in the household. Our conversations were held in the informants' homes or in their courtyards, or *concessions*, and most (91.8%) were conducted in Sara, the primary local language, with the remainder conducted in French.

The study did not make use of clinical measures of fertility status; no attempts were made to provide a medical diagnosis by conducting physical exams, and no inferences were made about a respondent's physical capacity to reproduce on the basis of birth histories or other demographic data. Rather, the intent was to capture the subjective experiences of the women interviewed and to examine their own conceptions of fertility problems. To that end, open-ended queries were used in the course of the household surveys, and less structured conversations were conducted with women who described their fertility as problematic.

Sociodemographic data for all 170 women interviewed as well as for the 21 women who reported being unable to conceive or bear a child when desired are presented in table 2 and are similar, apart from the proportions of women ever and currently married. All but one of the women with a self-defined fertility problem had been previously married. This subgroup of 21 women represents 12.4 percent of all the women interviewed and 17.1 percent of all ever-married women. The latter figure may serve as a more meaningful indicator of the prevalence of subjectively defined fertility problems in this community, where extramarital childbearing, although becoming increasingly common, is neither encouraged nor expected.

FERTILITY PROBLEMS OF THE SARA

Of the twenty-one women with self-defined fertility problems, five had never conceived and one conceived but miscarried. Thus the majority of the women ($n = 15$) who described themselves as currently or previously having a fertility problem had successfully produced at least one live-born child. Women's narratives incorporated several features of reproductive lives that render them problematic. These include (1) the need to prove one's fertility shortly after marriage; (2) reproductive mishaps (Bledsoe, Banja, & Hill, 1998) or the loss of reproductive potential through miscarriage, stillbirth, abortion, or accident; and (3) small completed family size. Each of these features is described in some detail below. Although presented as distinct categories, these experiences are by no means mutually exclusive and, indeed, in many instances occurred either simultaneously or sequentially.

Proving Fertility

Informants in the household survey reported that fertility needs to be proven very shortly after marriage or the establishment of a stable relationship. More than 40 percent of the women interviewed said they would expect a newly married woman to get pregnant within one month, while recognizing that factors such as the timing of her menstrual cycle, the compatibility of the couple's blood, and the husband's opinion could extend, slightly, the length of that interval. Women who failed to demonstrate their fertility early in a marriage found themselves in a precarious position: in-laws insulted, ignored, and ridiculed them while pressuring their sons to get divorced or to take other, more fertile wives. In-laws' constant surveillance of and commentary on the couple's fertility created tension in the household, leading women to concur that, regardless of the strength of the

TABLE 2   Sociodemographic Characteristics of the Study Sample

	All Women (n = 170)	Women with Self-Defined Fertility Problems (n = 21)
Mean age	28.7	30.9
	(15–74)	(16–72)
Attended school (%)	75.3	71.4
Mean years of education	4.4	4.4
	(0–14)	(0–13)
Religion (%)		
Christian	80.0	76.2
Animist	14.7	14.3
Muslim	5.3	9.5
Ever married (%)	72.4	95.2
Currently married (%)	58.8	85.7

marital bond, the odds of the relationship lasting in the absence of a child were small.

Thirteen of the twenty-one women who considered their fertility problematic talked about difficulties related to proving their ability to bear children following marriage or, in one case, the establishment of a stable relationship. Women who had been married more than once described this problem in relation to one or both relationships; indeed, the failure to demonstrate one's fertility often resulted in a cyclical pattern of marital dissolution, partner change, and renewed pressure to demonstrate reproductive capacity. Five of the women who talked about these pressures had not yet succeeded in conceiving and six had not delivered a child, although four of them had attempted it with more than one partner. Women who eventually got pregnant and carried the pregnancy to term described first waiting for periods that ranged from one to six years—well beyond the expectations of most. Four of these women considered their fertility problems resolved at the time of our interview; the remaining three described renewed problems related to having too few children or to the loss of reproductive potential.

Losing Reproductive Potential

The notion that women are born with a fixed number of children–some have few, some have many, and some have none at all—was reiterated with frequency in the household interviews and has been reported by ethnographers working in other parts of the continent (Bledsoe et al., 1998; Sargent, 1982). The Sara describe potential children as existing "in the stomach" or "on the back"; injuries or even blows to these areas elicit concern about or accusations of "killing" a woman's children. Given a quota of potential children, abortions, miscarriages, stillbirths, or other mishaps are seen as irrevocably reducing possible fertility and impeding women's goals to maximize their family size or have as many children "as God gives."

One-third ($n = 7$) of the twenty-one women who talked about their fertility as problematic mentioned the loss of children through miscarriages when discussing their problems. While most of these women had few or no children, several had "large" families, both by their standards and by the standards of the larger group of women interviewed. One woman, for instance, had given birth to ten children, eight of whom were living. However, her first pregnancy resulted in a miscarriage, as did two consecutive pregnancies occurring exactly in the middle of her reproductive career. Although she continued to reproduce "until there [weren't] any more children," the loss of three potential children prevented her from realizing her God-given endowment.

Bearing Too Few Children

Extended periods of barrenness following marriage, the loss of potential children through miscarriage, abortion, accidents, or other misfortunes, and infant deaths result, ultimately, in small families composed of "too few" children. While quantifying fertility desires and family size ideals is not a problem-free exercise (van de Walle, 1992), attempts to do so may provide general clues about adequate and inadequate levels of fertility. On average, women responding to the household survey wanted a minimum of three to four children and a maximum of six to seven. Slightly less than 15 percent of the sample provided non-numeric responses, indicating that they would have children "until there aren't any more," that these estimates were "up to God," or that they did not know or could not answer the question. Responses to questions about family size ideals varied substantially, both in form and in content, by the age of the informant; younger women were much more likely to provide numeric responses to the queries and to report wanting fewer children. Yet even fifteen- to nineteen-year-old women wanted, on average, 2.8 children; thus two-child families remain largely inadequate, even for those who want the smallest families.

Nearly three-fourths ($n = 15$) of the twenty-one women who reported a problem with their fertility indicated that they had fewer children than they desired. Women who talked about having too few children represented a range of fertility experiences: five had never conceived, one had a stillbirth but never a live birth, and nine had given birth but were subsequently unable to have more children. In addition to problems with conception and childbearing, child loss contributed to women's perceptions that their families were too small; only six of the fifteen women had any living children at the time of our interview, and none had more than two.

With few exceptions, the parities of the women who wanted more children were well below the age-matched averages for women in the sample, and the number of children these women had at the time of our interviews fell far short of the number they desired. Most women who talked about the desire for more children were still of reproductive age, and all but the two eldest women in this group continued to actively seek treatment for their problem and to hope for more children. Yet their optimism was tempered by the fact that, in all but three cases, at least five years had elapsed since they had last given birth.

WOMEN'S NARRATIVES

Each of the twenty-one women whose experiences are encapsulated, and necessarily condensed, in the preceding paragraphs has her own story and her own way of problematizing fertility. What follows is a re-presentation of the experience of one woman, Solkem, whose story is not meant to be representative or archetypal but to give voice to the experience of problems with fertility. This story was chosen for inclusion here because it illustrates all three features of problematic fertility described in this chapter.

Solkem's Story

When I interviewed Solkem, she was living with her family in a small house near the center of town. She was thirty-one years old and had been divorced recently. Not employed in the formal sector, Solkem supported herself and her son and contributed to the household economy through occasional small-scale trade. Relative to other Sara women her age, Solkem was well educated, having completed the eighth grade, and had married late, at the age of twenty-two.

During the first years of her marriage, to a man she referred to as her "friend," Solkem suffered two miscarriages, both of which were treated at the public hospital. Her slow start and initial reproductive difficulties elicited comment, concern, and disapproval from friends and family. Within one year of her marriage, her in-laws began "creating problems" and spreading the word that Solkem could not have children. Friends "continued to remind [her] that she [couldn't] have children" and drew unfavorable comparisons between Solkem and her mother, who had given birth to thirteen sons and daughters. In response to her attempts to help "educate" her nieces and nephews, Solkem's brothers and sisters told her that because she "didn't know what it was like" to give birth, she had no right to discipline their children. Solkem, who expected to get pregnant in the month following her marriage, reported that she wasn't "calm," and she worried, along with her parents, that she would have no one to "replace" her.

Although she was disheartened and desperately wanted a child, Solkem did not seek help—apart from the treatment she received after her miscarriages—for her problem. As a devout member of the local Baptist mission church that forcefully denounces all "traditional" practices, including the use of non-Western medicine or healing rituals, she chose instead to "just wait for the child to come." After four years of marriage, Solkem finally gave birth to a son. However, her problems were not resolved. Another four years passed during which Solkem never conceived, and this time her husband decided to divorce her rather than wait for another child.

Approximately one year after her divorce, Solkem talked of wanting more children but not being in a position to have them, because she wasn't "with a man." She thought she might like to have five children but given her situation felt that even one more would be acceptable. In the absence of a man and additional children, she was counting on her son to "take good care of [her]" and was watching over him carefully.

"SCIENTIFIC" VOICES AND THE VOICES OF WOMEN: AREAS OF OVERLAP AND DISJUNCTURE

Are the experiences of Solkem and the other less-than-fertile Sara women who formed part of this study incorporated, captured, and reflected in the scientific discourse on fertility problems in sub-Saharan Africa? Perhaps the simplest way to answer the question and to assess the degree of correspondence between etic and emic perspectives on problems is to examine women's self-diagnoses in light of the classification criteria—some of which are outlined in table 1—used in previous investigations. The questions asked as part of the three standardized studies described in the table undoubtedly permit additional formulations of problems. Nevertheless, the comparisons here rely on the widely cited conceptualizations displayed in the table that have been published in summary reports of the WFS (Vaessen, 1984) and DHS (Arnold & Blanc, 1990) studies and in journal articles and scientific reports describing the WHO clinical investigation (Cates et al., 1985; Rowe, 1984).

Most of the twenty-one Sara women with subjectively defined fertility problems would be labeled "infertile," "infecund," or "childless" by the standards of one or more of the featured studies. Thirteen would have been eligible to enroll in the clinical investigation sponsored by the WHO at the time of our interview, and an additional six, reporting retrospective difficulties, would have qualified at an earlier point in their reproductive careers. Using WFS standards, two-thirds ($n = 14$) of the twenty-one women would have been judged to have some type of fertility problem; however, this proportion drops to only one-third ($n = 7$) when DHS classification criteria are applied. Women who had never been pregnant or had no living children—the most extreme cases—exhibit the greatest degree of overlap in terms of their respective diagnoses. Yet, based on their marital statuses at the time of our interviews, not even all of these women would consistently be counted among those with problems.

The stories that fail to be recognized as problematic are perhaps most instructive. Solkem, for example, could not be categorized as "childless," "infecund," or "infertile" using most of the WFS and DHS definitions outlined in the table. Not only was she unmarried, making her, de facto, ineligible to have many of the problems captured by these assessments, but she exhibited, even during her marriage, a pattern of fertility not deviant enough—with only a couple of exceptions—to be labeled problematic. For the first four years of her marriage, Ndadnouba, a thirty-five-year-old woman who had two small children at the time of our interview, traveled throughout the country, from one medical center to another, looking for help for what was eventually diagnosed as "stenosis." Her struggle would be barely perceptible in the scientific accounts. Even more extreme is the experience of Moudiare, a never-married eighteen-year-old woman who had tried to conceive with a succession of suitors over a number of years. Her troubles were invisible, appearing nowhere in the scientific story of Africa's fertility problems.

How do these women's stories add to our knowledge of fertility problems in Central Africa, and where do they point us in terms of reproductive health policy and practice? First, the narratives raise questions about how to read and interpret estimates of the prevalence of fertility problems for the region, as well as how to read and interpret the derivative, scientific story: that is, that problems, while of importance historically, have diminished in frequency to the extent that sub-Saharan Africa now resembles any other region of the world with regard to levels of infertility. Instead, women's accounts impel us to ask *what* the estimates of "infertility" capture and how the pictures they portray are circumscribed by limiting our gaze to specific outcomes and to specific women. Sara women's narratives suggest that subjectively defined problems are relatively common—certainly more common than demographic and epidemiological reports emanating from the region would suggest—and that women (and men) in any of a variety of sociodemographic categories are affected.

The stories also serve as a window on indigenous models of fertility, allowing us to see the range of scenarios perceived locally as problematic. The narratives collected in the course of this and other studies reveal that sex and numbers are important (though well-established thresholds such as those described by Sangree are perhaps rare), that high parity does not necessarily preclude women from interpreting pregnancy loss as problematic, and that the expected rhythm and tempo of reproduction, particularly at critical junctures (e.g., marriage) in a woman's life, may diverge from "normal" or even probable biological functioning.

Why do these indigenous models—particularly those that stand in contrast to the biomedical model and are perhaps not even reflective of physical impairment, infection, or problems—merit attention? The answer to this question is located in the narratives as well. Women's, and men's, stories reveal the meaning and impact of subjectively defined fertility problems on lives. Their stories link reproductive trouble with sexual mobility, partner change, and the use of potentially iatrogenic treatments, all of which, paradoxically, place women at increased risk of sterilizing infections. They also suggest that self-defined problems may be better predictors of marital disruption, abuse, poverty, social isolation, treatment seeking, and resource use than problems defined by others.

In addition, the narratives compel us to recognize variations in social standards or expectations pertaining to reproduction and family composition. Reproductive problems are to some extent local, in that they are defined differently in different contexts. In her village in eastern Kenya, a Tiriki woman with two sons may suffer through old age without the support of her in-laws, whereas, as the mother of two sons, she may be revered elsewhere. The local—central to women's narratives but missing (by design) from the scientific accounts—is a key ingredient in the development of effective public health programs and policies.

In fact, the juxtaposition of scientific and local narratives highlights some of the gaps and disjunctures on which interventions could effectively be focused. For example, Sara women talk about the tremendous pressure they experience to become pregnant within one or two months of marriage, and physicians describe as common instances in which worried women or couples seek help for problems before they might be expected, based on clinical criteria, to conceive. If women are seeking help for fertility problems at clinically inappropriate times, the implementation of educational programs may save scarce health care resources as well as allay unwarranted fears and anxieties. Similarly, a greater awareness of the range of reproductive options considered acceptable in a particular community may help service providers to better understand their clients' reproductive, including contraceptive, needs and their room for maneuvering with respect to the timing, spacing, and number of births.

The influence of subjective accounts of fertility problems is absent especially from population and reproductive health policy. In many African settings, a large percentage of obstetric and gynecological outpatient services are devoted to treatment of the infertile (Belsey, 1983; Frank, 1983).

Indeed, to accommodate the demand, the family planning clinic in N'Djaména, Chad's capital, has reserved Thursdays for the exclusive consultation and care of women presenting with fertility problems. Yet, despite recognition of this demand, family planning services in most African settings are narrowly focused on the delivery of contraceptives (Bergstrom, 1992; Gerrits, 1997) and are undergirded by the construction of African women as "overproducers" (Kielmann, 1998) and the concomitant philosophy of population control. Such policies and their implementation are subscribed to by insiders (e.g., indigenous medical personnel) (see Inhorn, 1994b), as well as by development agencies and Western funding bodies.

Sara women's stories affirm that reproduction, like other biological processes, is shaped and interpreted by social and cultural processes. The fertility of women in Sarh, as in other Central African communities, is regulated by women's physiological capacity for childbearing but is also regulated by social forces. The influence of the latter is not always captured through clinical exams, the analysis of birth histories, or the use of standardized conceptualizations of problems derived from probabilistic, biomedical models. The realities revealed by women's stories are not wholly reflected in the scientific literature on African fertility problems, past or present. Women's voices expand this work and provide the means for a more inclusive and complete narrative, telling different but equally compelling stories.

NOTES

Funding for this study was provided by a J. William Fulbright Fellowship from the Institute for International Education, a Frederick Sheldon Traveling Fellowship from Harvard University, and a Population Council Fellowship. I would like to thank Nilesh Chatterjee and the editors of this volume for their very helpful comments on earlier versions of this chapter.

1. In this chapter, the terms "etic" and "emic" refer to the use of categories—in this case, ways of defining fertility problems—that derive from outside the culture studied ("etic") or that are based on concepts used by and meaningful to group members ("emic").

2. The bodies of work produced by demographers, epidemiologists, and clinicians are those labeled "scientific" in this chapter. However, the use of this terminology in reference to these literatures is not meant to imply that other types of knowledge are not scientific.

REFERENCES

Adadevoh, B. K. (1974). *Sub-fertility and infertility in Africa*. Ibadan: Caxton Press.

Allard, R. (1955). Contribution gynécologique à l'étude de la stérilité chez les Mongo de Befale. *Annales de la Societé Belge de Medecine Tropicale, 25,* 631–648.

Arnold, F., & Blanc, A.K. (1990). *Fertility levels and trends: DHS comparative studies no. 2.* Columbia, MD: Institute for Resource Development.

Belsey, M. (1983). Epidemiologic aspects of infertility. In K. K. Holmes & P. A. Mardh (Eds.), *International perspectives on neglected sexually transmitted diseases* (pp. 269–297). Washington, DC: Hemisphere Press.

Bergstrom, S. (1992). Reproductive failure as a health priority in the Third World: A review. *East African Medical Journal, 69,* 174–180.

Bledsoe, C., Banja, F., & Hill, A. (1998). Reproductive mishaps and Western contraception: An African challenge to fertility theory. *Population and Development Review, 24,* 15–57.

Boddy, J. (1989). *Wombs and alien spirits: Women, men, and the Zar cult in northern Sudan.* Madison: University of Wisconsin Press.

Bongaarts, J. (1978). A framework for analyzing the proximate determinants of fertility. *Population and Development Review, 4,* 105–132.

Bongaarts, J. (1982). The fertility-inhibiting effects of the intermediate fertility variables. *Studies in Family Planning, 13,* 179–189.

Bouquet, C. (1982). *Tchad: Genese d'un conflit.* Paris: Editions l'Harmattan.

Brass, W., Coale, A. J., Demeny, P., Heisel, D. F., Lorimer, F., Romaniuk, A., & van de Walle, E. (1968). *The demography of tropical Africa.* Princeton, NJ: Princeton University Press.

Bureau Central du Recensement. (1995a). *Recensement general de la population et de l'habitat 1993. Tome 2: Etat de la population.* N'Djaména: Bureau Central du Recensement.

Bureau Central du Recensement. (1995b). *Recensement general de la population et de l'habitat. Tome 3a: Fecondité.* N'Djaména: Bureau Central du Recensement.

Caldwell, J. C., & Caldwell, P. (1983). The demographic evidence for the incidence and cause of abnormally low fertility in tropical Africa. *World Health Statistics Quarterly, 36,* 2–34.

Cates, W., Farley, T. M., & Rowe, P. J. (1985). Worldwide patterns of infertility: Is Africa different? *Lancet, 2,* 596–598.

Central Statistical Office. (1975). *Inter-regional variations in fertility in Zambia. Population monographs no. 2.* Lusaka: Central Statistical Office.

Chauvet, J. (1984). *Atlas historique et geographique de Sarh, Tchad de 1899 à 1970.* Sarh: Centre d'Etudes Linguistiques.

Coale, A. J. (1968). Estimates of fertility and mortality in tropical Africa. In J. C. Caldwell & C. Okonjo (Eds.), *The population of tropical Africa* (pp. 179–186). London: Longmans.

Coale, A. J., & Lorimer, F. (1968). Summary of estimates of fertility and mortality. In W. Brass, A. J. Coale, P. Demeny, D. F. Heisel, F. Lorimer, A. Romaniuk, & E. van de Walle (Eds.), *The demography of tropical Africa* (pp. 151–167). Princeton, NJ: Princeton University Press.

Cohen, B. (1993). Fertility levels, differentials, and trends. In K. A. Foote, K. H. Hill, & L. G. Martin (Eds.), *Demographic change in sub-Saharan Africa* (pp. 8–67). Washington, DC: National Academy Press.

Collelo, T. (1990). *Chad: A country study.* Washington, DC: Library of Congress.

Devisch, R. (1985). Polluting and healing among the northern Yaka of Zaire. *Social Science & Medicine, 21,* 693–700.

Dunn, F. L., & Janes, C. R. (1986). Introduction: Medical anthropology and epidemiology. In C. R. Janes, R. Stall, & S. M. Gifford (Eds.), *Anthropology and epidemiology* (pp. 3–34). Boston: D. Reidel.

Ebin, V. (1982). Interpretations of infertility: The Aowin people of south-west Ghana. In C. P. MacCormack (Ed.), *Ethnography of fertility and birth* (pp. 141–159). New York: Academic Press.

Feldman-Savelsberg, P. (1994). Plundered kitchens and empty wombs: Fear of infertility in the Cameroonian Grassfields. *Social Science & Medicine, 39*, 463–474.

Feldman-Savelsberg, P. (1999). *Plundered kitchens, empty wombs: Threatened reproduction and identity in the Cameroon Grassfields.* Ann Arbor: University of Michigan Press.

Frank, O. (1983). Infertility in sub-Saharan Africa: Estimates and implications. *Population and Development Review, 9*, 137–144.

Gerrits, T. (1997). Social and cultural aspects of infertility in Mozambique. *Patient Education and Counseling, 31*, 39–48.

Headrick, R. (1990). Studying the population of French Equatorial Africa. In B. Fetter (Ed.), *Demography from scanty evidence: Central Africa in the colonial era* (pp. 273–298). Boulder: L. Rienner.

Henry, L. (1961). Some data on natural fertility. *Eugenics Quarterly, 8*, 81–91.

Inhorn, M. C. (1994a). Kabsa (a.k.a. Mushahara) and threatened fertility in Egypt. *Social Science & Medicine, 39*, 487–505.

Inhorn, M.C. (1994b). *Quest for conception: Gender, infertility and Egyptian medical traditions.* Philadelphia: University of Pennsylvania Press.

Inhorn, M. C. (1996). *Infertility and patriarchy: The cultural politics of gender and family life in Egypt.* Philadelphia: University of Pennsylvania Press.

Kielmann, K. (1998). Barren ground: Contesting identities of infertile women in Pemba, Tanzania. In M. Lock & P. A. Kaufert (Eds.), *Pragmatic women and body politics* (pp. 127–163). Cambridge: Cambridge University Press.

Larsen, U. (1995). Differentials in infertility in Cameroon and Nigeria. *Population Studies, 49*, 329–346.

Larsen, U. (1996). Childlessness, subfertility, and infertility in Tanzania. *Studies in Family Planning, 27*, 18–28.

Magnant, J. P. (1986). *La terre Sara terre tchadienne.* Paris: Editions L'Harmattan.

Mammo, A., & Morgan, S. P. (1986). Childlessness in rural Ethiopia. *Population and Development Review, 12*, 533–546.

Mollion, P. (1992). *Sur les pistes de l'Oubangui-Chari au Tchad, 1890–1930: Le drame du portage en Afrique centrale.* Paris: Editions l'Harmattan.

Ouagadjio, B., Nodjimadji, K., Ngoniri, J. N., Ngakoutou, N., Ignégongba, K., Tokindang,

J. S., Kouo, O., Barrère, B., & Barrère, M. (1998). *Enquête démographique et de santé, Tchad 1996–1997.* Calverton, MD: Bureau Central du Recensement and Macro International.

Page, H. J., & Coale, A. J. (1972). Fertility and child mortality south of the Sahara. In S. H. Ominde & C. N. Ejiogu (Eds.), *Population growth and economic development in Africa* (pp. 51–66). London: Heinemann.

Retel-Laurentin, A. (1967). Influence de certaines maladies sur la fécondité: Un example Africain. *Population, 22*, 841–860.

Retel-Laurentin, A. (1973). Fecondite et syphilis dans la region de la Volta Noire. *Population, 28,* 793–815.

Retel-Laurentin, A. (1978). Evaluation du rôle de certaines maladies dans l'infécondité: Un exemple Africain. *Population, 33,* 101–119.

Reyna, S. P., & Bouquet, C. (1975). Chad. In J. C. Caldwell (Ed.), *Population growth and socioeconomic change in West Africa* (pp. 565–581). New York: Population Council.

Romaniuk, A. (1968). Infertility in tropical Africa. In J. C. Caldwell & C. Okonjo (Eds.), *The population of tropical Africa* (pp. 214–224). London: Longmans.

Romaniuk, A. (1980). Increase in natural fertility during the early stages of modernization: Evidence from an African case study, Zaire. *Population Studies, 34,* 293–310.

Rowe, P. (1984). Workshop on the standardized investigation of the infertile couple. In *Fertility and sterility: The proceedings of the XIth World Congress on Fertility and Sterility.* Lancaster: MTP Press.

Sala-Diakanda, M., & Lohlé-Tart, L. (1982). *Social science research for population policy design: Case study of Zaire. IUSSP Paper No. 24.* Liege: Belgium.

Sangree, W. H. (1987). The childless elderly in Tiriki, Kenya, and Irigwe, Nigeria: A comparative analysis of the relationship between beliefs about childlessness and the social status of the childless elderly. *Journal of Cross-Cultural Gerontology, 2,* 201–223.

Sangree, W. H. (1992). Grandparenthood and modernization: The changing status of male and female elders in Tiriki, Kenya, and Irigwe, Nigeria. *Journal of Cross-Cultural Gerontology, 7,* 331–361.

Sargent, C. F. (1982). *The cultural context of therapeutic choice: Obstetrical care decisions among the Bariba of Benin.* Boston: Kluwer.

Service de Coopération. (1966). *Enquete demographique au Tchad, 1964: Resultats definitifs.* Paris: Service de Coopération.

Sundby, J. (1997). Infertility in The Gambia: Traditional and modern health care. *Patient Education and Counseling, 31,* 29–37.

Tambashe, O. (1992). Infecondite et politique de population en Afrique Centrale. *Vie et Santé, 12,* 3–7.

United Nations. (1991). *The world's women, 1970–1990: Trends and statistics.* New York: United Nations.

Vaessen, M. (1984). *Childlessness and infecundity. World Fertility Survey, Comparative Studies No. 31.* Voorburg, the Netherlands: International Statistical Institute.

van de Walle, E. (1992). Fertility transition, conscious choice, and numeracy. *Demography, 29,* 487–502.

van de Walle, E., & Page, H. (1969). Some estimates of fertility and mortality in Africa. *Population Index, 35,* 3–17.

ELEVEN

Is Infertility an Unrecognized Public Health and Population Problem?

The View from the Cameroon Grassfields

Pamela Feldman-Savelsberg

Many women in Cameroon, a sub-Saharan country located on the "hinge" between West and Central Africa, experience impediments to bearing healthy children. Results from the 1998 Demographic and Health Survey (DHS) demonstrate that despite recent decreases, 5.5 percent of married women between the ages of thirty-five and forty-nine still suffer primary infertility. In addition, 29 percent of Cameroonian women have had an "unproductive pregnancy" (i.e., miscarriage [22%], stillbirth [6%], or abortion [5%]) (Fotso et al., 1999, pp. 47–49). All of the approximately two hundred fifty diverse ethnic groups that constitute Cameroon's population highly value children and women's childbearing. Thus childlessness consistently causes emotional, social, economic, and sometimes physical suffering, particularly for women. Nonetheless, in Cameroon infertility receives only cursory attention as a public health concern.

This lack of attention to infertility may seem surprising. Based on post–World War II sample surveys and censuses, demographers have identified an "infertility belt," or geographic area of low fertility, in Central Africa, including Cameroon (Cordell & Gregory, 1994; Retel-Laurentin, 1974; for a fuller description, see chap. 10, this volume). Long before the infertility belt was identified, German, French, and British researchers and colonial administrators were concerned with low or decreasing fertility in Cameroon, especially in regions from which laborers were recruited for colonial public works projects (e.g., Cartron, 1934; Farinaud, 1944, p. 79; Ziemann, 1904, pp. 150–153).[1] The most recent DHS, compared to earlier survey data, suggests declines in childlessness in Cameroon and other countries in the Central African infertility belt (Larsen, 1995; chap. 10, this volume). Nonetheless, fertility remains lower here than in the rest of sub-Saharan Africa. And sub-Saharan Africa, particularly Central Africa, still exhibits the highest infertility rates in the world (Ericksen & Brunette, 1996; Larsen, 1994; Sciarra, 1994).

Despite the documented prevalence of infertility, local and international governmental and nongovernmental organizations have identified "hyper-fertility" and birth spacing, rather than infertility and threatened repro-duction, as "population problems" in Cameroon. These foci may grow from a demographic prejudice. Most demographers of sub-Saharan Africa have focused on its exceptionalism, its position as the only world region still characterized by high levels of fertility despite improvements in biomedical health care (e.g., Caldwell & Caldwell, 1987). The possibility of a nascent demographic transition has recently captured the attention of scholars and policy makers interested in population control (National Academy of Sci-ences, 1993; United Nations, 1998). Decreasing fertility is hailed as a suc-cess story, as the triumph of modernity, especially of the expansion of ed-ucation and economic development, over a pretransition, "natural" pronatalism.

The Bamiléké of the Cameroon Grassfields hold an important place in this fertility/infertility paradox. The Bamiléké, making up roughly 25 per-cent of the Cameroonian population, have higher rates of fertility than their average Cameroonian compatriots—6.8 Bamiléké versus 5.4 national average completed fertility (Wakam, 1994). The Bamiléké also exhibit lower rates of infertility than all other ethnic groups in Cameroon (4.9 % primary infertility and 22.2% secondary infertility; the Bamiléké combined infertility rate is 26%, whereas the national average combined infertility rate is 43.9%) (Akam, 1990, p. 180). Demographers note that Bamiléké fertility is higher than would be predicted by economic demographic mod-els (Wakam, 1994). Folk demographic discourse in Cameroon also focuses on high Bamiléké fertility. The often-heard comment, "Central Hospital's maternity ward is full of Bamiléké babies," indicates a reputation for high fertility both among Bamiléké living in their rural homeland and the urban "exile" population of migrants and their descendants.

Nonetheless, rural Bamiléké women fear infertility, and the social and psychological consequences of infertility are grave (Feldman-Savelsberg, 1999). Infertile and subfertile women in rural polygynous households may be less favored with access to land and material resources than their more fertile cowives. They risk divorce because they cannot contribute children to their husbands' patrilineage, and their natal families may become re-sentful at the need to repay the bridewealth of a divorced infertile bride. In addition, an infertile woman has not contributed children to her mother's matrilineage in the complex dual-descent kinship system (Feld-man-Savelsberg, 1995).

Infertility is a collective concern in the Cameroon Grassfields. Its cause is most commonly attributed to witchcraft practiced by envious peers in a situation of increasing competition and the partial breakdown of expected patterns of reciprocity. Bamiléké consider women to be more vulnerable to witchcraft attack because of the weakening power of their chiefs (Feldman-Savelsberg, 1999). Bamiléké assumptions about changing demographic trends (in this case, increased threat to women's reproductive capacity) are closely tied to a rhetoric of threatened cultural and political identity in the face of modern and state institutions.

Thus the local perceptions of one group of Cameroonian women, the Bamiléké and their related Grassfields neighbors, contrast sharply with official views of infertility at the global and national levels. This chapter explores global, national, and local understandings of public health, population, and infertility. It contrasts a global focus on population control to both shifting national concerns and consistent local concerns with enhancing fertility. The "local" section of this chapter focuses on women of the Grassfields region and in this grouping, on the Bamiléké. It is based on research in the rural Bamiléké chiefdom of Bangangté during the mid-1980s (a period of relative plenty) and among urban Bamiléké migrants in 1997, 1999, and 2001 (years of political and economic crisis). Placing local concerns in their cultural and social contexts reveals a multidimensional "ethnodemography." Its attention to issues of politics, morality, and cultural identity, in addition to sexual intercourse and to physical impediments to fertility, has significant implications for local reproductive practices.

ETHNOGRAPHIC SETTING AND METHODS

Cameroon is a west-central African country of great cultural, linguistic, and geographic diversity. It is also affected by a complex colonial history. From 1884 to 1916 Cameroon was subject to German colonial power. After World War I, from 1920 to 1960, 80 percent of Cameroonian territory was ruled by France and 20 percent by Britain under League of Nations mandates (followed by United Nations Trusteeships). Cameroon gained independence in 1960 and underwent a series of transformations in its federated political system, with implications for language, legal, and educational policy. The diverse geographic, cultural, and linguistic areas have been held together since that time by an authoritarian state centered on a powerful presidency (Bayart, 1979, 1993).

Currently, the Republic of Cameroon has two official European languages, English and French. The primary ethnographic research on which this chapter is based was conducted in the Grassfields, a region spanning the border between Anglophone and Francophone Cameroon. "Grassfields" is a term that describes both a geographic location and a group of culturally and politically related peoples in the West and Northwest Provinces. Eastern Grassfields peoples include the Francophone Bamiléké and Bamoun, living mostly in the West Province; western Grassfields peoples live in the Anglophone Northwest Province and include the chiefdoms of Nso, Bafut, and Bangwa-Fontem. "Bamiléké" refers to the roughly one hundred chiefdoms of the eastern Grassfields, culturally and linguistically distinct but sharing many features of politico-religious and social organization. Among these features are a sacred chiefship, a distinction between nobility and commoners, and opportunities for achievement through ranked title societies. Palace life and the office of sacred chiefship have served as focal points for the demonstration of cultural and political distinctiveness, often in opposition to the central state of Cameroon, since independence (Goheen, 1996). During the growth of multiparty politics in the 1990s, this Grassfields self-conscious reference to sacred chiefs was strengthened in those polities whose chiefs supported opposition politics. In those polities whose chiefs were considered clients of the state, traditional rulers' sacrosanct legitimacy was severely weakened (Jua, 1997).

The research on which this chapter is based spans nearly two decades and includes fourteen months of ethnographic field research conducted in the Bamiléké chiefdom of Bangangté, Cameroon, in 1983 and 1986. Data collected through participant observation and interviews with women, their husbands, and popular healers indicated that the disturbance of human reproduction was a prominent theme in everyday conversation. Discussion about infertility and threats to human reproduction were closely tied to perceived threats to the political and cultural integrity of Bangangté—in other words, to threatened social reproduction. The results of a survey of 53 medical personnel and the content analysis of 230 essays from schoolchildren confirmed the persistence of links between reproductive problems and sociocultural change but revealed divergent visions of social reproduction.

Additional field research in Yaoundé and in Bangangté chiefdom since 1997 has focused on Bamiléké women's reproductive concerns and urban-rural support systems in a period of economic crisis. As in 1986, women perceived cultural, political, and economic threats to themselves as members of the often oppositional Bamiléké. They expressed these feelings of vulnerability through an idiom of reproductive problems, including infertility.

HISTORICAL CONCERN WITH INFERTILITY

Contemporary anxiety regarding infertility is rooted in the early colonial period, when politico-religious African leaders as well as colonial labor recruiters, missionaries, and administrators were concerned about infertility in the Cameroon Grassfields. In fact, population and fertility have long been public concerns in African states, including precolonial, colonial, and postcolonial polities (e.g., Feeley-Harnik, 1985; Fernandez, 1982; Hunt, 1993). In Cameroon, the precolonial polities of the region that now encompasses the Anglophone Grassfields and the Francophone Bamiléké plateau were sacred kingdoms or chiefdoms, best glossed as "fon-doms." *Fons* (paramount chiefs), their royal retainers, and ritual experts organized royal rituals meant to ensure the dual fertility of land and people. Fertility was (and remains) both a sign and the basis of economic, political, and spiritual strength. This fertility was threatened by social disruptions and the spread of sexually transmitted diseases through labor recruitment in the Grassfields during the early colonial era. As early as the 1890s, Grassfields fons throughout what now includes both the West and Northwest Provinces traded "medicines" and "fetishes," performed cleansing rituals, and struck "blood friendships" between fon-doms in attempts to safeguard human and social reproduction (e.g., Conrau, 1898, pp. 196–197).

As the colonial era progressed, first the German and then the French and British colonists attempted to establish medical hegemony. These colonists included both government and missionary medical practitioners; both groups were centrally concerned with enhancing fertility and treating infertility but for different reasons. Government medicine was aimed primarily at ensuring the labor capacity of African men and focused on nutrition, epidemics, and enumerating populations. Women were seen as fertile producers of laborers, of rural traditional order, and of food (Guyer, 1987; Vaughan, 1991, p. 22). Official colonial reports expressed repeated concern with reproductive strength in the Grassfields. Government medical attention to fertility was supported by the interests of colonial trading firms, which wanted sufficient numbers of laborers and consumers (Diehn, 1956).

Missionary medicine aimed to create a new type of African, an individual who would resist the collective will of "tradition" to embrace Christianity. Missionaries found that African ideas about fertility, childbirth, and child rearing were "the locus of the reproduction of many strongly-held beliefs" (Vaughan, 1991, p. 66) and sought to replace traditional birth attendants with hospital birth. The pioneer Protestant mission doctor, Josette Debarge (1934, p. 112), found sterility and infant mortality to be among the most serious problems in the Bamiléké chiefdoms surrounding Bangwa and Bangangté. Recognizing that infertility was devastating to women because "children are their reason for living" (1934, p. 28), Debarge made midwifery, fertility, and child care the focus of Protestant mission work at the Bangwa mission hospital. Other mission establishments followed suit in the 1930s, 1940s, and 1950s.

Following independence, maternity services remained a centerpiece of both church-run and government medical services in the Grassfields of

Cameroon. While the Cameroonian government encouraged population growth as "the motor of development," the attention of policy makers and academics in the former metropoles shifted from a need for a fertile labor force to concern with high fertility and population growth. Thus the Cameroon Grassfields was faced with three sets of views regarding population, fertility, and infertility. Local, emic models of fertility and "reproductive problems" diverged from the models and concerns of demographers and policy makers in the "global" world of former colonizers and international organizations (for comparative views, see Bledsoe [1997]; Ginsburg & Rapp [1995]; chap. 10, this volume). These emic views also differed from the interests and views of the Cameroonian government. The policies of the Cameroonian government at first diverged from and later converged with global views of fertility and infertility. These three views are contrasted below, as different "publics" concerned in different ways with infertility as a public health problem.

WHEN IS FERTILITY, OR INFERTILITY, A PUBLIC HEALTH PROBLEM? THE VIEWS OF THREE "PUBLICS"

By treating public health as a set of culturally embedded practices, we can best explore who recognizes, or fails to recognize, infertility as a public health problem. In contemporary multiethnic African countries, such as Cameroon, several publics define public health problems in various ways. In the Cameroon Grassfields, these publics are constituted by a series of states within a state (local fon-doms, embedded in the United Republic of Cameroon). Cameroon itself is embedded in global political and public health structures (e.g., the Organization of African Unity, the United Nations, and the World Health Organization).

In her work on public health in precolonial Africa, Waite (1992, p. 213) defines public health as "all illness which affects the public as well as all activity that [the public] undertakes to influence its health status"; public health is "the meeting ground between politics and medicine." Politics are evident in the ways that each of the publics above, from local Grassfields polities to the World Health Organization, exert some measure of control over the social conditions of health, fertility, and infertility. In a recent study of responses to contagion in the Anglophone Grassfields polity of Kedjom (Babanki), Maynard (1998, p. 1) points out that popular medicine in sub-Saharan Africa (both intervention and prevention) is "quintessentially a matter of public health, bound to the political economy of public life." In the Cameroon Grassfields public health reflects a "moral polity . . . premised on centralized structures of authority" (Maynard, 1998, p. 1). When we pose the question, Is infertility an unrecognized public health problem? we generally think of recognition and definition of public health problems by nation-states and international organizations. Even the most nuanced studies analyzing the relationship between global and local views of fertility and reproduction tend to emphasize the effect of global and national public health policies on "local" cultures and individual women (Ginsburg & Rapp, 1995; Greenhalgh, 1995). Policy, as well as public health, is located in the state and in formal, international organizations. Observations of the public health concerns of the "moral polities" of the Cameroon Grassfields, however, remind us to look beyond state and national policies and to recognize multiple publics concerned with infertility.

Global Policy

Global policy regarding fertility and infertility is ambiguous. The 1994 Cairo document (emerging from the United Nations Conference on Population and Development) retains an ongoing global focus on fertility control (Cliquet & Thienpont, 1995), and this is the major thrust of global policy. This emphasis is reflected in current internationally funded population research in Cameroon. For example, research by demographers at the Institut de Formation et Recherche Démographique (IFORD), an organization of the United Nations, investigates the relationships among development, women's status, rural-urban migration, and family planning practices (e.g., Wakam, 1994). The United Nations Population Fund (UNFPA), the Gesellschaft für Technische Zusammenarbeit (GTZ), and the United States Agency for International Development (USAID) have provided funds to reinforce family planning services in maternal-child health centers (Yana, 1998, p. 7).

The Cairo document, however, reaches beyond concern with population control to place a new emphasis on women's health. Inspired by the growing concerns expressed in it, both the World Health Organization and the Population Council have funded studies on induced abortion and the impact of postabortion infection on future fertility (R. Leke, pers. com.). As the messages of the Cairo document filter through the media, Cameroonian women, as health clients intimately concerned with the devastating impact of infertility, may perceive the emphasis on women's health as a promotion of fertility. Many of the urban Bamiléké women with whom I spoke in 1997, 1999, and 2001 expressed their frustrations that health care aiming at the promotion of their reproductive capacity was a right that remained unfulfilled because of the economic crisis and shifting national priorities.

National Policy

National policy on population, fertility, and infertility in Cameroon historically has contrasted with global policy and experienced a dramatic shift in the 1990s. During the first twenty-five years of independence, Cameroon had no comprehensive population policy. Throughout the 1970s, presidential and ministerial pronouncements proclaimed that Cameroon's "underpopulated" state "justif[ied] its pronatalist policy" (UNFPA, 1980, p. 32). Contraceptive services were few, generally run as pilot projects with foreign aid. For the first two decades after independence, sale of contraceptives on the free market (in pharmacies) was a criminal offense. Contraception was legalized but not actively encouraged when President Ahidjo called for "responsible parenthood" at a party congress in Bafoussam in 1980. In 1985 the National Commission on Population met for the first, and only, time. It emphasized birth spacing rather than population control as the road to better health and development (National Population Commission, 1993). Thus Cameroonian population policy contrasted sharply with the population control recommendations of international organizations such as USAID, UNFPA, and the Futures Group (Futures Group, n.d.; Ndzinga, n.d.; UNFPA, 1980).

National population policy changed in response to the economic crisis that began in 1986 (National Population Commission, 1993:1). This extended period of negative economic growth (from 1986 through the late 1990s) was exacerbated by political instability and general strikes in 1990. In June 1990 President Biya warned about the "economic and social consequences of an unplanned increase in the birth rate" and urged the extension of family planning services (National Population Commission, 1993, p. 3).

Does infertility get lost in this context of shifting policy on fertility control? In the domain of medical practice, Cameroon is unique in being the first sub-Saharan African country to open an infertility clinic (in 1972, at the University Centre of Health Sciences in Yaoundé) (UNFPA, 1980, p. 22). This specialized clinic no longer exists, but infertility services are available as part of general OB-GYN services in teaching hospitals. Nonetheless, new reproductive technologies, such as artificial insemination by donor, have not achieved much success in Cameroon. They are financially out of reach and culturally incompatible to most Cameroonian couples (Njikam Savage, 1992). In addition, the legal status and regulation of new reproductive technologies is uncertain in bijural Cameroon (Ngwafor, 1994). As of July 1999, ten babies have been born (to wealthy parents) in Douala with the help of assisted reproduction by a team of private physicians. Such services have been available at General Hospital of Yaoundé since 1998 but have yet to produce a live birth (R. Leke, pers. com.). Needless to say, this high-tech infertility treatment barely scratches the surface of a public health problem widely affecting "average" Cameroonian couples.

Considering the domain of policy, infertility does not appear prominently in any of the national population policy documents of the 1970s,

1980s, or 1990s. For example, the 1993 document of the National Population Commission (1993, p. 12) mentions that sterility levels remain high
and expresses concern about the "resurgence of sexually transmitted diseases and AIDS" but does not propose targeted programs.

Thus infertility appears as an insignificant blip, a nonproblem, in the
high birthrate and densely populated (and far from docile) Grassfields
region of the West and Northwest Provinces. It is in these provinces that
family planning and prenatal vaccination programs have been launched,
beginning almost immediately after President Biya's public linking of the
economic crisis and the need for family planning. As a result of long-
standing and recently exacerbated political animosity between the Grassfields and the central Cameroonian government (Nkwi & Socpa, 1997),
such programs have been greeted with intense mistrust. For example, in
1990–1991, Grassfields schoolgirls climbed out of school windows to flee
public health workers, prompted by a rumor that the government was plot-
ting to sterilize the young women of its political opponents under the guise
of a vaccination campaign (Feldman-Savelsberg, Ndonko, & Schmidt-Ehry,
2000). The timing of the change in population policy—during a period of
political turmoil—was highly suspect and led to the grassroots response to
global and national projects in the population arena.

Local Concerns

In contrast to global and national concern with high fertility, the Bamiléké
of the Cameroon Grassfields fear infertility and population decline.
Throughout the 1980s and 1990s, both rural and urban Bamiléké women
used the rhetoric of reproductive threat in negotiations over cultural identity and gender relations (Feldman-Savelsberg, 1994, 1999). Two issues
seem to provide important contexts for the emergence of this idiom of
infertility. The feminization of rural poverty contributes to women's feelings of vulnerability and diminishes their ability to seek therapies for reproductive problems. Relations between local polities and the state in the
Grassfields of Cameroon appear to play a crucial role as well. These two
contexts are linked through the symbolism of fertility and infertility. Bamiléké use idioms of food, cooking, and provisioning to talk about and connect women's human reproduction and royal social reproduction. In this
way, women's complaints about the apparently physical matters of infertility
are conditioned by and also comment on political, social, and economic
change.

Symbolism of Infertility.   The symbolism of procreation, and of reproductive threat, centers on the kitchen and cooking. In the Bamiléké kingdom
of Bangangté, the fon-dom I know best, the word for marriage is *na nda,*

"to cook inside." Women cook meals for their husbands inside the kitchen built as a requirement for marriage. Women also metaphorically "cook" children inside the contractual boundaries of bridewealth marriage. This imagery is extended to express the stages of conception, gestation, and birth. Procreation occurs when diverse elements ("ingredients") from man and woman are measured *(mfi')*, mixed *(nu'u)*, and transformed through the cooking *(na)* of sex and gestation to form a new being, a fresh person *(men fi)*. The womb is simultaneously the cooking pot and the warm hearth around which matrifocal families gather, sharing ties of commensality and sentiment. These culinary metaphors are particularly elaborate in women's depictions of the process of gestation. Fetal growth is likened to the swelling of cooking beans and fetal movement to the bubbling of maize porridge slowly cooking in the pot. Pregnant women closely monitor the "cooking" of gestation, applying their culinary skills to promote reproductive health. For example, women decide when to "add a little water" (semen) and "stir" through sexual intercourse, believed to be beneficial to fetal development. While men and women contribute equally to the ingredients of procreation, the metaphoric emphasis on women's skills makes fertility an arena of particularly female accomplishment (Feldman-Savelsberg, 1995).

The converse of fertility-as-accomplishment, infertility, is a great misfortune for Bamiléké women. The imagery of infertility is rife with tales of misfortune caused by the "wrong ingredients" (e.g., poorly matched marriages), "stolen ingredients" (e.g., through witchcraft), and "poor cooking" (e.g., breaking taboos of pregnancy). Ingredients can even fight; when a pregnant woman has sexual intercourse with someone other than her fetus's father, the two men's "waters" fight in the womb, causing birth defects. The most commonly cited causes of infertility and pregnancy loss refer to interference, through witchcraft, in the flow, mixing, and cooking of the ingredients of procreation.

Royal social reproduction shares much of this culinary imagery. For example, during installation rites, the Bangangté fon ceremoniously feeds his populace a mixture of white beans and palm oil, potent symbols of the "swelling" of pregnancy and the blood of childbirth. Social integration, the responsibility of the fon (sacred king), is created through the balanced mixing and mingling of ingredients: genders, ranks, titles, and forms of spiritual or magical strength. Just as procreation is the physical and spiritual achievement of women, the constitution of society in Bangangté is, or should be, the political and spiritual achievement of the fon (Feldman-Savelsberg, 1999).

Infertility and Polity.   Among the Bamiléké, local conceptions of public health and fertility are linked to the physical and spiritual strength of their sacred king. The fon is responsible for creating a strong polity, for keeping occult, or extraordinary, forces in balance, and thus for protecting human and agricultural fertility from the threat of witchcraft. But the fon is no longer the overwhelming reference point for Bangangté (and Bamiléké) identity and life strategies. World religions, schools, the market, and national politics create new reference groups, modes of action, and definitions of self and belonging. Christian churches (especially Calvinist, Baptist, and Roman Catholic congregations in the Grassfields) remain important both in health care and in schooling. Mission and government schools teach "universal" values of Christian or national identity, values that can undermine the particularism of ethnic and kinship allegiances. Seeking wealth through commerce rather than through the acquisition of traditional titles provides many Bamiléké and other Grassfielders with opportunities for advancement and power independently of the regulation of palace associations. Often, this wealth is then legitimized through the buying of neotraditional titles (Fisiy & Goheen, 1998) and through the creation of new elite associations (Nyamnjoh & Rowlands, 1998). Party politics and the civil service provide yet another avenue for mobility and identity independent of palace life. The fon must share political, spiritual, and economic power with other institutions and is thus weakened. Nonetheless, he remains a powerful symbol of politico-ritual force and is deemed ultimately responsible for filling the bellies and wombs of his subjects. This context of historical transformation reveals a tension between a continuing and a diminishing relevance of the sacred kingship in matters of reproduction. Issues of politics and identity have demographic consequences (Kreager, 1997) and are central to an understanding of Bamiléké women's complaints about reproductive risk and failure.

Growing from these Bamiléké beliefs in the relation of the polity to public health, fertility and infertility are much-discussed indicators of the fortunes of and threats to this polity. For example, many rural Bangangté women told me they worried that there were "too few children in the royal household." Rural Bangangté women are careful "royalty watchers," because they believe that the well-being of the royal family affects their own well-being, including their reproductive health. And the symbolic, material, political, and reproductive roles of the fon's wives are what make royal power, and thus royal safeguarding of citizens' fertility, possible (Feldman-Savelsberg, 1999).

Fertility and infertility are also indicators of personal well-being and tragedy. Fertility and infertility reveal individuals' psychological states (e.g., tranquillity required for conception vs. anger and agitation associated with infertility), their physical and nutritional health (e.g., having a full belly vs. being hungry or empty), and the state of their social relations (e.g., properly achieved bridewealth transactions vs. disputes between wife givers and wife takers). Infertility is an indicator of women's vulnerability to witchcraft, to occult powers used to harm rather than to enhance health and good fortune.

Infertility and Occult Powers.   Bamiléké women fear that their kings can no longer keep social forces in balance and thus can no longer protect their wombs from witches. Witches, like fons, twins, and certain categories of healers, possess *kà,* occult or extraordinary power. Witches use kà for nefarious, greedy purposes rather than for the public good. There are many types of witches; they may manipulate powders, potions, or fetishes; use poison; or transform themselves into birds or animals at night to consume the organs of their victims. Rather than share food and nourish others, witches "eat" people and nourish themselves at others' expense. Witches may be jealous kin and neighbors, competing for ever scarcer resources, or may be the greedy new elite or the state, seeking to "eat" their vulnerable compatriots in pursuit of personal gain (Geschiere, 1998). Bamiléké women perceive witchcraft to cause infertility by interfering at various points in the culinary process of procreation (Feldman-Savelsberg, 1994). The mixture of male and female ingredients may be prevented through anger and jealousy or by witches spoiling a woman's insides, giving her "bad water" or "bad blood." Cooking may not work, as envious witches may cause a fetus to stick to the sides of the womb or may steal the fetus.

For example, Josette,[2] the *mabengoup,* or first queen, of the Bangangté royal household, accused a number of her cowives of destroying her alleged pregnancy in 1986. Her troubles culminated in the accusation that a junior cowife had stolen her unborn child. Her case, described briefly below, illustrates the idiom of theft of cooking ingredients in symbolic explanations of the causes of infertility.

> Josette's cowives often giggled and repeated stories about her imaginary, invisible pregnancies. They said she had claimed to be pregnant between the births of her two daughters in 1974 and in 1981. When asked by one of her cowives where the baby was, Josette allegedly answered that someone had hidden the child in her buttocks. . . . Again in 1986 Josette claimed to be pregnant, contrary to the results of an examination at the mother-child clinic of Bangangté Hospital and to any observable signs. . . . [In late March 1986] Josette expressed fear for the safety of her fetus if she should have intercourse with the king, who was ill. In April and again in June . . . , when Paulette, [Josette's] weakest cowife, made sarcastic references about her motherhood, Josette accused her of . . . stealing her unborn child.

Josette exhibited what a Bangangté obstetric nurse termed "hysterical pregnancy," resulting from the enormous psychological and social pressures many Bangangté women feel to bear children frequently. Josette, officially the most powerful of the royal wives but in fact ridiculed by her cowives, blamed her cowives for damaging or stealing her fetus and thus denying her the pride of once again bearing a child (Feldman-Savelsberg, 1999, pp. 118–119).

Infertility and Rural Female Poverty

Many of the social and economic transformations discussed above have left rural Grassfields women in a vulnerable position. Bamiléké women are closely tied to the traditional, local polity as carriers of local politico-religious traditions. They gain status and self-esteem as guardians of "country fashion." On the other hand, Grassfields women, including Bamiléké women, are largely alienated from decision-making bodies in national politics and bureaucracies. As a result, they find it increasingly difficult to maintain a viable standard of living for themselves and their families.

Rural female poverty in Bangangté and in other Grassfields communities is rooted in the gendered division of labor, the monetarization of the economy, and patterns of labor migration. It has been exacerbated by the economic crisis of the 1980s and 1990s. Most of the rural inhabitants of the Bamiléké fon-doms are agriculturalists. Women gain access to land on which to grow their food crops (maize, beans, and groundnuts) through their husbands and, less often, through their natal families. Men grow cash crops (coffee and cocoa) and hunt intermittently. Men tend to have more formal education than women, to have easier access to credit, and to find greater economic opportunities in nonagricultural sectors. Because prices for coffee and cocoa have been depressed and because not all men inherit land, Grassfields men have been migrating in search of wage labor for many generations. Their rural wives now need cash to pay for health care and schooling for their children and to pay for treatment for reproductive problems. Food, so closely associated with female labors, plays an important role in women's strategies to meet cash needs and in their overall struggle for economic survival. When cash is short, women sell foodstuffs even when they do not have a surplus. Women also use the exchange of food to maintain support networks. Deeply impoverished women's support networks shrink when they cannot exchange cooked food and sacks of beans or peanuts with their network compatriots. A very poor woman would thus be at particular risk should she face a health crisis, such as infertility.

To add to these economic difficulties faced by rural Bamiléké women, patterns of reciprocity within kin groups as well as patterns of migration between the countryside and cities have been transformed by the economic crisis (Eloudou-Enyegue, 1992; Timnou, 1993). Even such cultural obligations as death celebrations (marking the achievement of full ancestorhood by the deceased) have been adapted to new, often desperate economic conditions (Mouafo, 1991). Rural women face increasing burdens to feed their urban kin. Cash outlays for such things as medical treatment have been severely reduced. Although not a part of my study, the relationship among female poverty, prostitution, and sexually transmitted diseases must be significant with regard to secondary infertility.

Infertility can also induce poverty. An infertile wife is likely to receive fewer gifts and poorer plots of land from her dissatisfied husband. Should she be divorced, a childless woman would lose her access to land and thus to her means of livelihood. Thus Bamiléké women have good reason to link poverty, and worries about food, to their fear of infertility. And they often blame the degree of poverty that they face on one or the other of two states: the traditional polity of their fon-dom or the Republic of Cameroon.

CONCLUSION: INFERTILITY AS A PUBLIC HEALTH PROBLEM

Demography examines the ultimate and proximate causes of fertility and infertility, of population growth and decline, and of the movement of peoples. This exposition of indigenous views of infertility in the Grassfields of Cameroon, both the western, Anglophone Grassfields and the eastern, Francophone Bamiléké Grassfields, takes us closer to defining an ethnodemography of ultimate and proximate causes of fertility and infertility. This ethnodemography is constituted by folk theories about procreation and the forces that enhance or undermine fertility. In a Grassfields ethnodemography, proximate causes of fertility include many of the elements of standard demography (identified as "scientific" discourse by Leonard, chap. 10, this volume). How often couples have sex (to allow their respective ingredients to "touch" and "mix") is crucial. Physical impediments to the mixing of the ingredients of procreation, such as blocked fallopian tubes, have their parallel in clinical assessments of infertility (e.g., tubal occlusion). However, among the Bamiléké, fallopian tubes can be blocked through witchcraft, and emotions such as anger and agitation can prevent ingredients (blood and semen) from mixing properly. Notions of the proper mix of ingredients, and socially appropriate coupling, are closely tied to the kinship system.

In a Bamiléké ethnodemography, ultimate causes include these kinship relations, the goodwill of ancestors, and appropriate fulfillment of marriage and bridewealth transactions. They also include aspects of the moral polity, especially the spiritual, physical, and political state of the fon. When a sacred king of a local Grassfields polity does not follow the spiritual strictures of his office, is physically ill, or is politically weakened by the constraints of the central state of Cameroon, his populace is vulnerable to a variety of misfortunes. These misfortunes threaten the reproductive capacity of individual women and of the population as a whole.

Bamiléké ethnodemography is far-reaching and multifaceted. It encourages us to expand our vision of demography and of infertility as issues of central concern to the public's health. Among the local Bamiléké polities of the Cameroon Grassfields, infertility has long been recognized as a major "public health" issue. These groups perceive infertility as an indicator of social disruption and misfortune and take steps to ameliorate it through royal ritual aimed at reestablishing the balance of social statuses and powers.

The Cameroonian government, however, is preoccupied with political survival. For several decades it has received messages from international health and development organizations about "population pressure." In addition, Cameroon has suffered more than a decade of economic crisis. Government health services have faced severe cutbacks. Thus, despite recent decreases, it would not be surprising if infertility rates increase in the context of economic and political crisis, the spread of sexually transmitted diseases, and the continuing degradation of public health services. In this context, infertility takes low priority; its status as a public health problem is defined away. Women and families suffering infertility remain in the shadows, struggling with a purportedly private affliction.

These contrasting perspectives on infertility have practical consequences. Fear of reproductive threat, perceptions of high infertility, and perceptions of demographic competition with other ethnic groups make women resist lowering fertility and thus bring the Bamiléké into conflict with global and national population goals. It would be too simple to identify this divergence as one of differing belief systems, or as a contrast between a rational future-oriented population control ideology and a traditional, pronatalist ideology rooted in the conditions of rural poverty and the institutions of the past. The picture is much more complex, involving economic and political change in a multiethnic state. Central to this are relations between local polities and the central government. The current climate of mistrust has already had dramatic effects on public health projects in Cameroon, given the suspicions that government public health services threaten the highland Grassfields region's most culturally valued resource—human fertility.

NOTES

This research was supported by grants and fellowships from the International Education Institute (Fulbright), the National Science Foundation (Graduate Fellowship, 1982–1985, and POWRE grant, 2000–2002), the Wenner-Gren Foundation, the Andrew W. Mellon Foundation, Sigma Xi, Johns Hopkins University (graduate research grants), and Carleton College (Faculty Development Endowment). I am grateful to each of these organizations. I am deeply indebted to my Cameroonian hosts and collaborators for so openly welcoming a foreigner into their midst. This chapter was first presented at the session "Interpreting Infertility" at the 1998 annual meeting of the American Anthropological Association and was later presented at a Department of Anthropology colloquium, University of Yaoundé I. It has benefited greatly from the astute comments of participants at that panel, as well as from Marcia Inhorn, Frank van Balen, Alma Gottlieb, Flavien Ndonko, Laure Ndonko, and Jean Wakam. As always, I am grateful to Joachim Savelsberg, who with good cheer and in practical, emotional, and intellectual ways continues to make my work on three continents possible.

1. Only one dissenting voice appears in the colonial commentary on "population decline" in Cameroon. Kuczynski (1939, p. xvi) introduces his extensive demographic study of Cameroon and Togo by criticizing French concern with population decline in the Cameroon Grassfields (a labor reserve area and the geographic focus of my research) as revealing the "administrator's lack of sense for figures."

2. A pseudonym, as are all Bangangté names (other than fons) in this chapter.

REFERENCES

Akam, E. (1990). *Infécondité et sous-fécondite: Evaluation et recherche des facteurs. Le cas du Cameroun.* Yaoundé: IFORD.

Bayart, J.-F. (1979). *L'état au Cameroun.* Paris: Presses de la Fondation Nationale des Sciences Politiques.

Bayart, J.-F. (1993). *The state in Africa: The politics of the belly.* London: Longman.

Bledsoe, C. (1997). Numerators and denominators. Unpublished manuscript.

Caldwell, J. C., & Caldwell, P. (1987). The cultural context of high fertility in sub-Saharan Africa. *Population and Development Review, 13,* 409–438.

Cartron, Médecin Commandant. (1934). Étude démographique comparée des pays Bamiléké et Bamoum (Cameroun). *Annales de Médecine et des Pharmacies Coloniales, 37,* 350–363.

Cliquet, R., & Thienpont, K. (1995). *Population and development: A message from the Cairo conference.* Dordrecht: Kluwer Academic Publishers.

Conrau, G. (1898). Einige Beiträge über die Voelker zwischen Mpundu und Bali. *Wissenschaftliche Beihefte zum Deutschen Kolonialblatte . . . , 11,* 194–204.

Cordell, D., & Gregory, J. (1994). *African population and capitalism: Historical perspectives.* Madison: University of Wisconsin Press.

Debarge, J. (1934). *La mission médicale au Cameroun.* Paris: Société des Missions Evangéliques.

Diehn, O. (1956). *Kaufmannschaft und deutsche Eingeborenenpolitik in Togo und Kamerun von der Jahrhundertwende bis zum Ausbruch des Weltkrieges.* Unpublished doctoral dissertation, Universität Hamburg. Found in Staatsarchiv Bremen.

Eloudou-Enyegue, P. M. (1992). Solidarité dans la crise ou crise des solidarités familiales au Cameroun? *Les Dossiers du CEPED, 22.*

Ericksen, K., & Brunette, T. (1996). Patterns and predictors of infertility among African women: A cross-national survey of twenty-seven nations. *Social Science & Medicine, 42,* 209–220.

Farinaud, Médecin Colonel. (1944). *Rapport annuel, année 1944.* Yaoundé: Cameroun Français, Service de Santé.

Feeley-Harnik, G. (1985). Issues in divine kingship. *Annual Review of Anthropology,* *14,* 273–313.

Feldman-Savelsberg, P. (1994). Plundered kitchens, empty wombs: Fear of infertility in the Cameroonian Grassfields. *Social Science & Medicine, 39,* 463–474.

Feldman-Savelsberg, P. (1995). Cooking inside: Kinship and gender in Bangangté idioms of marriage and procreation. *American Ethnologist, 22,* 483–501.

Feldman-Savelsberg, P. (1999). *Plundered kitchens, empty wombs: Threatened reproduction and identity in the Cameroon Grassfields.* Ann Arbor: University of Michigan Press.

Feldman-Savelsberg, P., Ndonko, F. T., & Schmidt-Ehry, B. (2000). Sterilizing vaccines or the politics of the womb: Retrospective study of a rumor in Cameroon. *Medical Anthropology Quarterly, 14,* 159–179.

Fernandez, J. (1982). *Bwiti.* Princeton, NJ: Princeton University Press.

Fisiy, C., & M. Goheen (1998). Power and the quest for recognition: Neo-traditional titles among the new elite in Nso', Cameroon. *Africa, 68,* 383–402.

Fotso, M., R. Ndonou, Libité, P. R., Tsafack, M., Wakou, R., Ghapoutsa, A., Kamga, S., Kemgo, P., Kwekam Fankam, M., Kamdoum, A., & Barrère, B. (1999). *Enquête démographique et de santé, Cameroun, 1998.* Yaoundé: Bureau Central des Recensements et des Etudes de Population; Calverton, MD: Macro International.

The Futures Group. (N.d.). *Cameroon: The Interrelation of population and development.* Washington, DC: Office of Population, Agency for International Development.

Geschiere, P. (1998). *The modernity of witchcraft: Politics and the occult in postcolonial Africa.* Charlottesville: University of Virginia Press.

Ginsburg, F., & Rapp, R. (1995). Introduction: Conceiving the new world order. In F. Ginsburg & R. Rapp (Eds.), *Conceiving the new world order: The global politics of reproduction* (pp. 1–17). Berkeley: University of California Press.

Goheen, M. (1996). *Men own the fields, women own the crops: Gender and power in the Cameroon Grassfields.* Madison: University of Wisconsin Press.

Greenhalgh, S. (1995). Anthropology theorizes reproduction: Integrating practice, political economic, and feminist perspectives. In S. Greenhalgh (Ed.), *Situating fertility: Anthropology and demographic inquiry* (pp. 3–28). Cambridge: Cambridge University Press.

Guyer, J. I. (1987). *Feeding African cities: Studies in regional social history.* Bloomington: Indiana University Press.

Hunt, N. (1993) *Negotiated colonialism: Domesticity, hygiene, and birth work in the Belgian Congo.* Madison: University of Wisconsin Press.

Jua, N. (1997). Contested meanings: Rulers, subjects and national integration in post-colonial Cameroon. In P. N. Nkwi & F. B. Nyamnjoh (Eds.), *Regional balance and national integration in Cameroon* (pp. 62–66). Leiden: African Studies Centre; Yaoundé: ICASSRT.

Kreager, P. (1997). Population and identity. In D. Kertzer & T. Fricke (Eds.), *Anthropological demography* (pp. 139–174). Chicago: University of Chicago Press.

Kuczynski, R. R. (1939). *The Cameroons and Togoland: A demographic study.* London: Oxford University Press.

Larsen, U. (1994). Sterility in sub-Saharan Africa. *Population Studies, 48,* 459–474.

Larsen, U. (1995). Differentials in infertility in Cameroon and Nigeria. *Population Studies, 49,* 329–346.

Maynard, K. (1998). *"Blocking the road" and quarantines: Contagion and indigenous public health in a Grassfields society.* Paper presented at the annual meeting of the African Studies Association, Chicago, IL.

Mouafo, D. (1991). *L'économie des funerailles face aux mutations socio-economiques. L'exemple de quelques villages de la Mifi (Cameroun de l'Ouest).* Yaoundé: Seminaire OCISCA.

National Academy of Sciences. (1993). *Demographic effects of economic reversals in sub-Saharan Africa.* Washington, DC: National Academy Press.

National Population Commission. (1993). *Declaration of the national population policy.* Yaoundé: Ministry of the Plan and Regional Development, Republic of Cameroon.

Ndzinga, M. (N.d.). Brief history of the USAID Health, Nutrition and Population Office/Yaoundé. Unpublished manuscript.

Ngwafor, E. N. (1994). Childlessness in Cameroon: Artificially assisted fertility or the customary law solution. *Medicine and Law, 13,* 297–306.

Njikam Savage, O. M. (1992). Artificial donor insemination in Yaoundé: Some socio-cultural considerations. *Social Science & Medicine, 35,* 907–913.

Nkwi, P. N., & Socpa, A. (1997). Ethnicity and party politics in Cameroon: The politics of divide and rule. In P. N. Nkwi & F. B. Nyamnjoh (Eds.), *Regional balance and national integration in Cameroon* (pp. 138–149). Leiden: African Studies Centre; Yaoundé: ICASSRT.

Nyamnjoh, F., & Rowlands, M. (1998). Elite associations and the politics of belonging in Cameroon. *Africa, 68,* 320–337.

Retel-Laurentin, A. (1974). *Infécondité en Afrique Noire: Maladies et consequences sociales.* Paris: Masson.

Sciarra, J. (1994). Infertility: An international health problem. *International Journal of Gynecology & Obstetrics, 46,* 155–163.

Timnou, J.-P. (1993). Migration, urbanisation et développement au Cameroun. *Les Cahiers de l'IFORD, 4.*

UNFPA (United Nations Population Fund). (1980). United Republic of Cameroon. *Report of mission on needs assessment for population assistance.* New York: UNFPA.

United Nations. (1998). *Revision of the world population estimates and projections.* Http://www.popin.org.

Vaughan, M. (1991). *Curing their ills:Colonial power and African illness.* Stanford: Stanford University Press.

Waite, G. (1992). Public health in precolonial East-Central Africa. In S. Feierman & J. M. Janzen (Eds.), *The social basis of health and healing in Africa* (pp. 212–231). Berkeley: University of California Press.

Wakam, J. (1994). *De la pertinence des théories "économistes" de fécondité dans le contexte socio-culturel Camerounais et Negro-Africain.* Yaoundé: IFORD.

Yana, D. (1998). *Environnement institutionnel et transition de la fécondité au Cameroun.* Paper presented at Troisièmes journées du reseau demographie sur le thème "Les transitions démographiques des Pays du Sud." Rabat, December 9–12..

Ziemann, H. (1904). Zur Bevölkerungs- und Viehfrage in Kamerun. Ergebnisse einer Expedition in die gesunden Hochländer am und nördlich vom Manengubagebirge. *Wissenschaftliche Beihefte zum Deutsche Kolonialblatte . . . , 17,* 11–48.

TWELVE

Infertility and Matrilineality

The Exceptional Case of the Macua of Mozambique

Trudie Gerrits

In the scarce literature on infertility in Africa, negative consequences for the infertile couple—in particular for the infertile woman—are generally stressed. Anthropological studies on social and cultural aspects of infertility in Botswana (Mogobe, 1998), Egypt (Inhorn, 1994, 1996), The Gambia (Sundby, 1997), and Nigeria (Koster-Oyekan, 1998; Okonofua, Harris, & Odebiyi, 1997; Onah, 1992) show that when pregnancy does not occur, it leads to many problems at the personal, conjugal, family, and community levels. Infertile women, and sometimes infertile men as well, describe their lives without children as meaningless, fruitless, miserable, shameful, or unhappy. Moreover, they speak about feelings of guilt and loss of self-esteem (Inhorn, 1996; Koster-Oyekan, 1998; Sundby, 1997). Childless women and men fear lack of social security and support from their children when they themselves grow old (Inhorn, 1996; Koster-Oyekan, 1998). In addition, they are worried because they will not have a child to bury them when they die (Koster-Oyekan, 1998).

All the studies mentioned above, as well as others from around the world (e.g., many of those in this volume), find that the woman is generally blamed as the main cause for the lack of conception. This is the reason many childless women suffer from physical and mental abuse, including disrespectful treatment and neglect by their husbands and often his relatives (Inhorn, 1996; Okonofua et al., 1997). Many women also fear being separated from or divorced by their husbands or ending up as a second wife in a polygamous marriage (Inhorn, 1996; Okonofua et al., 1997; Sundby, 1997). Unfortunately, for many, these fears become reality. Often (female) relatives of the husband force him to divorce or to take a second wife, because his children are needed to guarantee the continued existence of his extended family and lineage. In this context, women, especially moth-

ers- and sisters-in-law, are described as being hostile to, instead of supportive of, infertile women (Inhorn, 1996; Mogobe, 1998). In some societies,
furthermore, it is reported that the divorced infertile woman becomes an
outcast and is excluded from inheriting property and from decision making
in the family (Inhorn, 1996; Okonofua et al., 1997). For example, a case
study in Nigeria reports that the stigmatization extends even beyond the
childless couple: unmarried male and female family members of the infertile couple are suspected of harboring an infertility problem as well and
are therefore not considered eligible for marriage (Onah, 1992).

Problems do not exist only at the family level. Both infertile men and
women may be seriously offended, denigrated, and stigmatized by community members (Inhorn, 1996; Onah, 1992) or bothered by negative
gossip (Sundby, 1997). Infertile women, more often than infertile men,
are accused of being witches (Koster-Oyekan, 1998; Okonofua et al., 1997)
or casting the evil eye (Inhorn, 1996). As a result, children are warned not
to seek their company, because at best the infertile women are thought to
be incapable of properly caring for children (Mogobe, 1998; Okonofua et
al., 1997) and at worst may be considered harmful to children's health
(Inhorn, 1996) or may be thought to exploit them for illicit ceremonies
(Koster-Oyekan, 1998). For all of these reasons, infertile women are often
stigmatized and excluded from certain social events (Inhorn, 1996; Okonofua et al., 1997).

These examples summarize how the lives of infertile African women are
generally depicted in the anthropological literature: as marked by suffering
and exclusion. That in most African societies women primarily gain status
by having children and caring for their families—and consequently childless women do not have the opportunity to gain this status—is generally
provided as a cultural explanation for this phenomenon.

But there are clearly exceptions to this depiction (e.g., Inhorn 1996;
Okonofua et al., 1997), and the study described here provides a case in
point. Among the matrilineal Macua of Mozambique, the inability to have
children is also a considerable problem for women. However, cultural ideas
about who is to blame for the infertility, and subsequent consequences and
coping strategies, are clearly different from those in the patrilineal societies
that are the subject of the reports cited above. In a society with a matrilineal
kinship system, the children born to a woman belong to her descent group.
When a man marries a woman, he does not gain rights over her children.
Matrilineal systems tend also to be correlated with matrilocal residence: a
man goes to live with or near his wife's kin after marriage. This means that
in the domestic group, it is the man who is among "strangers," whereas his
wife is surrounded by her supportive kin (Nanda, 1987).

In this chapter, the beliefs, experiences, and coping strategies of infertile
Macua women are described in the context of this matrilineal kinship sys-

tem. My main argument is this: In a matrilineal African society such as the Macua, matrilineality itself may be somewhat protective of women who find themselves in the potentially stigmatizing situation of infertility.

THE STUDY AND ETHNOGRAPHIC SETTING

The research findings presented here are based on an anthropological study conducted among the matrilineal Macua in the north of Mozambique from July to October 1993. The study was undertaken in Montepuez, a district capital in the northern province of Cabo Delgado. Of the 46,000 inhabitants, only 1,100 lived in the center of the capital, the Bairro Cimento (Cement Town); the others lived dispersed in several neighborhoods. The majority of the inhabitants in the capital belong to the ethnic group Macua, a minority are Maconde, and a few have a Portuguese or Indian background. About 60 percent of the Montepuez population are Muslim, and about 10 percent are Catholic. There are also a small number of Protestant churches in the area.

Montepuez district is rural, and the main source of income is agriculture, mainly small-scale. Some people have jobs as seasonal laborers in cotton production, either in the fields or in the factory. The Bairro Cimento has a mosque, a Catholic church, one primary and two secondary schools, and a rural hospital. A provincial hospital is located in Pemba, the provincial capital, at a distance of two hundred kilometers.

The study was conducted in two neighborhoods in Montepuez: Nacate (8,600 inhabitants), adjacent to the Bairro Cimento; and Nicuapa (2,000 inhabitants), in fact, a separate village six kilometers from the center of Montepuez. During the fieldwork, I was assisted by two women, thirty-eight and forty-five years of age, both residents of Nacate, who were well educated by local standards (both had six years of primary school). Both spoke fluent Portuguese and the local language, Macua, and had good communication skills. Data were collected by means of semistructured interviewing, normally conducted at the compounds of informants. In-depth interviews were undertaken with thirty-four infertile women, six "cured" infertile women, and ten fertile women.

As the study focused on the experiences and perceptions of the women involved, definitions such as primary and secondary infertility, generally used in biomedically or demographically oriented studies, were avoided as selection criteria for inclusion in the study. Instead, the study methodology privileged individuals' own definitions and criteria (see chap. 10, this volume). In this study, an "infertile" woman is one who wants to get pregnant but does not succeed, irrespective of the length of time during which she tries to become pregnant or the number of children she already has. The determining factor is that the woman herself considers her inability to become pregnant undesirable. It is possible that from a biomedical point of view the condition is caused by her husband. In this study, twenty-five infertile women without any living children were interviewed, as were nine infertile women with one or more children. A "cured" woman is one who experienced infertility but resolved it in one way or another. She may have received treatment, but she may also have managed to conceive with another man. Finally, a "fertile" woman is a woman who has never experienced any infertility problem.[1]

In addition to the interviews with the women, interviews were conducted with traditional healers; *nankossi* (female advisers in initiation rites and pregnancy ceremonies); members of the *tribunal do povo* (local tribunal);[2] a group of elderly men; and a physician and a nurse from the rural hospital in Montepuez.[3] Data were also collected through observations at initiation rites, pregnancy ceremonies, sessions of traditional healers, and ordinary compound life.

I contacted informants through the snowball method. The assistants proved to be very valuable in contacting infertile women. From the moment interviewing started, the rumor of my presence and the topic of the research spread and attracted the attention of the people involved. Again and again, I was approached by infertile women or their husbands with requests to be interviewed. In Nicuapa, the Mozambican Women's Organization (OMM) recruited informants. In both research sites, more women offered themselves as interview candidates than were possible to include. Care was taken to not include only those women who offered themselves, and only a few informants were contacted through the local hospital so as to avoid the sampling biases involved in hospital-based studies. It was constantly stressed to the assistants and to the infertile women who participated in the study that no solution to their problem was being offered, to avoid creating false expectations.

All informants in the study belonged to the Macua and hence spoke Macua-meto. Most of them were Muslim; a small minority were Catholic. Their ages varied from nineteen to fifty. Almost 50 percent never attended school; only 6 informants finished primary school. With the exception of 4 women, all of those interviewed were small farmers. At the time of the interviewing, 28 (80%) of the 34 infertile women were married, 9 of them in polygynous unions.[4] Of the 6 cured and 10 fertile women, 11 (68%) were married, and 2 had polygynous husbands. The majority of the women in all three categories had been divorced once or more.

FERTILITY-ENHANCING RITUALS

Among the Macua, the way in which women cope with their infertility is very much related to their matrilineal kinship system. Having children is an important event in Macua culture, not only for the parents and other direct relatives, but also for all the members of the matrilineage, as children guarantee the continued existence of the matrilineage as a whole (Martinez, 1989). Childlessness is a problem that needs to be prevented; thus, during initiation rites and pregnancy ceremonies, women and men are taught how they can improve their chances of having healthy offspring.

Initiation rites are held for a group of girls when they have had their first menses. During these rites, which last four days, nankossi initiate the *namwali* (girls to be initiated) into the secrets and life of an adult and fertile woman. After having passed through this ceremony, the namwali are ready to marry and to have children; some girls already live with their husbands before the initiation rites.

The future fertility of the namwali is an important theme during these rites. Prophecies are uttered on the fertility status of the girl. For that reason, on the second day of the rites, all women involved go to the field to collect medicinal plants. Each *ananku* (a female relative of the girl who accompanies her throughout the initiation rites) selects a plant for her *amwali* (singular of *namwali*) and covers it with a piece of cloth. On the second or third day, the plant is dug up: if the roots have small bulbs, it is predicted that the girl will be infertile; if the roots are sound, fertility is thought to be guaranteed.

During the initiation rites, the amwali has to prove that she can perform the sexual act, and at the same time the sperm of her (potential) husband is tested. Therefore, the couple has to perform the sexual act in the presence of the girl's ananku. The boy is asked to ejaculate on a piece of cloth, which is taken to the namwali's mother, who studies the sperm carefully. She returns the cloth to the ananku, who buries it in a secret place. The women judge the substance of the sperm: white and thick sperm is considered to be of good quality; if it is watery, reddish, and/or warm, the man is deemed to have a disease and incapable of impregnating the girl. In such cases, relatives of the namwali might reject the boy as a future husband. If the (potential) husband is not even able to ejaculate, or, in Bairro Nicuapa, if the girl does not yet have a husband, another man is requested to perform the sexual act with her, because the amwali has to prove during the initiation rites that she can withstand the act. In Bairro Nacate, however, it is more common today for girls to undergo the initiation rites when they do not yet have a husband; in these cases, the sperm test is postponed until the girl has found a man.

On the last day of the initiation rites, infertility can be caused. The girls have to remove their pubic hair, wrap it in a cloth, and bury it in the earth. If a *feiticeira* (witch) digs up this cloth, treats it with some medicinal plants, and buries it again, the concerned girl is thought to remain childless.

Another important ceremony to enhance the chance of having healthy children is the *nthaára*, organized when a Macua woman—often still a teen-ager—is pregnant for the first time for about four or five months. In the nthaára, the nankossi instruct the pregnant woman how to behave during pregnancy and labor. By following these rules, she is thought to avoid risks and problems at these times. Only women who have been pregnant and gone through the nthaára themselves may assist in this ceremony. With the exception of the husband of the pregnant woman, no men are allowed to attend. The nthaára is considered a happy social event, involving lots of dancing, singing, drama, and laughter. After the birth of the baby, another ceremony, *nthaára no mwana,* is held. On this occasion, usually held after the umbilical stump has fallen off, the parents receive advice on how to behave now that their child is born.

PERCEPTIONS OF INFERTILITY: CAUSES AND CURES

But what happens to women in Macua society who are confronted with the fact that they cannot conceive? Typically, they make use of the services of the local rural hospital and of three kinds of traditional healers: *akulukanos* (herbal healers), *majini* (spiritual healers), and *xehes* (Islamic healers).[5] In this study, all of the infertile women except one had sought treatment from at least one of these types of healers, and many had visited different types of traditional healers more than once. In contrast, only half had visited the hospital. The intensity of treatment seeking varied considerably, especially with regard to the number of visits paid to the traditional healers. For example, more women visited akulukanos than majini; xehes were not often consulted about infertility problems. Most women first visited traditional healers and only later went to the hospital. In reality, the local rural hospital could offer very few means of diagnosing the cause of infertility or providing treatment.

Half of the husbands had accompanied their wives once or more to a traditional healer or had encouraged their wives to go. More women were accompanied by their mothers or other female relatives than their husbands. Clearly, women's families were interested in helping their daughters or sisters to have children.

Not surprisingly, given the high number of visits to traditional healers, explanations the women themselves had for their infertility more often originated from the traditional healers than from the hospital. Explanations most often mentioned were spirit possession, witchcraft, *norro* (the local term for gonorrhea), "incompatibility of blood," and poor-quality sperm.

The last two explanations are extremely interesting, because they tell us something about who, in the context of Macua culture, may be blamed for the infertility. When a woman suffers a lot of pain after sexual contact or during her menses, she and her family interpret this as a sign that the blood of the man does not combine with that of the woman. In these cases, the man is accused of causing the infertility, an etiological explanation that is widely recognized in Macua culture. For example, all informants mentioned "incompatibility of blood between spouses" as a legitimate reason for divorce, initiated by the woman or her relatives. In some cases, the concerned woman may not even fully agree with this attribution. As one woman told it, "I am not in favor of it [the divorce], but because I am always ill when I have sexual intercourse with this man, and the family already decided it, I have to divorce. But it is not my wish!"

The perceived quality of a man's sperm is another important factor. The fertilizing capacity of a man's sperm may be tested by a traditional healer in the process of determining the cause of infertility in a couple. But it is also a standard procedure during initiation rites. Both perceptions ("incompatibility of blood" and "bad quality of sperm") provide evidence that in Macua culture, the continuity of the matrilineage is considered to be crucial, and hence the contribution of the man—a "foreign element" to the matrilineage—is critically observed and judged. This is because he might harm or even destroy the fertility of a matrilineal daughter or sister.

The idea of a woman producing offspring for her own lineage is also apparent in another fertility-seeking strategy. Besides seeking medical care with spiritual and herbal healers and at the rural hospital, many infertile women in Montepuez "try their luck" with other men. Sometimes they do this explicitly on the advice of traditional healers to check whether the blood of another man is more compatible. In other cases, they do this while the husband is temporarily absent or simply to take revenge if the husband has taken a second wife. According to the women, their husbands do not know that they have committed adultery. If they become pregnant by another man, women are not very likely to tell their husbands. If the husband finds out, women say they do not fear the consequences, even if this means divorce. Their main goal is to have a child, not to remain with their husbands. And, once again, the influence of the matrilineal kinship system is clear in that the child stays with the mother after a divorce. Thus, to a considerable extent, women can and often try to influence their own reproductive life courses.

Almost all of the married infertile women interviewed were convinced that their husbands had sexual contact with other women. Some women simply complained about their husbands' infidelity; others got really angry, saying, "He is bringing diseases to our homestead," and were even considering leaving their husbands; still others considered it "normal" and understood the man's wish to try to impregnate another woman.

Evidently, having unprotected sex with multiple partners *as a fertility-seeking strategy* may lead to infection (or reinfection) with sexually transmitted diseases (STDs), some of which are, paradoxically, sterilizing. In an epidemiological study in Montepuez, conducted among one hundred infertile women and two hundred proven fertile women one year before this anthropological study was undertaken, it was found that 76 percent of the infertile women were suffering from long-term exposure to repeated gonorrheal infection, whereas the corresponding proportion among fertile women was 40 percent (Samucidine, Barreto, Lind, Mondlane, & Bergstrom, 1999). The researchers emphasized that this markedly elevated prevalence figure of gonorrhea may reflect either that tubal blockage (and thus infertility) occurs frequently as a consequence of STD infection or that the need to engage in risky behavior is increased for infertile women in order to achieve a much-desired pregnancy, or both. In addition, it might be possible that STD infections worsen a preexistent subfertility caused by previous tubal disease.

It must be noted here that having multiple sexual partners is very common in Montepuez for men and for women, married or unmarried, fertile or infertile. Women interviewed for this study described having sex with men in exchange for goods or money, especially to support themselves financially when their husbands were absent for long periods. Earning money for sex was referred to as *ajuda de sal* (help with salt). During the initiation ceremony, older women sang a song in which they stressed the economic value of women's sexuality. Moreover, in the period of sexual abstinence after delivery, which traditionally lasts until a child can walk, the man is allowed to have sexual relations with other women.

CONSEQUENCES OF INFERTILITY
Sadness and Jealousy

Childlessness and infertility affect a Macua woman's life in various ways and at various levels. At the personal or psychological level, all women interviewed expressed strong feelings of sadness and jealousy. Sadness derives from living without the joyful company of children: "A compound without children is a place without pleasure." Some women referred to the uselessness of a life without the capacity to bear and rear children. They sometimes described themselves as "a pumpkin [plant] without fruits." One infertile woman said that she sometimes felt so useless and unfulfilled that she had considered committing suicide.

However, being childless in Montepuez does not necessarily mean living a life without children. Quite a few of the infertile women in this study lived in compounds with other relatives and their children, and they felt at least assured of the company of children in their daily lives. About half of the infertile women interviewed were taking care of the children of others (or had done so in the past). Some of the foster children were orphans; civil war in Mozambique had ended only in 1992. Fostering was found to decrease the extent to which the women suffered from their childlessness. But most women did not see fostering as a permanent solution, and it could cause problems as well. For example, sometimes biological parents accused foster parents of mistreating or exploiting their children. Other women described problems with the conduct of the children themselves; for example, the children did not want to obey a woman who was not the "real mother." On the other hand, a few women were extremely positive about being able to take care of the children of relatives, and others expressed the strong wish to do so. For example, one infertile woman reported an exceptionally loving relationship with her husband's daughter (from his former wife, who was still alive), and an infertile couple who took in four war orphans (her sisters' children) found their own biological childlessness easier to bear as a consequence of having these foster children in the household.

Feelings of jealousy were expressed strongly, especially by young women when they compared themselves with their sisters and friends from the same age group, with whom they had passed the initiation rites. Seeing them caring for their children was painful. Women whose husbands had one or more children with other women also expressed their jealousy strongly. Generally, infertile women who had at least one child compared themselves favorably to those who had no children at all, describing themselves as less jealous and better off. They argued that at least they had someone to care for, and their family would not die out—a concern often mentioned by childless women, especially in cases in which siblings also suffered from infertility.

Lack of Support

Childless women, as well as women with only one child, most often emphasized the problem of lack of support from their children, now and in the future. Women without children have to perform all household tasks by themselves when they return from the fields, including fetching water and firewood, cleaning the compound, and preparing the food. Elderly childless women in particular experience this as a heavy and time-consuming daily burden. They are scared and feel uncertain about their futures: Who will construct a new house or improve the existing one when they are too old? Who will feed them or give them a new *capulana* (wraparound cloth)? Who will care for them when they are sick? Who will mourn them, and who will bury them, in a society where funerals and other ceremonies for the dead are very important?

Women who have only one child foresee comparable problems for that child when they themselves die, for the only child will be left without a network of brothers and sisters who can support him or her when needed.

Exclusion from Ceremonies

Besides practical worries and concerns, the consequences of infertility include exclusion from important activities and ceremonies. Generally, women who have never been pregnant suffer the most problems. They are not allowed to assist the nth, or assist deliveries, or be involved in conversations about these events. Also, a few informants mentioned that these women are not allowed in places where the bodies of the dead are washed or placed on a bier.

Exclusions are less severe for two other categories of infertile women. Women who have gone through the nthara themselves (this means that they have been pregnant for at least four months) are allowed to assist in the nthara of other pregnant women, even when their pregnancy ended in miscarriage; but they are not allowed to attend a delivery. The same principle applies to women who have had a delivery and gone through the nthara no mwara themselves: they may assist deliveries and attend these ceremonies (even if their child or children died afterward).

Women excluded in these ways say they feel enormously isolated and miss the gatherings and the conviviality with other women. Although the *fertile* women interviewed realize that infertile women feel this way, they say that these cultural taboos have to be respected. If infertile women do not follow these cultural rules, they or their relatives will develop serious health problems or even die.

Fear of Divorce: Threat or Reality?

Fear of divorce over infertility was often mentioned by infertile women, many of whom had been married and divorced before. Some women explained the reasons for divorce with expressions such as: "No man likes not having children" and "A man does not like to work for nothing." This idea that infertility leads to divorce was confirmed by various fertile and infertile informants who said they knew couples who were divorced because of infertility. Examples were also provided of couples who divorced over infertility and subsequently one of them managed to have children with another partner.

On the contrary, some infertile women who knew that their husbands were trying to procreate with other women said this did not necessarily signal the end of their marriage, even if the husband succeeded in impregnating someone else. Two women said that their husbands would never leave them because of their childlessness; one of these women was, in fact, extremely positive about her relationship with her husband.

Indeed, despite the perceived threat of divorce, the actual reasons for earlier divorces among women in this study do *not* appear to be related largely to infertility. Twenty-six of the thirty-four infertile women interviewed had divorced at least once, but, according to the infertile women themselves, their husbands had generally not left them because of their infertility. Many other motives for divorce were mentioned. In fact, only five infertile women mentioned their childlessness as the reason for a former divorce. Moreover, it was not only men who wanted to leave their wives. Under certain conditions—mainly perceived incompatibility of blood and an unacceptable degree of promiscuity on the part of the husband—women or their relatives were the ones to seek a divorce. To summarize, although the threat of divorce as experienced by infertile Macua women is real, not having children does not automatically mean that a man will repudiate his wife.

Moreover, although some women wished that they received more financial and moral support from their husbands in their search for infertility treatments, none of them complained about domestic violence because of their infertility. The only woman who had suffered physical and mental maltreatment at the hands of her husband and his family was married to a man from a patrilineal ethnic group in the south of Mozambique. In that part of the country, a brideprice (*lobolo*) is paid to the parents of the bride, to compensate for the lost labor potential and the children the woman shall bear for the husband's lineage (Sachs & Honwana Welch, 1990). In the matrilineal north, such a transaction does not take place and consequently the husband's family has less interest in the offspring of their daughters-in-law.[6] Moreover, Macua residence patterns are dominantly matrilocal, meaning that the wife remains with or close by her parents, while the husband joins his family-in-law. The woman then enjoys the protection of her own relatives, which may explain to a certain extent why few women complained of physical or mental harassment from husbands or their husbands' family members.

CONCLUSION

This study among the Macua of Montepuez, Mozambique, shows that the way in which women experience and cope with their infertility is indeed highly dependent on the social and cultural context. In the cultural setting described here, matrilineality–in combination with matrilocality—is in some ways protective of women who find themselves in the difficult position of being infertile.

Children in Macua society are of great value to the woman's family. Thus an infertile woman's family generally supports her in her search for a solution. Moreover, because the woman remains in or near her parents' house, she enjoys the protection of her own relatives, should she face difficulties with her husband or his family. But, given that children do not affiliate in the same way with husbands' families, husbands and husbands' family members generally do not mistreat and repudiate infertile women in the ways described in other patrilineal societies in Africa.

Furthermore, Macua men may be considered the cause of infertility in any given case—a rare finding in the literature on infertility in "traditional" African societies. In the case of suspected male infertility, the woman and/ or her relatives may even initiate divorce. However, women who enjoy happy relationships with their husbands resist this eventuality, even in the face of family pressure. Similarly, some women stated that their husbands would never leave them (cf. Inhorn, 1996), or as they put it: "We love each other and therefore he will never leave."

Despite the protective effects that matrilineality and matrilocality seem to provide for infertile Macua women and the happiness of some infertile women in their marriages, many women nonetheless seem to feel the constant threat of divorce or polygamy as a result of their childlessness. Yet the main concern of many of these women is clearly not to maintain their marriages with their current husbands but rather to have a child. In the hope of conceiving, most of the infertile women in this study had had several sexual partners, a fertility-seeking strategy almost unheard of for women in patrilineal African societies. Unfortunately, this strategy—having unprotected sex with multiple partners—may lead to infertility (and even death from AIDS) instead of resolving the problem.

Another strategy for overcoming childlessness in Macua society is child fostering, which is commonly accepted and practiced. Fostering may decrease the extent to which women experience their infertility as a problem, but most women do not see this as an absolute solution. The quality of the relationship with foster children obviously is of great importance.

To summarize, infertile women in this matrilineal society are able to use strategies that to some extent help them to cope with their infertility. However, Macua culture is also hard on them. Infertile women are stigmatized and excluded from certain social events and ceremonies. There is no way to escape this exclusion, and women feel deeply saddened by it. Infertile women see themselves constantly and "for life" stigmatized by their infertility. Macua society currently provides no alternatives to the highly valued role of mother, and there are no organized support mechanisms for infertile Macua as reported in some other African societies. Infertile Macua women reported that they rarely spoke about their feelings with other women in the same condition, and in the few cases in which this occurred, they felt they could give little support to each other.

Obviously, besides cultural factors and the particular situation of each individual infertile woman, the prevailing health care system also has an enormous impact on the coping strategies of infertile women. Because of the very limited number and poor quality of diagnostic and treatment facilities for infertility in the rural hospital in Montepuez, infertile women continue to seek traditional remedies, usually without success. Without denying possible positive effects of traditional medicine and without exaggerating the effectiveness of modern health services regarding the treatment of infertility, it is nonetheless clear that infertile couples in the Montepuez district of Mozambique could be helped by better medical services, even of a "low-tech," inexpensive kind. Improving the quality of biomedical infertility services for Mozambican as well as other African women and men is clearly a need that has yet to be met and contributes to the suffering described in the opening of this chapter, as well as in other chapters in this volume.

NOTES

1. Elsewhere (Gerrits, Boonmongkon, Feresu, & Halperin, 1999) I have shown that professionals and lay people have different viewpoints about the definition of infertility, so that women may see themselves as having an infertility problem while not being recognized in this way by biomedical services and in demographic statistics.

2. Each bairro has a tribunal do povo, with seven or eight members, chosen by the local population. The inhabitants of the bairro can present problems that they have not managed to deal with themselves, for example, cases of adultery, divorces, conflict, and aggression. Members can be male and female. In this study, only male members were interviewed.

3. I planned to interview some of the husbands of the infertile women as well. The female research assistants recommended making use of a male research assistant. The husband of one of the female assistants seemed appropriate for this task. However, because of seasonal labor in the cotton fields, he was available only during the last weeks of the fieldwork period. When this male assistant and I finally tried to contact the men, none were willing to participate in the study, because, as they said, they had to prepare the fields.

4. It must be noted here that in the study area the term "married" is commonly used when a man and woman live together; this form of cohabitation is rarely formalized by a traditional, religious, or legal ceremony. Consequently, divorce in these cases often means simply packing one's personal goods and leaving.

5. In the early 1990s, the Mozambican minister of health recognized that the national health system reached only 30 percent of the population and that the other 70 percent had to rely on self-care, on the services delivered by churches, and especially on traditional healers (Jurg 1993).

6. This does not mean, however, that the husband's relatives are not at all concerned with the lack of children in their son's or brother's homestead. Some infertile women said that their in-laws expressed their sorrow over their misfortune.

REFERENCES

Gerrits, T., Boonmongkon, P., Feresu, S., & Halperin, D. (1999). *Involuntary infertility and childlessness in resource-poor countries. Experiences and needs: An exploration of the problem and an agenda for action.* Current Reproductive Health Concerns. Amsterdam: Het Spinhuis.

Inhorn, M. C. (1994). *Quest for conception: Gender, infertility, and Egyptian medical traditions.* Philadelphia: University of Pennsylvania Press.

Inhorn, M. C. (1996). *Infertility and patriarchy: The cultural politics of gender and family life in Egypt.* Philadelphia: University of Pennsylvania Press.

Jurg, A. (1993). Traditionele genezers in Mozambique in ere hersteld (Traditional healers in Mozambique rehabilitated). *Medische Antropologie, 5,* 38–49.

Koster-Oyekan, W. (1998). Olorun a shi e ni inu. God will open your womb: Causes, treatment and consequences of infertility among Yoruba women in Nigeria. *Medische Antropologie, 10,* 43–58.

Martinez, F. L. (1989). O povo e a sua cultura. Lisbon: Ministerio da Educação/ Instituto de Investigação Cientifica Tropical.

Mogobe, K. D. (1998). Denying and preserving self: Batswana women's experiences of infertility. Ph.D. dissertation, University of Washington.

Nanda, S. (1987). *Cultural anthropology.* 3d ed. Belmont, CA: Wadsworth.

Okonofua, F. E., Harris D., & Odebiyi A. (1997). The social meaning of infertility in southwest Nigeria. *Health Transition Review, 7,* 205–220.

Onah, N. (1992). The sociocultural perception and implications of childlessness in Anambra State. In M. N. Kisekka (Ed.), *Women's health issues in Nigeria* (pp.183–190). Nigeria: Tamaza Publishing Company.

Sachs, A., & Honwana Welch, G. (1990). *Liberating the law: Creating popular justice in Mozambique.* London: Zed Books.

Samucidine, M., Barreto, J., Lind, I., Mondlane, C., & Bergstrom, S. (1999). Serological evidence of gonorrhoea among infertile and fertile women in rural Mozambique. *African Journal of Reproductive Health, 3,* 102–105.

Sundby, J. (1997). Infertility in The Gambia: Traditional and modern health care. *Patient Education and Counseling, 31,* 29–37.

THIRTEEN

Infertility and Health Care in Countries with Less Resources

Case Studies from Sub-Saharan Africa

Johanne Sundby

To what extent will the meaning, causes, consequences, and treatment of infertility differ according to culture, context, and socioeconomic environment? And what are the challenges if the aim is to promote a more equitable world, including better care for those couples who are affected by infertility? In the developed part of the world, infertility has become an important issue in the public debate. In the developing countries, infertility is still an issue that receives little public policy attention. One reason for this is the developed world's preoccupation with increasing population growth; infertility has been seen as one way of reducing fertility that is estimated as "too high" in Africa, Asia, and South America. But "too high" for whom? Even if current population growth rates and migration patterns are serious environmental and global problems, one of the challenges of formulating appropriate population policies is to address the needs of individuals, including those coping with childlessness. Some countries, such as China, have strict reproductive policies that regulate individuals' fertility, while other countries, such as Norway, have policies that promote childbearing through a series of incentives. Infertility presents a paradox, because its psychosocial consequences in high-fertility settings may often be worse than in countries where women have more flexible models of expressing femininity and fulfilling societal roles (Gerrits, 1997; Sundby, 1997). And where women may expect to lose children because of high child mortality risks, low fertility may be a serious economic concern.

In this chapter, I discuss developing-country perspectives on the definition of, health care for, and social consequences of infertility. The entry point is public health, and a core issue is the need for better infertility health care policy in developing countries. This chapter is based on large-scale case studies carried out in The Gambia (Sundby, 1997; Sundby,

Sonko, & Mboge, 1998) and Zimbabwe (Runganga, Sundby, & Aggleton, 1999; Sundby & Jacobus, 2001). Our study in The Gambia was a two-step representative survey on the prevalence, social consequences, and treatment of infertility in that country. In Zimbabwe, we carried out a case-control study of infertile and fertile couples in the Harare hospitals. The different methodologies applied in these studies are described in detail elsewhere (Runganga et al., 1999; Sundby, 1997; Sundby & Jacobus, 2001).

In this chapter I draw on findings from the qualitative elements of the studies, including interviews and discussions with infertile patients and care providers. My major focus is on the significant shortcomings in the delivery of comprehensive biomedical health care for infertile couples in developing countries, using these two sites as examples. I argue that even if the agendas of the two large health- and population-related conferences of this century (in Cairo and Beijing)[1] emphasized the need for comprehensive reproductive health care, including for infertility, health services in developing countries have a long way to go to accomplish this goal.

PROBLEMS WITH INFERTILITY DEFINITIONS: THE CASES OF ZIMBABWE AND THE GAMBIA

Both sub-Saharan African countries, Zimbabwe and The Gambia are nonetheless quite different. The Gambia is a small, Muslim, West African country of one million people representing four major ethnic groups, with an agriculture-based economy. Zimbabwe is in the southern African region, has about 10 million people from two major ethnic groups, and is more developed from a socioeconomic point of view than The Gambia. While women in The Gambia still seem to have a very high fertility rate (i.e., total fertility rate of approximately 6), Zimbabwe has started to experience a fertility decline (i.e., total fertility rate of between 4 and 5). Both countries have developed a good standard of decentralized primary health care in rural areas, and infertility is an issue for health care management in both countries.

Infertility is commonly defined in biomedicine as "one (or two) years of unprotected (by contraceptives) intercourse without conception" (Schmidt & Munster, 1995; Sundby, 1994). "Primary infertility" means that pregnancy has never been achieved, and "secondary infertility" means that pregnancy has occurred previously at least once but fails to occur again. In both biomedical definitions, the assumption is that intercourse occurs on a regular basis.

As shown in a number of studies in this volume, these definitions have limited applicability in Africa. In The Gambia, any failure to have children or to have them survive childhood is seen as infertility (Skramstad, 2000). In Zimbabwe, a "reproductive failure" is someone who fails to fulfill any reproductive ambition, including getting children of only one sex or not becoming pregnant more than once or twice (Runganga et al., 1999). Because of culturally different definitions of unions, marriage, and mating patterns, it may be unclear what definitions to use when investigating infertility in a developing country. Once family planning becomes widespread, it becomes more difficult to estimate the level of involuntary infertility as determined by traditional demographic and health surveys (Larsen, 1994). In The Gambia, a country with a low contraceptive prevalence rate, the most recent contraceptive prevalence study (WB/MOH/UNFPA, 1993) found that among women at the end of the reproductive period, up to 3 to 4 percent had no children, suggesting that a diagnosis of infertility could be made for these women. In demography, however, subfecundity is defined as a longer than expected time since last birth—five years or more in developing countries with low contraceptive prevalence rates (Larsen, 1994).

For many developing counties, there are no available data on the frequency of infertility. In the World Health Organization (WHO, 1991) tabulation of infertility worldwide, the definitions used for different settings vary considerably. The same applies to infertility estimations in more developed countries (Schmidt & Munster, 1995). The main difference between infertility in the developed and developing countries is that in developing countries, a higher proportion of infertile couples suffer from secondary infertility, reflecting the fact that they manage to become pregnant before they experience their first pelvic infection (WHO, 1991).

LACK OF ACCESS TO MEDICAL CARE AND REPRODUCTIVE TECHNOLOGIES

In both Zimbabwe and The Gambia, there is overwhelming evidence from our studies that infertile couples are massive users of many kinds of medicine and often mix biomedical and traditional approaches. Not only is biomedical treatment difficult to get; it may be difficult to get to. Sometimes attitudes by care workers, embarrassment on the part of the patient, failure to cope with recommendations, and problems with the spouse break treatment contracts even before they get started. Sometimes health care workers ask for more (or informal) payment to continue an investigation, and the patient, usually a woman, does not have the money or is embarrassed to ask someone for it. Negative attitudes by health workers may also hamper patients' ability to cope with a definite negative outcome.

Lack of control of the treatment process is another dimension. This lack of control is bilateral. Patients do not control their reproductive ability. Doctors cannot control their patients' access to care. Overburdened clinics, lack of skilled manpower, lack of structure in the working day, competition with physicians' financial drive to work in the private sector after hours, and increasing patient fees for services outside the minimal package are reasons that many patients discontinue their investigations once started.

Even if health care is available, its content may be inadequate. Only 40 percent of the 243 women classified as infertile in our survey in The Gambia (Sundby et al., 1998) had sought care in the formal health care system for their problem. The most frequently visited health care institutions were primary health centers, the referral hospital in the capital, Banjul, and other hospitals or doctors. Most women had experienced health interventions that, in biomedical terms, are ineffective in overcoming infertility (see Inhorn, 1994). For example, more than 10 percent of women reported having a dilatation and curettage (D&C), and 25 percent were given some kind of medicine, most often oral contraceptives. Only a few had had a tubal patency test (hysterosalpingogram) or reported that the husband had had a sperm test, even though those two procedures are a necessary minimum. Less than 5 percent of women were examined together with the husband (Sundby & Jacobus, 2001).

Thus, to summarize, biomedical forms of diagnosis and treatment, for those who are successful in gaining access to them, may be of limited success. Even in a fairly comprehensive reproductive health service in the tertiary teaching hospital in Harare, Zimbabwe, where specialized infertility services were offered, many patients never conclusively overcame their infertility.

Clearly, in this setting, where biomedical health services are of limited quality and scope, traditional care comprises an important alternative among different ethnic groups, who may use this form of care in various ways. For example, some women in The Gambia become members of a supportive women's group called the Kanyaleng. In our study in The Gambia, the most frequently mentioned form of traditional care was to consult a Muslim doctor, or *marabout*, or to visit a sacred place, such as a crocodile pool, the grave of a famous marabout, or sacred tree. Nonetheless, traditional caregivers may not be confident about their ability to provide satisfactory care. As one marabout who was also the relative of an infertile woman said: "It is difficult to help infertile people; myself, I have not been able to cure this relative, even if I am a *marabout*" (Sundby et al., 1998).

In both The Gambia and Zimbabwe, many infertile women and sometimes their husbands seek alternative sources of care, and they spend considerable amounts of time and money in their healing quests. Indeed, traditional healers and their practices are widely accepted, even among the educated. Before the AIDS epidemic, the majority of those who sought traditional healers in Zimbabwe were people with procreative problems.[2] In Zimbabwe, traditional healers called *n'gangas* are frequently consulted, and they offer remedies, advice, and discussion of possible explanatory factors. In addition, there are herbalists and several types of faith healers who belong to specific churches. Many healers claim the ability to communicate with ancestral spirits, and sometimes the infertility problem is interpreted as a consequence of the ancestors' dissatisfaction with the performance of certain tasks. Further, in Zimbabwe, beliefs in witchcraft are still prevalent, and some infertility problems are attributed to this cause (Aileen Jacobus, pers. com.).

INFERTILITY CARE AMID LIMITED RESOURCES: REALITIES OF REFERRAL

So what can be offered in a context with less than optimal resources for health care and limited access to formally trained doctors and nurses? At the village level in some countries, the backbone of primary health care is provided by laypeople with some formal training. Traditional birth attendants and village health workers have little to offer infertile patients other than referral. But, in reality, they are often the first ones to get involved, and they make use of what they have at hand. This may be oral contraceptive prescriptions, rituals performed with a "modern" birth attendant kit used as a kind of "child substitute," traditional herbs, or prayers, or a combination of these.

As our study demonstrated and as demonstrated by others (Inhorn, 1994), a supply-demand issue drives infertility treatment. This allows both biomedical and traditional health care workers at all levels to exploit the "desperate" infertile woman, her partner, and her family by offering many remedies with unknown benefits or, in worst-case scenarios, that may even be harmful (Inhorn, 1994). Indeed, even biomedical health care providers use a mixture of "traditional" and "modern" knowledge to justify their practice (Inhorn, 1994; Skramstad, 2000; Sundby, 1997). The cause of infertility may be explained as incompatibility between husband and wife, "tired" wombs, "bad" blood, blocked tubes, "weak" sperm, or hormonal disturbance. And biomedical treatment modalities may do more harm than good. Even in vitro fertilization (IVF) facilities set up by some private physicians in the developing world (see chaps. 14, 16, 17, this volume) offer more "magic" than live babies, as they perform the procedures without statistically sound outcomes. However, in places such as The Gambia and Zimbabwe, most infertile couples have access only to "lower" levels of care, in primary care or primary referral settings. Thus the question I pose here is: What kind of care can they can expect to find at different levels of referral?

Health Centers

The typical health care delivery site in rural Africa is variously known as the health post, the health clinic, or the health center. In these facilities in

The Gambia, we interviewed several nurses about their knowledge of infertility investigation and treatment. In Zimbabwe, we observed infertility patient "health promotion pep talks," as well as consultations in family planning mobile units. Although there was some knowledge of the different forms of infertility, as well as the difference between secondary and primary infertility, among nurses in the health centers, only those who ran family planning delivery units or were trained as nurse-midwives seemed to have a thorough understanding of how an infertility investigation should be conducted. Yet the Gambian nurses all claimed to have seen infertile clients within the last six months.

Screening and treatment for sexually transmitted diseases (STDs) is commonly done by trained nurse-midwives, both in Zimbabwe and in The Gambia. Most often, the nurse sees the woman alone. Some, but not all, trained nurses do adequate history taking, treat suspected STDs, and then refer the patients (including the husband) to a doctor. Others seem to have very little to offer.

In this setting, then, there is significant room for improvement. STD screening, counseling on menstrual cycle and intercourse, and a minimal level of counseling and referral follow-up could be done at this level, even with very little investment in infrastructure. This counseling could include information about the menstrual cycle and fertile period, about proper and improper investigation methods, and about the fact that infertility can be caused by problems in the male as well as in the female. Counseling could also include attention to the emotional distress of infertility and its effects on marital and sexual life.

Local Rural Hospitals: The Gambian Case

In The Gambia, there is only one hospital in the rural area. Here most of the outpatients are screened by trained nurses. The workload is heavy. In 1993, the first year of complete hospital statistics, a total of more than thirty thousand clients were seen. Thirty percent were referred to one of the more specialized clinics. The nurses in charge who were interviewed told us that most infertile clients do not initially reveal their problem but present it as "pain in the body" or "something wrong in the pelvis." Special skills are needed to identify those with no explicit complaint who are actually infertile. Only one nurse in this setting had a special interest in infertility. The expatriate doctors there were generalists and did not see infertility problems as a special priority for which they should offer specialized treatment.

The hospital kept no specific records of outpatient diagnoses. Thus it was difficult to obtain an estimate of the number of clients presenting with infertility. The nurse in charge of services for STDs thought he might see one to two infertile clients per day. In the records for the STD clinic for the period January through May 1993, 32 out of 170 (19%) female clients reported an infertility problem. For an additional five clients, infertility appeared to be a problem, but record keeping was less detailed. For the first half of 1994, the same figures were 15 out of 128 (12%), with 4 to 5 possible additional cases. Thus the infertility problem was clearly present in this setting, even though it was not receiving attention from a diagnostic and treatment perspective.

There were no reported cases of hospitalization for infertility, although it appears that there had been two operations for fallopian tube obstruction in 1993. The doctors were not in favor of doing tubal surgery, because of poor preoperative diagnoses and presumably poor results. Fortunately, they did not regularly undertake D&Cs for infertility in this hospital unless there was a severe menstrual problem. One doctor attempted to perform tubal patency tests by insufflation of carbon dioxide or saline, given that X-ray services were scarce. However, other doctors discouraged this practice. Laboratory-based hormonal tests of any kind would have to be sent to the capital and would take at least a couple of months to complete, so they were not being done. However, fourteen semen analyses were reported from the lab unit in 1993.

Our informants in this hospital felt that secondary infertility was seen more often than primary infertility. Most of the infertility clients were self-referred, and the clients had often bypassed the local health center. It was almost always women who took the initiative, but some men attended on request. (Elderly men were more likely to refuse, whereas younger men seemed to have fewer objections.) The one nurse with a special interest in infertility felt that most patients had very little basic knowledge about infertility, including an understanding of the fertile period in the cycle.

At rural hospitals such as this one in The Gambia, a number of basic tests, including vaginal examination, vaginal swab if symptoms of infection are present, syphilis testing after history taking, white blood cell counts, and sperm test if male infertility is suspected, could be undertaken in cases of infertility. This is a basic but nevertheless suitable diagnostic package, given the lack of expertise, heavy workload, and scarce resources.

Unfortunately, however, treatment options at rural hospitals will probably remain limited. In the hospital studied in The Gambia, there was no supply of the popular hormone-inducing agent, clomiphene. This was one reason why oral contraceptives had become a popular hormone treatment and were given out by some nurses and paramedics (doctors there rarely prescribed them).

Referral Hospital Care: Two Case Studies

In the only referral hospital in Banjul, the capital of The Gambia, most infertile couples come to the gynecology outpatient department. All gynecologists see infertility clients, but a few doctors seem to have a special interest in this problem, which is often related to STD-induced tubal problems (Mabey, Ogba Selassie, Robertson, Heckels, & Ward, 1985). One reason for this is that infertility is a potentially lucrative health problem, for which patients may be willing to pay extra fees. Doctors in public hospitals also work in private clinics, and they may refer public-hospital patients to their private practices for follow-up and more sophisticated treatment, if the patient is willing and able to pay (cf. Inhorn, 1994). Sometimes clients are referred *from* private clinics for specialized tests. The referral hospital offers screening for STDs, and semen analyses can be performed if the samples are delivered to the laboratory in a timely fashion. In The Gambia, the husband is most often asked to accompany his wife to the hospital, but some men do not comply with this request. There are no laparoscopic diagnostic technologies to assess the patency of fallopian tubes and no hormonal assay tests for detection of ovulation.

In The Gambia, occasionally timed D&Cs are performed with endometrial histology to determine ovulatory phase, but the hospital is well aware that this procedure has a limited place in modern infertility investigation. D&C is a procedure in which the cervical opening is dilated with instruments, and then mucosal tissue from the uterus is removed by a sharp curette. In developed countries, D&C is no longer a standard procedure for any gynecological problem, but it is often used in developing countries as a method to induce abortion or for menstrual irregularities. In some instances, it may harm more than help, especially if performed under less than hygienic conditions in a woman with recurrent infections. The World Health Organization has produced a document reviewing standard guidelines for infertility investigations (WHO, 1993). D&C is not a standard procedure according to these guidelines.

Indeed, the WHO guidelines call for a full clinical examination of both the male and the female, many laboratory tests, including hormonal assays and sperm analyses, and eventually invasive surgical (laparoscopic) examination of the female partner. These guidelines are advanced and would require infrastructure, skills, and financial resources that are out of reach for most public hospitals in the developing world. Thus they are seldom followed strictly. As shown in our two case studies, hysterosalpingograms and sperm tests seem to be the only routine tests for all clients.

Yet infertility is a common cause of admission to the outpatient unit of the referral hospital in The Gambia. Out of a total of 4,044 gynecological patients seen in 1993, 404 were new admissions for infertility, and 262 were follow-up clients. Infertility clients thus make up more than 16 percent of the gynecology workload. The ratio of new admissions to follow-up indicated that a majority of the clients are seen only once, which is inadequate from a clinical point of view, especially if review of tests or treatment options are to be discussed with clients.

In the wards, again in the referral hospital in The Gambia, 64 out of 1,448 gynecological cases were admitted for infertility in 1994, but only two tuboplasties were performed. Forty-nine cases underwent salpingectomy (removal of the tubes and sometimes the ovaries) because of severe damage to the tubes. Antesuspension of the uterus was performed five times. In contrast, there were more than eight hundred cases of abortion. The proportion of ward admissions for infertility was, then, between 4 and 5 percent. But considering that a tubal surgery patient stays on average up to a week in the hospital, while abortion cases are released within a few days, the burden is fairly high.

In contrast, in Harare, Zimbabwe, the reference for infertility investigation in the university teaching hospital is, indeed, the WHO manual (1993). Infertility services there were initiated through sponsorship from our project. But when key staff are on occasional leave, the process comes to a total halt. Nonetheless, this hospital has more sophisticated equipment and resources, including several specialists in gynecology, andrology, and infertility nursing. The main constraints to following the WHO manual for the investigation of infertility are that patients in general cannot afford to pay for the tests, public funding for health care is limited, and private insurance is almost nonexistent among the vast majority of the population. Hormone assays and laparoscopy are the tests that suffer most from lack of financial resources, and treatment options such as surgery and IVF are very limited.

Another constraint is the many other reproductive health problems that doctors and midwives must deal with, including abortion complications, maternal morbidity and mortality, complicated deliveries, and HIV/AIDS in pregnancy. Infertility ranks low on this list of urgent priorities. This and the constraints described above, along with the high cost and long waiting lists, may prevent many infertile couples from using the services, even in this public hospital. On a positive note, however, the hospital's andrology laboratory offers a special clinic day for men with fertility problems, who are also given health instruction. They seem to appreciate this special service, which has increased awareness of male infertility.

The Private Sector

In both Harare and Banjul, there are well-equipped private gynecological clinics that can do comprehensive infertility investigations. A considerable number of infertility clients from the more affluent sectors of the population are often seen in these clinics. Services may include hysterosalpingograms, semen analyses, endometrial biopsies, laparoscopies, and hormone treatment with clomiphene.[3] Many clients are reported to come to these private clinics after inadequate investigations elsewhere.

As noted above, the demarcation lines between the private and public sectors are not always clear, as many doctors work in both areas and refer back and forth between facilities. The private providers who were interviewed seemed to have a good understanding of standards of infertility investigation, but they could not offer gynecological surgery or advanced assisted reproductive technology.

A study of the practice of other, less specialized private facilities reveals some important issues. In The Gambia, it is evident that there is gross overuse of D&C when clients present with infertility. Why? First, doctors can charge for this procedure. Second, there is little knowledge, even among physicians, about its limited value in the investigation of infertility. Third, a public demand for D&C has been created because of its overuse. The Gambia is not the only country where this is happening. Inhorn (1994) has clearly demonstrated how some harmful practices such as electrocauterization and D&C are embedded in a contemporary clinical setting that contributes to massive overuse. Indeed, in other hospitals throughout the African subcontinent, the D&C is a "multipurpose" procedure performed secretly by paramedics and medical doctors at large. The indications are both to interrupt unwanted pregnancies and to enhance fertility.

CONCLUSION: THE DIFFICULTIES OF INCLUDING INFERTILITY ON THE GLOBAL REPRODUCTIVE HEALTH AGENDA

Around the world, people with infertility problems often look to health services to obtain a biomedical solution. Although the social and psychological dimensions of infertility are important, the problem, from a biomedical viewpoint, is often diagnosed and treated as a disease, with the goal being to "cure" infertility and give women babies. This is as true for Africa as the rest of the world and is a justified goal. On the other hand, a large proportion of infertile women may never be able to give birth, especially given the realities of health care delivery.[4]

As seen in this chapter, the treatment possibilities for infertility remain less than optimal, and health care resources may not be sufficient to provide full investigation and successful treatment for all. Crucial questions then become: Can infertility be prevented? And if it can, how? The answers to these questions are complex. A first response is that even if infertility is fairly common, little is known about the major factors leading to the condition. The ability to reproduce is a relatively robust biological function, and most people eventually conceive at least one child. Nonetheless, sexual behavior, including many partners before childbearing leading to sexually transmitted diseases, is a central risk factor for infertility that has significant potential for prevention. It has also been demonstrated that extreme obesity or extreme thinness (e.g., from starvation or anorexia nervosa) influences sex hormone regulation negatively and thus contributes to subfertility (Sundby, 1994). Information about associations and risks is one component of health education, and health information could focus on infertility, as well as HIV/AIDS and unwanted pregnancies, as a potential outcome of sexual behavior. Just as many women who are now mature adults past childbearing age were aware of the possibility for unplanned pregnancies when they were young, today's youth should be prepared for the possible risk of infertility. As some portion of every population will eventually experience this problem, it should be part of the reproductive health education of young people everywhere.

Still, health information does not always change behavior. Sexual (and eating) behaviors can be difficult to change, especially as they have a series of emotional and economic implications. Furthermore, current knowledge concerning public attitudes toward infertility in developing countries is scarce (Gerrits, 1997; Inhorn, 1994; Mogobe, 2000; Odejide, Ladipo, Otolorin, & Makanjuola, 1986; Sundby, 1997), and most studies report that infertility is a major social stigma.

From a biomedical standpoint, when it comes to health care in settings with scarce resources, a minimal package of infertility services cannot attempt to meet all criteria in the WHO manual (1993). A basic package could be to invite both a woman and her partner for STD screening and treatment; ordinary clinical evaluation; sexual, dietary, and emotional counseling; sperm tests; and menstrual cycle recordings. Access to more comprehensive infertility investigation may be available only to the wealthier part of the world. On the other hand, it is important to spend more resources on infertility treatment even in developing countries. As population growth can only be curbed by access to contraceptives and reproductive health care and the global message becomes "a small, healthy family," it is equally important to assure people that they can indeed have some children if and when they wish to. If women's fear of infertility and knowledge of poor outcome of infertility treatment is too high, population programs may fail to accomplish successful contraceptive delivery (Bledsoe, D'Allessandro, & Langerock, 1994; chap. 11, this volume).

The global ethical dilemma in infertility, as well as in many other issues of health care, is that the resources for care and cure are unevenly distributed worldwide. Thus infertility care will probably continue to be hampered by a severe scarcity of know-how and resources in places such as The Gambia and Zimbabwe, as well as in many other countries around the globe.

NOTES

1. In 1994 the United Nations Conference on Population and Development was held in Cairo, and in 1995 the United Nations Conference on Women and Development was held in Beijing. Both of them produced several documents and plans of action.

2. It is very common to seek traditional healers for infertility, and most clients do this before they seek formal care, according to several studies (Hellum, 1999; Runganga et al., 1999) and the current research of Aileen Jacobus, a nurse-midwife who is studying community perceptions of infertility in rural areas. Infertility is often attributed to problems related to bridewealth, sexual behavior, or in-laws, and most often the woman is blamed for the problem.

3. Hysterosalpingograms are X-rays taken with a contrast medium injected into the fallopian tubes to see if the tubes are patent, or open. Laparoscopies are small surgical procedures in which an instrument is inserted through the umbilicus to view the internal pelvic organs. Hormonal assays are blood samples taken to assess the function of the ovaries or testes. Clomiphene is a drug that induces ovulation in women with ovulatory problems.

4. The May 1999 issue of the journal *Reproductive Health Matters* contained several papers on living without children, in both developing and developed countries. The editor, Marge Berer, states that the papers from Africa certainly suggest that living without children in Africa is a problem "so shrouded in silence that many will not talk about it at all" (p. 9).

REFERENCES

Bledsoe, C., Hill, A., D'Allessandro, U., & Langerock, P. (1994). Constructing natural fertility: The use of Western contraceptive technologies in rural Gambia. *Population Development Review, 20,* 81–113.

Gerrits, T. (1997). Social and cultural aspects of infertility in Mozambique. *Patient Education and Counseling, 31,* 39–48.

Hellum, A. (1999). *Women, human rights and legal pluralism in Africa: Mixed norms and identities in infertility management in Zimbabwe.* Oslo: TANO.

Inhorn, M. C. (1994). *Quest for conception: Gender, infertility, and Egyptian medical traditions.* Philadelphia: University of Pennsylvania Press.

Jacobus, A., & Sundby, J. (1997). *Infertility: A guide for patients.* Oslo: Organon.

Larsen, U. (1994). Sterility in sub-Saharan Africa. *Population Studies, 48,* 459–474.

Mabey, D. C. W., Ogba Selassie, G., Robertson, J. N., Heckels, J. E., & Ward, M.E. (1985). Tubal infertility in The Gambia: Chlamydia and gonococcal serology in women with tubal occlusion compared with pregnant controls. *Bulletin of WHO, 63,* 1107–1113.

Mgobe, K. (2000). Traditional therapies for infertility: Implications for the brokerage role of the nurse in Botswana. In F. van Balen, T. Gerrits, & M. Inhorn (Eds.), *Social science research on childlessness in a global perspective* (pp. 111–117). Amsterdam: SCO-Kohnstamm Instituut.

Odejide, A. O., Ladipo, O. A., Otolorin, E. O., & Makanjuola, J. D. A. (1986).

Infertility among Nigerian women: A study of related psychological factors. *Journal of Obstetrics and Gynecology in Eastern and Central Africa, 6*, 613–617.

Runganga, A., Sundby, J., & Aggleton, P. (2001). What's love got to do with it? Culture, identity and reproductive failure in Zimbabwe. *Sexualities.*

Schmidt, L., & Munster, K. (1995). Infertility, involuntary infecundity, and the seeking of medical advice in industrialized countries, 1970–1992: A review of concepts, measurements and results. *Human Reproduction, 10(6)*, 1407–1418.

Skramstad, H. (2000). Are foster children a solution for infertile Gambian women? In F. van Balen, T. Gerrits, & M. Inhorn (Eds.), *Social science research on childlessness in global perspective* (pp. 15–27). Amsterdam: SCO-Kohnstamm Instituut.

Sundby, J. (1994). Infertility: Causes, care and consequences. Medical dissertation, University of Oslo.

Sundby, J. (1997). Infertility in The Gambia: Traditional and modern health care. *Patient Education and Counseling, 31*, 29–37.

Sundby, J., & Jacobus, A. (2001). Health and traditional care for infertility in The Gambia and Zimbabwe. In J. T. Boerma & Z. Mgalla (Eds.), *Women and Infertility in sub-Saharan Africa* (pp. 257–268). Amsterdam: KIT Publishers.

Sundby, J., Sonko, S., & Mboge, R. (1998). Infertility in The Gambia: Traditional and modern health care. *Social Science & Medicine, 31*, 29–37.

WB/MOH/UNFPA. (1993). *Contraceptive prevalence and fertility determinants in The Gambia.* Banjul, The Gambia.

WHO (World Health Organization). (1991). *Infertility: A tabulation of available data on prevalence of primary and secondary infertility.* Geneva: Programme on Maternal Health and Family Planning, Division of Family Health, WHO.

WHO (World Health Organization). (1993). *Manual for the standard investigation and diagnosis of the infertile couple.* Cambridge: Cambridge University Press.

PART IV

Globalizing Technologies

FOURTEEN

The "Local" Confronts the "Global"

Infertile Bodies and New Reproductive Technologies in Egypt

Marcia C. Inhorn

Since the birth in 1978 of Louise Brown, the world's first test-tube baby, new reproductive technologies (NRTs) have spread around the globe, reaching countries far from the "producing" nations of the West. Perhaps nowhere is this globalization process more evident than in the nearly twenty nations of the Muslim Middle East, where in vitro fertilization (IVF) centers have opened in small, petro-rich Arab countries such as Bahrain and Qatar and in much larger but less prosperous North African nations such as Morocco and Egypt. Egypt provides a fascinating locus for investigation of this global transfer of NRTs because of its ironic position as one of the poor, "overpopulated" Middle Eastern nations. With nearly 70 million citizens and an annual per capita GNP of $3,460 (Population Reference Bureau, 2001), Egypt has pursued population reduction goals through family planning since the 1960s, the first Muslim Middle Eastern nation to do so (Stycos, Said, Avery, & Fridman, 1988). Yet, as in the vast majority of the world's societies, infertility has never been included in Egypt's population program as a population problem, a more general public health concern, or an issue of human suffering for Egyptian citizens, especially women. This is despite the fact that a recent World Health Organization–sponsored survey placed the total infertility prevalence rate among married Egyptian couples at 12 percent (4.3% primary infertility and 7.7% secondary infertility) (Egyptian Fertility Care Society, 1995). Given the size of this infertile population and the strong culturally embedded desire for children expressed by virtually all Egyptian men and women, it is not surprising that Egypt provides a ready market for NRTs. Despite its regionally underprivileged position, Egypt has been on the forefront of NRT development in the Middle East—a legacy, perhaps, of its long history with colonially inspired biomedicine (Inhorn, 1994). In 1986 Egypt was one of two nations in the region to open an IVF center. By 1996, when the research for this chapter was carried out, there were ten Egyptian IVF centers in full operation or development. By the end of the decade, there were more than thirty-five IVF centers in Egypt—a greater than threefold expansion in only three years, placing Egypt ahead of even Israel, which alone boasts twenty-four IVF centers (Kahn, 2000). This explosion of IVF services in Egypt is perhaps surprising when one considers that a single trial of IVF can cost more than £E 10,000, or U.S. $3,000. This represents several times the annual income of a poor Egyptian and is an admittedly large sum for even the most affluent Egyptian patients. In other words, the new reproductive technologies would seem to be out of reach for most ordinary Egyptians; yet infertile Egyptian patients are inundating IVF centers, which face such great demand for their services that they are chronically short of the powerful drugs, supplies, and even competent technical staff necessary to carry out IVF procedures.

A critical question thus becomes: What factors explain the consumption of high-cost, high-tech reproductive technologies in a Third World country such as Egypt? Or, put another way, why are Egyptian consumers so powerfully motivated to try these costly, potentially risky, and often unsuccessful technologies? Certainly, to understand this demand for NRTs requires an analysis of pronatalism, or child desire, and the accompanying dread, severe stigmatization, and suffering that infertility brings for most Egyptian couples. These are subjects that I have taken up at length elsewhere (see Inhorn, 1994, 1996) and that provide the implicit background to this chapter.

But my primary goal here is to ask, not what motivates Egyptians to use these technologies, but rather what might prevent them from doing so. Namely, my research in Egypt shows that would-be Egyptian IVF consumers confront numerous "arenas of constraint," or various structural, social-cultural, ideological, and practical obstacles and apprehensions that may detract or deter them altogether from using NRTs. During two periods of research in Egypt, I have identified eight major arenas of constraint, ranging from local formulations of patriarchy, which privilege infertile Egyptian men in their marital relationships, to local versions of Islam and Coptic Christianity, which legislate the "appropriate" use of new reproductive technologies, thereby restricting who may benefit from them (Inhorn, 2001). I would argue that examining such arenas of constraint facing the infertile wherever these technologies spread is an extremely useful exercise, for it serves to deconstruct the myth that NRTs are some sort of panacea for infertility wherever it occurs. Such critical deconstruction stands in sharp contrast to various "pro-technology" modernist narratives, which argue that NRTs are a great boon to infertile couples around the world—providing them with an opportunity to overcome their stigma through the use of a "modern" technology representing the "cutting edge" of advances in Western science and medicine. By using such technologies, the infertile would therefore seem to be agents of their own reproductive futures, and issues of human suffering would be alleviated. Yet, as many feminist authors have argued (see chap. 3, this volume), such utopian scenarios are unrealistic and even dangerous, for they not only ignore the myriad obstacles and risks that consumers of these technologies face (Ginsburg & Rapp, 1995) but also fail to interrogate the notion of reproductive choice, particularly in pronatalist societies such as Egypt where motherhood, and thus infertility therapy seeking, are rarely if ever viewed as optional.

My second major line of argument in this chapter is that NRTs are not transferred into cultural voids when they reach places like Egypt. Rather, local considerations, be they cultural, social, economic, or political, shape and sometimes curtail the way these Western-generated technologies are both offered to and received by non-Western subjects. In other words, the assumption on the part of global producer nations that these NRTs—as purportedly value-free, inherently beneficial medical technologies—are "immune to culture" and can thus be "appropriately" transferred and implemented anywhere and everywhere is subject to challenge once local formulations, perceptions, and consumption are taken into consideration.

Indeed, the global spread of NRTs provides a particularly salient but little discussed example of what Appadurai (1996, p. 34) has termed a "technoscape," or "the global configuration, also ever fluid, of technology, and the fact that technology, both high and low, both mechanical and informational, now moves at high speeds across various kinds of previously impervious boundaries." Clearly, as with the global spread of other technologies, the NRT technoscape is an uneven terrain, in that some nations and regions within nations (e.g., major metropolises) have achieved greater access to these "fruits" of globalization than others. Furthermore, even in the West—and then on magnified terms in the non-Western world—lines of demarcation between gender, race, and class have been brought into great relief vis-à-vis access to these technologies. Ginsburg and Rapp (1995) have employed the term "stratified reproduction" in an attempt to get at these transnational inequalities, whereby some are able to achieve their reproductive desires, often through recourse to globalizing technologies, while others—usually poor women of color around the globe—are disempowered and even despised as reproducers. However, Ginsburg and Rapp are quick to point out that the power to define reproduction is not necessarily unidirectional—flowing from the West, with its money and technology, to the rest of the world. Rather, "people everywhere actively use their local cultural logics and social relations to incorporate, revise, or resist the influence of seemingly distant political and economic forces" (Ginsburg & Rapp, 1995, p. 1). Indeed, a growing number of studies asserting the voices and agency of non-Western peoples have challenged the image of Third World subjects, particularly women, as passive and powerless in the face of global forces (Mohanty, Russo, & Torres, 1991). It is useful instead to ask how Third World recipients of global technologies resist their application, or at least reconfigure the ways they are to be adopted in local cultural contexts (Freeman, 1999). In other words, globalization is not enacted in a uniform manner around the world, nor is it simply homogenizing—necessarily "Westernizing" or even "Americanizing"—in its effects (Appadurai, 1996; Hannerz, 1996). The global is always imbued with local meaning, and local actors mold the very form that global processes take, doing so in ways that highlight the dialectics of gender and class, production and consumption, local and global cultures (Freeman, 1999).

In this chapter, I intend to focus on how local Egyptian culture both accommodates and curtails the incorporation of globalizing reproductive technologies into the Egyptian landscape. In particular, I hope to show how Egyptian IVF patients and their doctors imbue the practice of IVF with an Egyptian sensibility—not to be found in the IVF laboratories and clinics of London, Los Angeles, Sydney, or other Western sites. This Egyptian sensibility, furthermore, has much to do with issues of embodiment (Bourdieu, 1977), or local, culturally embedded notions of infertile bodies and human reproductive bodies in general. As I show here, understandings of the reproductive body and its physiology are highly culturally variable, as are perceptions of bodily risk and vulnerability, safety and efficacy, and social stigmatization associated with "abnormal" bodies and births. Such culturally specific understandings and experiences of the reproductive body may shape the way the new reproductive technologies are to be used, curtailing their application in some cases. Thus, although demand for NRTs has grown dramatically in Egypt over the past decade, the case of NRTs clearly demonstrates how the "local" confronts the "global": how local cultural factors reshape and sometimes constrain how global technologies are to be used. Such local considerations speak to the need for greater historical and ethnographic grounding of bioethical, feminist, and technological debates over the various impacts of reproductive technologies. For, as my own ethnographic research suggests, the use of NRTs in Egypt involves not only a unique history, but different understandings of the body, the limits of science and technology, and the local "moral worlds" (Kleinman, 1992, 1995) in which the recipients of such global technologies and their high-tech offspring must live.

THE ETHNOGRAPHIC SETTING AND SUBJECTS

The research on which this chapter is based encompasses two distinct time periods and research settings, thereby capturing the historicity of the NRT globalization process in Egypt. The first period is 1988–1989, or the "early IVF period" in Egypt. The first Egyptian IVF center had just opened in an elite suburb of Cairo in 1986, and the first Egyptian "baby of the tubes" (as they are called in Egypt), a little girl named Heba Mohammed, was born in 1987 (Stephens, 1995). In these early days of NRT transfer to Egypt, I conducted fifteen months of anthropological research on the general problem of infertility in that country, basing my research in the public OB-GYN teaching hospital in Alexandria, Egypt's second largest city. This hospital, popularly known as "Shatby," was initiating Egypt's only government-sponsored IVF program, thereby drawing large numbers of lower-class, IVF-seeking patients for purportedly "free" NRT technology.[1] At Shatby, I conducted in-depth, semistructured interviews in the Egyptian dialect of Arabic with one hundred infertile women and a comparison group of ninety fertile women, most of whom were poor, uneducated, illiterate or only semiliterate housewives (see the appendixes in Inhorn [1994] for further details).

The second period of research took place in 1996, or what could be characterized as the "IVF boom period" in Egypt. In the midst of this NRT explosion, I spent the summer in Cairo conducting participant observation and in-depth, semistructured interviews with sixty-six mostly middle- to upper-class women; nearly all of them were undergoing IVF or related procedures at two of the major IVF centers in Cairo, Egypt's largest city of more than 10 million inhabitants. Both of these IVF centers were situated in private hospitals in Heliopolis and Maadi, elite neighborhoods on the outskirts of Cairo. They were among the three most established and respected clinics in the city and received a daily influx of new patients, especially during the summer months, which were the busiest and therefore ideal for my research. The patients presenting to these IVF clinics were generally (although not exclusively) well-educated, professional, comparatively affluent women, who were often accompanied by their husbands. Indeed, in 40 percent of the interviews conducted in these clinics (in marked contrast to my earlier research), husbands were present and participated, often enthusiastically, in discussions. Moreover, whereas interviews in my first study were conducted entirely in Egyptian Arabic, many of the women and men who participated in the second study spoke fluent, even flawless English in a Western argot as a result of their advanced education, and they chose to conduct the interview in their second language.

Thus my work on this subject incorporates both a longitudinal and a class-based comparison of infertile women seeking treatment in the two largest cities of Egypt. The findings presented here are based largely on the second period of research, but they are clearly informed by insights gained through the initial, longer period of research on the general problem of infertility.

ARENAS OF CONSTRAINT

"Reproducing" Knowledge and Belief

Perhaps the most fundamental cultural constraint to the practice of IVF and other NRTs in Egypt has to do with deeply embedded beliefs about the nature of the reproductive body—beliefs that have yet to be supplanted through widespread education in contemporary Western reproductive biology. What Martin (1991) has called the "romance of egg and sperm"— the now widely held Western version of duogenetic inheritance through equal contributions of egg and sperm—is not the cultural script of procreation imagined by most Egyptians. Instead, among the poorly educated, often illiterate Egyptian "masses" (i.e., the urban and rural poor), views of procreation are decidedly "monogenetic" (Delaney, 1991): that is, men are literally thought to create life vis-à-vis preformed fetuses that they carry in their sperm and ejaculate into women's waiting wombs. Since sperm are popularly referred to as *didan,* or worms, among the Egyptian masses, this masculinist, monogenetic, preformation model (Laqueur, 1990)[2] is typically glossed as: "men's worms carry the kids." Women, who are clearly marginalized in this procreative scenario, are thought of as mere receptacles for and nurturers of men's substantive input rather than as active contributors to the process of procreation per se. Among uneducated Egyptians, women are not deemed contributors of biogenetic substance but rather serve to carry, "cushion," or perhaps "nourish" the growing fetus with menstrual blood (a substance that is nonetheless polluting and thus deemed troublesome as a source of fetal sustenance). Indeed, the notion of women having "eggs" is seen as ludicrous and unthinkable—equating, as it would, human females with chickens!

Given such differences in knowledge and belief, biomedically oriented infertility treatment is typically deeply disturbing and even threatening for both Egyptian men and women. It requires men to "bring," or ejaculate, their sperm into plastic containers and women to take powerful hormonal medications to stimulate their egg production. The new reproductive technologies such as IVF take such manipulation of procreative materials several steps further, requiring that both ova and sperm be removed from the body, sometimes surgically, and that embryos formed through in vitro fertilization in a laboratory be placed back inside a woman's body. This technology challenges the most basic precepts of monogenetic procreation and patrilineally based kinship envisioned by most uneducated Egyptians. Such challenges include the notions (1) that women have eggs that can be removed from and later returned to their bodies in a different form; (2) that women's eggs contribute material to the creation of offspring, thereby giving women biological "ownership" of their children in their own right; (3) that men do *not,* in fact, contribute "everything" to procreation if their sperm are made to "combine" with women's eggs; (4) that men's sperm and women's eggs may somehow be of equal weight in biogenetic inheritance, a form of equality questioned even by more educated Egyptians; and (5) that this combination of eggs and sperm can occur outside the body, separate from the "bringing" of children through male-orgasmic sex.

Indeed, questions about what happens to such procreative materials during the period in which they are "in vitro" (literally, outside the body) are deeply troubling to Egyptians of all social backgrounds. Among the less educated, wild, futuristic fantasy visions of babies lingering for months in aquariums or giant test tubes abound, making such "extracorporeal pregnancies" decidedly "unnatural" and against God-given plans for pregnancy and birth (Inhorn, 1994). Even among the most highly educated Egyptians, the in vitro nature of NRTs evokes widespread moral uncertainty, for they worry about inadvertent laboratory mixups of procreative materials. An accidental laboratory recombination of eggs and sperm outside the marital union—as has happened in Western IVF laboratories—is considered tantamount to adultery in this Muslim society, where donation of sperm, ova, embryos, and wombs (through surrogacy) are all strictly prohibited (Inhorn, 2000, 2001).

In the early IVF period, when I conducted my first research on this subject in Egypt, fears of this kind abounded, such that only the most desperate "moral pioneers" (Rapp, 1988) seemed willing to actually enter the brave new world of high-tech reproductive medicine. However, the past ten years have yielded dramatic changes in the realm of knowledge and hence belief. Patients who reached Egyptian IVF centers in the late 1990s were relative "experts" on the basic biology, mechanics, and religious permissibility of NRTs, easily reciting the differences between the various types of NRTs, as well as contemporary religious thinking on the subject. But this is largely a function of the educational level of IVF clientele; those who eventually overcome the various obstacles to using NRTs are generally affluent, highly educated women and men, who have received Western-style higher education including instruction in Western reproductive biology. In addition, most cope with the trials and tribulations of the IVF treatment process by seeking out information on NRTs both before and after they embark on this line of therapy. In many cases, this typically includes patient education received in IVF centers, as well as books and other printed materials, generally written by physicians for educated Arabic-speaking audiences.

Furthermore, gaining access to popular information on NRTs has been made much easier for potential Egyptian NRT consumers through the veritable information explosion in Egypt, a country that has long been receptive to global media forces and prides itself on being the "Hollywood of the Middle East." Each new development in the world of Egyptian high-tech medicine becomes big news and is covered by various forms of print and electronic media. In addition, movies and television soap operas about the human dilemmas of high-tech reproduction have been both imported and produced locally and broadcast to literally millions of curious Egyptians. Although "IVF for entertainment" has often been as misleading as it has been educational, the very fact that such movies are being watched by millions of Egyptians of all social backgrounds has served to inform the public and to normalize NRTs to some extent.

Nonetheless, judging by the degree of stigma and secrecy still associated with IVF, it seems unlikely that all the media coverage in the world can alleviate and eliminate some of the widespread misunderstandings about high-tech baby making in Egypt. To do this will require, instead, unseating deeply held monogenetic cultural models of how babies are made. As I have argued elsewhere (Inhorn, 1996), it is these very models of monogenetic male procreation that serve as the ideological underpinning of Egyptian patriarchy, particularly as it is manifest in patrilineal kinship and family life. Thus I predict that no amount of media coverage will do away entirely with widely held, powerful beliefs about the nature of reproductive bodies, procreative substances, and the inherent "wrongness" of a technological innovation that tampers with these bodies and substances—in addition to the highly gendered notions of their relative importance. To that end, knowledge and belief themselves will probably continue to serve as one of the most fundamental impediments to the use of NRTs for many years to come, especially among more traditional segments of Egyptian society.

Embodiment and Efficacy

Given the uncertainties about reproductive bodies and the entire NRT enterprise, it is not surprising that questions of safety and efficacy are also of paramount concern to Egyptians, both men and women. Clearly, it is women who experience most powerfully the "embodiment" of the NRT process, and it is they who put their bodies on the line from the first injection of side effect–producing, ova-stimulating hormones to the typically cesarean birth of often multiple "babies of the tubes."[3] Thus Egyptian women, like women considering NRTs anywhere, are concerned with (1) the immediate risks and long-term safety of such procedures; (2) their individual somatic and psychic sensitivities to the debilitating aspects of such procedures; and (3) the efficacy, or the ultimate likelihood of success, of conception through such extraordinary means. These concerns are often shared by women's husbands, particularly in cases of male infertility. In the latter cases, a perfectly "healthy" wife must nonetheless experience the psychosomatic risks and discomforts of the NRT procedure, while her infertile husband's only psychosomatic suffering may involve the tension of time-sensitive, masturbatory ejaculation of his "weak" sperm into a plastic cup.

The very embodiment of NRT procedures is experienced by Egyptian women and men in culturally specific ways—ways that often magnify the psychic costs of this type of treatment and that in some cases may prevent Egyptian couples from going forward with IVF or a related procedure. Even well-informed couples who decide to visit an Egyptian IVF clinic have deep concerns about the embodiment of a potentially risky and not necessarily successful form of high-tech therapy. And these concerns are exacerbated by real structural tensions having to do with the availability of supplies and competent personnel to perform effective IVF in a Third World setting that is on the perceived receiving end of global technological transfer. In fact, Egyptian patients' anxieties about this related set of issues are well founded, for a number of reasons.

"Weakness."   First, Egyptian women are often fundamentally ambivalent about taking the powerful hormonal agents required before any trial of IVF, because of deep culturally entrenched beliefs about the bodily "weakness" produced by hormones of any kind. "Weakness" is a common cultural illness idiom in Egypt (DeClerque, Tsui, Abul-Ata, & Barcelona, 1986; Early, 1993), one that is viewed both as a general condition of ill health and as a problem localized to specific parts of the body (e.g., "weak heart," "weak lungs," and "weak blood"). The idiom of weakness is rife in popular Egyptian reproductive imagery, and it is given further support by Egyptian gynecologists, who tend to use the adjective "weak" to describe reproductive processes to laypersons. Thus *mibāyiḍ da'īf,* or weak ovaries, is a term used by both Egyptian physicians and patients to describe ovarian problems, particularly anovulation (Inhorn, 1994). And such "weakness" is often translated into more condemnatory terms by patients themselves, who refer to their own ovaries as "lazy" and in need of "activation."

The hormonal medications that women are given before an IVF cycle are generally viewed as "strengtheners," capable of stimulating ovarian function even in the "weakest" ovaries. However, the paradoxical problem with these agents is that they may overcome weakness in one set of organs, the ovaries, only to produce a more generalized bodily weakness apparent in the noticeable list of side effects that they produce. Indeed, in the minds of Egyptian women, IVF hormones belong in the same category as contraceptive hormones, including oral contraceptives, Depo-Provera injections, and NORPLANT, all of which are widely available in Egypt. Although their mechanisms of action and desired effects are different, all reproductively related hormonal agents are viewed as powerful drugs, which, over time, produce a long list of potential side effects, including a condition of generalized weakness characterized by enervation, loss of muscular strength and appetite, and even fainting. Furthermore, women taking pre-IVF hormones generally complain of other, more immediate debilitating side effects, including pain, bruising, and swelling at the site of injections; abdominal bloating, fluid retention, and weight gain; breast enlargement and tenderness; nausea and vomiting; and headaches, dizziness, lightheadedness, and general feelings of moodiness and depression. Women are understandably concerned about whether such bodily weakness is temporary, lasting, or even permanent, and they wonder aloud whether even worse problems, such as grave diseases like reproductive cancers, may be produced by these agents in the long term. Such concerns are especially pronounced for women who have undergone repeated cycles of ovulation induction before IVF.

In part because many women undergoing IVF feel weak and sick, they take to their beds during periods of therapy. This is especially true following embryo transfer, when successful fertilization has occurred in the laboratory, and the embryos are transferred back into the woman's uterus in the hope that at least one of them will implant. Women who pass the stage of embryo transfer virtually immobilize themselves, barely moving from bed during the two-week period until the pregnancy test is performed (or menses occurs, indicating a "failed" cycle). Basing their immobility on popular notions of pregnancy loss caused by overexertion, women hope that by remaining still and inactive, the pregnancy will "stick" or "hang" (i.e., implant) and will not "fall down," resulting in miscarriage. Women maintain this belief even though Egyptian IVF doctors usually inform patients that movement and activity have little to do with the success of implantation and that bed rest beyond the day of embryo transfer is therefore unnecessary. Indeed, those days spent in bed are rarely restful for women, who tend to brood excessively about whether the IVF trial has been successful and are thus prone to the ill effects of excessive stress (see chap. 4, this volume). The emotional devastation that follows a failed trial, furthermore, is often experienced in relative isolation, for reasons to be described below; hence it often takes women months to muster sufficient courage to repeat the procedure, assuming financial resources are available.

Success Rates.   Given the physical and emotional rollercoaster associated with IVF, Egyptian women are clearly concerned about whether their efforts will be fruitful—whether placing one's body at risk and enduring periods of immobilization will lead, ultimately, to a successful pregnancy and birth of a precious "baby of the tubes." Consequently, patients are keen to know percentages of success, and, once informed of the lower-than-average odds, they debate whether undergoing IVF is worth the physical risks, the worry, and the money, which may end up being gambled and then lost. Conscious of their position in the global arena, many Egyptian patients also wonder whether the percentages they are quoted by their physicians are equivalent to the best centers in the West. Unfortunately, because of various technical obstacles and lack of training and technique on the part of most NRT providers, local success rates in Egypt—except in the very best centers—are comparatively poor. But they are rarely presented as such to patients. Instead, patients are routinely quoted inflated success rates—generally in the 30 to 40 percent range—in order to maintain patients' hope and willingness to undergo NRT procedures. Yet such percentages are high, even by Western standards, and do not represent the take-home-baby rate, which in the West is rarely higher than 20 percent.[4]

Furthermore, many patients are given false hope that a first trial of IVF will be successful. Given all the hardships described above, it is not surprising that patients ardently hope to avoid repeated trials of IVF and are usually devastated when pregnancy is not achieved on the first attempt. With very few exceptions, most Egyptian patients also hope that the first trial of IVF will yield multiple births—ideally twins or triplets. Because of the cultural unacceptability of a one-child family, low-order multiple births mean that the "ideal" urban Egyptian family size of at least two but not more than three children can be achieved without having to resort to future IVF trials. For this reason, four to six embryos are usually transferred in any given IVF trial, and occasionally, when most of these embryos "take," so-called selective reductions through the "therapeutic" abortion of "excess" embryos are advised and performed. Nonetheless, fascination with higher-order births can be found in Egypt, as in the West, and the rare birth of IVF quadruplets and beyond generally makes headline news in the Egyptian media.

Test-Tube Babies' (and Women's) Futures

But what about these Egyptian babies of the tubes? Do their parents fear for their future well-being? The answer to this question is definitely yes. But the concerns and apprehensions of Egyptian IVF parents may be considerably different from those of their counterparts in the West.

First, concerns about the physical well-being of offspring conceived through NRTs continue to be in the forefront of Egyptian patients' minds, especially those couples who are undergoing the newest variant of IVF called intracytoplasmic sperm injection (ICSI) for cases of severe male-factor infertility. Since its introduction in the early 1990s, ICSI has created a revolution in the treatment of male infertility, which contributes to more than half of all infertility cases and has traditionally been intransigent to standard treatment protocols (Inhorn, 2002). With ICSI, men with very poor semen profiles—even true azoospermia, or lack of sperm in the ejaculate—are now able to produce a "biological" child of their own. As long as a single viable spermatozoon can be retrieved from a man's body—even through epididymal aspiration or testicular biopsy—it can be injected vis-à-vis laboratory micromanipulation techniques directly into an ovum, thereby increasing the chances of fertilization. Thus men whose only chances for having children would have been through adoption or donor insemination—both of which are prohibited on religious grounds in Egypt—are now able to conceive children "of their own" with the help of this revolutionary technology. Not surprisingly, since ICSI's arrival in Egypt in the mid-1990s and its subsequent heralding in the Egyptian media, Egyptian IVF centers have been virtually flooded with cases of often long-term, male-factor infertility—for example, 70 percent of those couples participating in my study in 1996. But the arrival of ICSI has itself generated new sets of culturally based dilemmas and constraints.

"Weakness Revisited."   Many of the men who have lived with the fact that their sperm are "weak" are clearly concerned about the biological transmission of "weakness" to their children. As with "weak ovaries," weakness is the cultural idiom used to describe male infertility in Egypt. Among the less educated, who conceptualize sperm as worms, men suffering from infertility are seen as having weak worms, incapable of carrying fetuses to women's wombs. Among the more educated clientele at Egyptian IVF centers, male infertility problems, of which there are more than ten different types, are understood in more nuanced terms as problems of sperm count or motility. Nonetheless, such male infertility problems are routinely glossed as "weakness," even in Egyptian IVF clinics, and it seems that many infertile Egyptian men take this cultural idiom to heart, feeling that they are somehow weak, defective, and even unworthy as biological progenitors. Many men in Egyptian IVF centers are openly concerned about whether they will "pass their weakness" on to their children, and this is especially pronounced among men with spermatic deformities, who wonder if their children will suffer from congenital malformations. Given the growing evidence that ICSI offspring are just as "normal" as any other population of children conceived through NRTs, Egyptian physicians attempt to reassure their male patients that their offspring will be healthy and normal. But these lingering doubts about the general health and well-being of offspring conceived from "weakness" plague many men—up to and even beyond the birth of their own evidently physically normal ICSI babies.

Aging Wives.   The wives of infertile men may share their anxieties but are also confronted with additional serious concerns of their own. For one thing, many of the women who eventually arrive at Egyptian IVF centers are "reproductively elderly," approaching or having passed the age of forty.

Some of these are women with their own infertility problems, who eventually resort to NRTs after many failed attempts at less invasive therapies. Others are the wives of infertile men who have stood by their husbands after many years of childless marriage. Unfortunately for both groups of women, the age of forty marks a key watershed, in that they themselves are no longer viewed as acceptable candidates for IVF or ICSI therapy. Because of significantly declining success rates for IVF and ICSI in women aged forty and older, most Egyptian IVF centers refuse to accept these women into their patient populations. Some Egyptian IVF doctors argue that this is a compassionate restriction, because it prevents older women from suffering the economic, physical, and psychic hardships of likely futile attempts at repeated NRT trials. Furthermore, technologies such as amniocentesis for genetic testing of fetuses are virtually undeveloped in Egypt. Although this may seem ironic, given the enthusiasm for other forms of high-tech reproductive medicine, the lack of prenatal testing clearly reflects at least three factors: (1) physicians' extreme reluctance to intervene invasively in a "God-given" pregnancy; (2) greater cultural tolerance than in the West for disability and family care giving of the disabled; and (3) the continuing criminalization of abortion in the country (Lane, 1997). Hence older women who end up conceiving through IVF or ICSI have fewer means of guaranteeing that their children will be genetically "normal," and midtrimester abortion of children with maternal age–related genetic defects is not an option anyway. In fact, many infertile Egyptian women believe that they or their husbands may be infertile precisely because God is sparing them from the birth of such a "defective" child.

However, female age restrictions in the midst of an ICSI revolution have proved particularly devastating for Egyptian wives of infertile husbands. Because contemporary Islamic, as well as Egyptian Coptic Christian, religious opinion forbids any kind of egg, embryo, or semen donation, as well as surrogacy arrangements, couples in which the wife is reproductively elderly face four difficult options: (1) to remain together permanently without children; (2) to raise orphaned foster children; (3) to partake in a polygynous marriage; or (4) to divorce so that the infertile husband can try his luck with a younger, more fecund woman. Polygyny is unacceptable to most Egyptian women today; yet the options of permanent involuntary childlessness or permanent fostering are unacceptable to a significant proportion (although not necessarily the majority) of Egyptian men, including the highly educated ones presenting to Egyptian IVF centers. Thus, sadly, cases of male-initiated divorce—between infertile men in their forties and fifties and the once-fertile but now reproductively elderly wives who stood by them, for decades in some cases—are increasing.

For their part, Egyptian physicians who perform ICSI realize this potentially untoward outcome but remain divided in their approach. Some believe that these scientific developments give infertile men the God-given right to conceive their own biological children, regardless of the marital repercussions; thus they inform their patients about ICSI, regardless of a wife's age or marital vulnerability. Others argue for a less scientific but more "compassionate" approach, refusing to inform *either* partner in such marriages that ICSI is an option. But given the way such information quickly spreads in the urban Egyptian landscape, it seems likely that men turned away at one clinic may simply seek another clinic that will accept them— with a new, more fertile second wife. Thus the gendered dimensions of this "newest" new reproductive technology reveal the ongoing nature of Egyptian patriarchy and the ways in which Egyptian Muslim women continue to remain vulnerable to Islamic personal status laws that allow relatively easy divorce when initiated by men—including infertile ones.

Envy, Secrecy, and Stigma.   Yet, even among Egyptian couples who avoid these marital outcomes and who succeed in bearing a baby of the tubes, completely happy endings are never to be assumed. For very few Egyptian parents of test-tube babies are willing to admit to anyone, outside of perhaps their closest family members, that conception occurred in anything but an "ordinary" fashion. Despite widespread public knowledge that babies of the tubes are in fact being "made" in Egypt, the actual production of such children remains in the realm of the extraordinary and is a subject of wild speculation and moral uncertainty among ordinary "fertile" Egyptians. The vast majority of patients undergoing NRT procedures are extremely concerned about issues of confidentiality, because of the social stigma and ridicule that they anticipate may be directed toward them or their baby of the tubes as the child grows up.

Moreover, widespread cultural notions of envy—resulting in harm to the pregnancy or the test-tube child itself—come into play even among the "modern," educated elite. Egyptians of all social backgrounds abide by the notion that those who covet one's success or material possessions, including one's children, may direct an envious glance—the so-called evil eye— thereby harming or "ruining" another's good fortune. As a result, most Egyptians place protective amulets on prized possessions, such as automobiles, and are never too boastful—even hiding or lying about particular accomplishments, good health, and good fortune. As has been widely documented throughout the Middle East (Inhorn, 1994), *hasad,* or envy, is considered a major etiological factor in childhood illness, and envious infertile women are considered major perpetrators of the evil eye. Although they may not intend to harm a child, they are seen as incapable of controlling their feelings of envy and are sometimes accused of causing childhood illness and even death. As a result, infertile women are often avoided by others with children, and infertile women themselves are often sensitive about attending rituals and celebrations where many children are present (Inhorn, 1996).

Given that infertile Egyptian women know all too well how society views them, they are likewise concerned about revealing their own good fortune when they eventually become pregnant through IVF or ICSI. Many women who achieve IVF or ICSI pregnancies attempt to hide the pregnancy for as long as possible. Moreover, they ask to see their physicians at their private OB-GYN clinics rather than in their IVF centers where high numbers of potentially covetous infertile patients are to be found.

In this local moral world marked by fear, envy, paranoia, and stigma, women and men who attempt NRT procedures must go it alone, that is, in relative emotional isolation. The pervasive fear of others' envy clearly militates against the formation of patient coalitions, as most Egyptian couples are reluctant to disclose their IVF or ICSI successes to other hopeful patients. Furthermore, although some patients admit that professional psychological support services or patient-led self-help groups, such as RESOLVE in the United States, would be extremely beneficial, they are quick to point out that these will never happen in Egypt, primarily because of these fears of envy and the desire to prevent stigmatization by keeping one's identity as an IVF or ICSI patient a true secret.[5] Thus those Egyptian men and women, such as Mohammed and Shahira, whose telling case is described below, experience both their hopelessness and their exaltation in silence. For they live in a society that, like many others, has yet to come to terms with the myriad implications of the new reproductive technologies being so rapidly exported around the globe.

THE CASE OF INFERTILE MOHAMMED, HIS TWO WIVES, AND HIS ICSI TWINS

Many of the issues described above are clearly revealed in the case of Mohammed,[6] a forty-three-year-old Egyptian man with a long history of infertility. Mohammed is a lawyer whose father was once a powerful politician. By Egyptian standards, Mohammed is affluent; in addition to his legal practice, he rents a villa to a foreign embassy and owns a "business center" for photocopying and office supplies. For seventeen years Mohammed was married to Hala, a woman now in her forties whom he divorced two years ago as a result of their childlessness. Relatively early in his marriage to Hala, Mohammed was told by physicians that he suffered from rather severe malefactor infertility, involving both low sperm count and poor motility. He underwent repeated courses of hormonal therapy, none of which was successful in significantly improving his sperm profile. Ultimately, he and Hala underwent several cycles of intrauterine insemination using concentrates of his sperm, as well as five cycles of IVF, three times in Germany and two times in Egypt. Each trial was unsuccessful.

According to the Egyptian physicians who undertook one of the failed trials in Mohammed's home country, it was obvious to them that Mohammed and Hala's marriage was deteriorating during the course of therapy— a deterioration they blamed on Hala's "very strong personality." After the second failed IVF trial in Egypt, Mohammed divorced Hala, who herself was never infertile but is now unlikely to remarry as her reproductive clock runs out. Mohammed, meanwhile, was remarried within a year to Shahira, a Christian woman approximately half his age. Mohammed was less interested in Shahira's "pedigree" (her college degree in tourism, with fluency in both French and English) or in her differing religious background (a Muslim man is allowed to marry a Christian woman) than in her youth, her potential fecundity, and her acceptance of his infertility problem, including her willingness to try ICSI with him.

Within a few months of their marriage, Mohammed took Shahira to one of the two Egyptian IVF clinics where he had also taken his first wife, Hala. The physicians there confirmed that because Shahira was young, with no known reproductive impairments, her chances of conceiving with ICSI were significantly greater than in Mohammed's previous IVF attempts with the aging Hala. Mohammed was delighted with the news that he and Shahira were candidates for ICSI. However, Shahira's reaction was fear. She said, "I'm very afraid of *any* operation, or anything. . . . I was *so* afraid, and I was not thinking it was going to be successful. But [the doctor] told me, 'Don't be afraid. It's easy. A small operation. It will be successful.' But I was convinced it was *not* going to be successful."

Shahira suffered from uncomfortable side effects from the hormones used to stimulate her ovulation. Her gastric ulcer symptoms were exacerbated, and she felt abdominal cramping and pain at various points in the treatment cycle. "It's too difficult doing this ICSI," Shahira explained. "*I* take all these injections, *I* come to the hospital every day, *I* prepare for the operation, *I* see the anesthesia, the doctors. It's frightening. My husband— they just take the semen from him."

Once the ICSI embryo transfer was completed, Shahira was still unconvinced of its possible efficacy. She stayed in her house and refused to go out to take the pregnancy blood test scheduled at a nearby laboratory. Finally, Mohammed had a doctor sent to their home to draw the blood sample. The pregnancy test, which was followed by more blood tests and ultrasounds, confirmed that Shahira was indeed pregnant—with twins in separate amniotic sacs.

Now it is Mohammed who is in disbelief. Every day he looks at Shahira's expanding belly and says, "Now I can't believe I will have children. I will believe it if I touch my son or daughter by myself." Shahira hopes that the birth of his ICSI twins will make Mohammed stop smoking three packs of cigarettes a day, which may be implicated in his ongoing infertility problems. For her part, Shahira is concerned about the potential difficulties associated with a twin pregnancy and a mandatory cesarean. She is also concerned about keeping the ICSI conception of her twins a secret, to be carefully guarded by Mohammed and her brother and sister. She hopes that both twins will be born live and healthy and that at least one of them will be a girl, although Mohammed hopes for a son who he can name Ahmed. If God wills and both twins survive and are normal, Shahira says she will not do ICSI again. "Once is enough," she says. "One operation, one delivery. It's too difficult and too frightening."

CONCLUSION

Mohammed and Shahira are among the "lucky" ones, for whom the fruits of globalization are literally the test-tube children they bear. But many other cautionary tales could be written of the ways in which infertile Egyptian women and men confront the realities of the NRTs currently flooding into their country. Such stories would tell of class-based barriers to NRT access among the Egyptian lower and middle classes; the necessity of income-generating labor migration even among the upper classes and the search for NRT solutions on month-long holidays "back home"; the unavailability of drugs and the creation of pharmaceutical "suitcase trading" across national borders; the greed and arrogance of physicians who are in it for the money and treat their NRT-seeking patients like furniture; and morally based anxieties about the handling of biogenetic substances in behind-the-scenes places like IVF laboratories.

In this chapter, I have focused primarily on one aspect of NRT treatment seeking in Egypt, namely, on issues of embodiment, or how local, culturally shaped knowledge of, beliefs about, and experiences of the human body serve as constraints on the practice and use of NRTs in this country. In so doing, I have attempted to highlight the cultural variability inherent in perceptions of the reproductive body and its physiology, as well as notions of bodily risk and vulnerability, safety and efficacy, and the social stigmatization associated with "abnormal" bodies and births.

As the NRTs become further entrenched in the urban Egyptian landscape and other forms of high-tech reproductive technology become available in this setting, new dilemmas and new local cultural responses to these forms of globalization are likely to arise. Indeed, the pace of change evident in the production of NRTs themselves—and the rapidity of their globalization and penetration into far reaches of the so-called Third world—is certain to engender much that is "new": new social imaginaries, new forms of cultural production, and new utopias, as well as new dystopias, new forms of local resistance, and new arenas of cultural constraint.

For all of these reasons and for others as well, following the globalization of NRTs into the new millennium—in places such as Egypt and elsewhere around the globe—seems a worthy endeavor. For, the examination of these Western technologies in non-Western places offers an illuminating case study of local-global intersections and particularly the importance of inter-rogating what is "local" in an increasingly "global" world.

NOTES

The research on which this chapter is based was supported by grants from the National Science Foundation, the Fulbright Institute of International Education, and the U.S. Department of Education's Fulbright-Hays Research Abroad Program (the latter of which provided separate grants for each field period). I am grateful to these granting agencies for their support and to the hospitals in Egypt, including Shatby University Hospital, Nozha International Hospital, and Nile Badrawi Hospital, where I was allowed to conduct my research. I am also grateful to the many physicians at Shatby Hospital who facilitated my early field research and to Drs. Gamal Serour, Mohamed Yehia, and Salah Zaki, who were instrumental in allowing me to undertake my later research in Egyptian IVF centers. My research in these centers was immeasurably aided by my able and sympathetic research assistant, Tayseer Salem. Finally, and most significantly, I could not have conducted this research without the goodwill, patience, and extraordinary candor of my many infertile Egyptian informants, who opened up to me despite their desires to remain anonymous as IVF seekers. My feelings of gratitude toward them are profound.

1. Shatby Hospital's IVF center opened in 1991, and the first Alexandrian "baby of the tubes" was born and heralded in the Egyptian media in early 1992. However, since those early publicity-driven days of "free," government-sponsored IVF, fewer and fewer test-tube babies have been born to poor Egyptian women. As Egypt's one and only *public* IVF program, the Shatby Hospital IVF clinic continues to run but on such a low volume that very few patients receive treatment and success rates are compromised. For the most part, the physicians charged with running this public clinic put their energies into their private IVF practices, which, as is typical for Egyptian physicians working in the public sector, they run on the side.

2. Such "preformation" models also dominated early European biomedical thinking after Antonie van Leeuwenhoek discovered sperm through the microscope and declared that he found a homunculus, or little person, folded inside the head of the sperm (Laqueur, 1990). Such ideas were probably brought to Egypt in the nineteenth century with the advent of British colonial medicine (Inhorn, 1994). However, a monogenetic theory of procreation has an indigenous origin as well, which can be traced back to the pharaonic period in Egypt (Inhorn, 1994).

3. Prescheduled cesarean deliveries are now widely touted by Egyptian gynecologists to IVF patients as the easiest and "safest" form of childbirth, avoiding as they do the potentially harmful exertions of natural labor and vaginal delivery. Thus

mothers of IVF babies uniformly consent to cesareans without ever questioning their value or necessity.

4. In summer 1996, for example, it became known to me that one Egyptian IVF center had prepared more than thirty patient couples for the IVF variant called intracytoplasmic sperm injection (ICSI), with no pregnancies achieved by summer's end (i.e., yielding a 0 percent "un-success rate").

5. Furthermore, psychotherapy of any kind is generally associated with severe forms of mental illness. Thus it is highly stigmatized and rarely do Egyptians go into therapy, as is relatively common in the West. When one Egyptian IVF clinic advised psychological counseling before patients' enrollment in IVF/ICSI, few patients could be convinced to attend sessions with a psychologist. Thus the effort was dropped.

6. This name and all others used here are pseudonyms.

REFERENCES

Appadurai, A. (1996). *Modernity at large: Cultural dimensions of globalization.* Minneapolis: University of Minnesota Press.

Bourdieu, P. (1977). *Outline of a theory of practice.* Translated by Richard Nice. New York: Cambridge University Press.

DeClerque, J., Tsui, A. O., Abul-Ata, M. F., & Barcelona, D. (1986). Rumor, misinformation and oral contraceptive use in Egypt. *Social Science & Medicine, 23,* 83–92.

Delaney, C. (1991). *The seed and the soil: Gender and cosmology in Turkish village society.* Berkeley: University of California Press.

Early, E. A. (1993). *Baladi women of Cairo: Playing with an egg and a stone.* Boulder, CO: Lynne Rienner.

Egyptian Fertility Care Society. (1995). *Community-based study of the prevalence of infertility and its etiological factors in Egypt: (1) The population-based study.* Cairo: Egyptian Fertility Care Society.

Freeman, C. (1999). *High tech and high heels in the global economy: Women, work, and pink-collar identities in the Caribbean.* Durham, NC: Duke University Press.

Ginsburg, F. D., & Rapp, R. (1995). Introduction: Conceiving the new world order. In F. D. Ginsburg & R. Rapp (Eds.), *Conceiving the new world order: The global politics of reproduction* (pp. 1–17). Berkeley: University of California Press.

Hannerz, U. (1996). *Transnational connections: Culture, people, places.* London: Routledge.

Harvey, D. (1989). *The condition of postmodernity: An enquiry into the origins of cultural change.* Cambridge, MA: Blackwell.

Inhorn, M. C. (1994). *Quest for conception: Gender, infertility, and Egyptian medical traditions.* Philadelphia: University of Pennsylvania Press.

Inhorn, M. C. (1996). *Infertility and patriarchy: The cultural politics of gender and family life in Egypt.* Philadelphia: University of Pennsylvania Press.

Inhorn, M. C. (2000) . The quest for conception in Egypt: Gender, class, and religion in infertility therapy decisions. In F. W. Twine & H. Ragone (Eds.), *Ideologies and technologies of motherhood.* London: Routledge.

Inhorn, M. C. (2001). Money, marriage, and morality: Constraints on IVF treatment seeking among infertile Egyptian couples. In C. M. Obermeyer (Ed.), *Cultural perspectives on reproductive health.* Oxford: Oxford University Press.

Inhorn, M. C. (2002). "The worms are weak": Male infertility and patriarchal paradoxes in Egypt. Special issue on Islamic masculinities, L. Ouzgane (Ed.). *Men and Masculinities.*

Kahn, S. M. (2000). *Reproducing Jews: A cultural account of assisted conception in Israel.* Durham, NC: Duke University Press.

Kleinman, A.M. (1992). Local worlds of suffering: An interpersonal focus for ethnographies of illness experience. *Qualitative Health Research, 2,* 127–134.

Kleinman, A. M. (1995). *Writing at the margin: Discourse between anthropology and medicine.* Berkeley: University of California Press.

Lane, S. D. (1997). Gender and health: Abortion in urban Egypt. In M. E. Bonine (Ed.), *Population, poverty, and politics in Middle East cities* (pp. 208–234). Gainesville: University Press of Florida.

Laqueur, T. (1990). *Making sex: Body and gender from the Greeks to Freud.* Cambridge, MA: Harvard University Press.

Martin, E. (1991). The egg and the sperm: How science has constructed a romance based on stereotypical male-female roles. *Signs, 16,* 485–501.

Mohanty, C. T., Russo, A., & Torres, L. (Eds.). (1991). *Third World women and the politics of feminism.* Bloomington: Indiana University Press.

Population Reference Bureau. (2001). *World population data sheet: Demographic data and estimates for the countries and regions of the world.* Washington, DC: Population Reference Bureau.

Rapp, R. (1988). Moral pioneers: Women, men and fetuses on a frontier of reproductive technology. In E. H. Baruch, A. F. D'Adamo, Jr., & J. Seager (Eds.), *Embryos, ethics, and women's rights: Exploring the new reproductive technologies* (pp. 101–116). Special issue of *Women & Health, 13(1–2).* New York: Haworth Press.

Stephens, A. (1995). Fertile ground. *Egypt Today (February),* 73–80.

Stycos, J. M., Said, H. A. A., Avery, R., & Fridman, S. (1988). *Community development and family planning: An Egyptian experiment.* Boulder, CO: Westview Press.

FIFTEEN

Rabbis and Reproduction

The Uses of New Reproductive Technologies among Ultraorthodox Jews in Israel

Susan Martha Kahn

What are the contemporary attitudes toward new reproductive technologies (NRTs) among ultraorthodox Jews in Israel? Ultraorthodox Jews have embraced the practical and theoretical challenges presented by NRTs and have created innovative if often contradictory rulings about their appropriate use. That they inhabit a world governed by ancient traditions and rooted in a two-thousand-year-old legal system has not prevented them from adapting the newest technologies to their way of life, including the latest techniques to conceive persons.

In this chapter, I argue that the phenomenon of NRT use among ultraorthodox Jews in Israel is instructive on many levels. We learn something about how the Jewish legal system works and how it has evolved to allow for innovation (provided the impulse toward innovation preserves and reinforces foundational assumptions, in this case, about the Jewish family). We learn how rabbinic attitudes toward these technologies have created remarkable applications for the treatment of infertility among ultraorthodox Jews, applications that embody innovative and counterintuitive understandings of reproductive genetic material. And we also learn from what is absent from this rabbinic discussion: namely, the voices and experiences of ultraorthodox women. Specifically, we must ask what happens to ultraorthodox Jewish women, whose bodies bear the brunt of most high-tech reproductive interventions, when law and technology converge to make fertility treatment all but inevitable. Finally, an examination of the social uses of NRTs by ultraorthodox Jews reveals how these can be adapted in highly specific ways to achieve highly specific outcomes—in this case, to assist ultraorthodox Jews to realize the biblical commandment to "be fruitful and multiply."

This study is based on my analysis of the Halakhic (Jewish legal) literature regarding infertility and on fieldwork I conducted in Jerusalem-area infertility clinics, one of which caters almost exclusively to ultraorthodox Jews.[1] I include in this sphere of fieldwork conversations with patients and interviews with Israeli rabbis, infertility doctors, and clinic staff who counsel infertile ultraorthodox Jews.

NEW REPRODUCTIVE TECHNOLOGIES AND PRONATALISM IN ISRAEL

It is important to understand the social context in which ultraorthodox Jews in Israel gain access to the new reproductive technologies, for these technologies are widely available to all segments of the population in Israel, both religious and secular, Jewish and non-Jewish. There are more infertility clinics per capita in Israel than in any other country in the world (at least four times the number per capita in the United States), and Israeli fertility specialists are global leaders in the research and development of these technologies. In addition, Israeli lawmakers have created legislation that guarantees insurance coverage for these treatments at unprecedented rates: not only are less invasive technologies and their associated treatments heavily subsidized, so are in vitro fertilization (IVF) and other advanced treatments. Indeed, every Israeli citizen is entitled to receive unlimited rounds of IVF, up to the birth of two live children, as part of their basic basket of health services.[2] Moreover, these subsidies are available to Israelis regardless of marital status, which means that even unmarried women may receive the equivalent of thousands of dollars of infertility treatment at the state's expense. In March 1996 Israel became the first country in the world to legalize surrogacy agreements that are regulated by a publicly appointed government commission; since that time, numerous surrogacy contracts have been successfully negotiated and carried out (Shalev, 1998).

Contrast this extraordinary state support for reproductive technology with the striking degree to which treatments that limit family size remain unsubsidized in Israel. Family planning services do not receive state support and are funded on a voluntary and charitable basis. Moreover, contraceptives, unlike fertility treatment, are not included in the basic medical services broadly subsidized by Israeli health insurance. Officials from the Ministry of Health explain that contraceptives are not subsidized because of lack of funds. Rather, funds earmarked for reproductive services are simply allocated to treatments and programs that encourage and enable women to give birth rather than to those that limit reproductive productivity (Reminnick, 1996). This attitude is reflected in the regulation of abortion in Israel as well. Abortion is legal, although it is subsidized only for those under the age of seventeen or over forty, for those whose pregnancies were the result of rape or incest, for those for whom pregnancy would endanger the woman's health, or in cases in which the fetus is suspected to be malformed physically or mentally. These regulations make it difficult for healthy, married women to receive abortions.

There are many explanations for this overt pronatalism in Israel. Since the establishment of the state of Israel in 1948, there have been a range of state policies explicitly aimed at increasing Jewish birthrates, from Ben Gurion's rewards to "heroine mothers" to present-day economic incentives to have large families.[3] This interest in increasing Jewish birthrates has historic roots in early propaganda about the need to produce soldiers to defend the fledgling state; it also comes from perceived demographic concerns about maintaining parity with Palestinian and Arab birthrates. For some Israeli Jews, having children is a direct response to the loss of the six million Jews in the Holocaust and reflects a desire to "replace" those who were killed. Other Jews have immigrated to Israel from traditional cultures that are very child centered. And finally, many Israelis bear a range of historical sensitivities to practices designed to limit the number of Jewish births, given that such policies were often employed in various diasporic contexts as part of other anti-Semitic measures.

WHO ARE ULTRAORTHODOX JEWS?

There are approximately thirteen million Jews in the world; of these, close to 600,000 are ultraorthodox.[4] About one-half, or 300,000 ultraorthodox Jews, live in Israel, a country in which the Jewish population is approximately six million. This means that ultraorthodox Jews make up just over 5 percent of the Israeli Jewish population (Heilman, 1992, p. 12). Ultraorthodox Jews are largely descended from Jews who fled eastern Europe in the years before and after World War II. They maintain strict adherence to Jewish law, and those who live in Israel make every effort to limit their interactions with the secular Israeli society in which they live.[5] They often live in semi-isolated enclaves and neighborhoods; they wear distinctive clothing that clearly sets them apart, and most speak the traditional European language, Yiddish, instead of the modern Israeli language, Hebrew. They are largely non-Zionist, in that they do not believe in the legitimacy of a secular Israeli state that is not governed by Jewish law. The vast majority do not serve in the Israeli army, which is mandatory for other Israeli Jews—a fact that creates no small amount of resentment among the secular population. Indeed, negative myths and stereotypes about ultraorthodox Jews abound among secular Jews in Israel, myths and stereotypes that are derived from certain assumptions about the ultraorthodox way of life and are nurtured by their isolation from mainstream Israeli society. Hostility between secular and ultraorthodox Jews in Israel is also generated by the complex ways in which ultraorthodox Jews are economically dependent on the secular Jewish community. Many ultraorthodox educational and social institutions are heavily subsidized by the secular Israeli government through the taxes it collects from secular citizens.

Although generalizations about cultural similarities among different segments of the ultraorthodox population often obscure more than they reveal, they may be cautiously proffered, because all ultraorthodox Jews share certain central cultural ideals. The core values that inform ultraorthodox life are strict observance of Jewish law as interpreted by ultraorthodox rabbis, personal responsibility, and the giving of charity; continual efforts are made to actualize these values in daily life. Ultraorthodox men are meant to dedicate their lives to the study of Torah, and indeed, many ultraorthodox men do so in all-male institutions called yeshivas. In a recent study, the economist Eli Berman (2000) found that almost two-thirds of all working-age males in the ultraorthodox community are not gainfully employed. Ultraorthodox women are meant to dedicate their lives to bearing and raising children, and many also work outside the home to support their families. Financial assistance, either in the form of yeshiva stipends for the men or in the form of generous government subsidies for dependent children, also helps to support these families. Nevertheless, many ultraorthodox families in Israel live well below the poverty line.

According to Berman's (2000) study, ultraorthodox Jewish communities are the fastest-growing segment of the Israeli Jewish population and are increasing annually by 4 to 5 percent, or doubling every eighteen years. By 1993 the number of live births projected for the average ultraorthodox woman increased to 6.9, up from 5.8 in 1980. This contrasts markedly with the projected birthrates for other population groups in Israel. For the average Israeli Jewish woman in 1993, the projected number of births was 2.6, a decrease from the 1980 projection of 2.9. In other words, the average ultraorthodox woman in Israel can now expect to have three times as many children as her nonultraorthodox counterpart.[6] This high birthrate among ultraorthodox Jews helps to boost overall fertility among Israeli Jews to levels that are higher than any economically developed nation—twice as high as those in western Europe (Reminnick, 1998). When birthrates are so high, the desire to have children, let alone the social pressure to do so, is great. Unwanted childlessness in these communities is therefore as socially stigmatized as it is personally painful.

INFERTILITY TREATMENT: PRACTICAL CONCERNS
FOR ULTRAORTHODOX JEWS

It is in this broader social context that ultraorthodox Jews in Israel seek out infertility treatment.[7] Unlike their secular counterparts, however, ultraorthodox Jews seek out infertility treatments only with explicit rabbinic guidance and in close consultation with rabbinic authorities. Many will seek treatment only in Israeli hospitals that operate under close rabbinic supervision, although some seek treatment at the larger secular hospitals that contract rabbinic supervision when necessary, as discussed below.

A Jerusalem-based organization called PUAH operates as the central clearinghouse for advice, information, and referrals for ultraorthodox Jews who wish to seek fertility treatment. The acronym PUAH, which stands for Poriyoot veRefuah Alpi HaHalakha (Institute for Fertility Treatment According to Jewish Law), is not coincidentally the name of one of the biblical midwives who saved Jewish babies from the Pharaoh's genocidal decree in Egypt. PUAH acts as the liaison between ultraorthodox couples seeking guidance for their fertility treatments, ultraorthodox rabbis who determine the appropriate uses of these technologies, and infertility doctors who provide treatments for ultraorthodox Jews. Because most infertility specialists in Israel are not ultraorthodox, PUAH maintains an active list of those infertility specialists known to be sensitive to the special needs and concerns of ultraorthodox Jews. PUAH performs an important function for these nonreligious doctors by translating rabbinic concerns and provisos about these technologies into medical language, thereby ensuring that rabbinic theory turns into medical practice.

Before beginning infertility treatment, an ultraorthodox couple must first obtain a letter from two doctors that diagnoses and confirms their infertility. Couples must then seek specific rabbinic advice about the appropriate treatment for their specific infertility problem from an authoritative rabbinic decisor. If a couple does not already have a relationship with an authoritative rabbinic decisor, PUAH refers them to well-known rabbis from the same ethnic and/or ultraorthodox subgroup for advice and assistance. In other words, an infertile couple of Ashkenazi (European) heritage would be referred to an appropriate rabbi of Ashkenazi heritage, and a couple of Sephardi (Spanish–Middle Eastern) heritage would be referred to a rabbi of Sephardi heritage.[8] Given that rabbinic rulings on the appropriate uses of NRTs vary widely, with some rabbis being significantly more lenient and permissive and others being significantly more restrictive, two couples with the identical infertility problem may receive entirely different directives about which infertility treatment they may use simply because they have sought advice from rabbis of different ethnic or religious subgroups. Moreover, because each couple's infertility problem is evaluated individually in its particular context, two couples from the same ethnic or religious subgroup with the same infertility problem may consult the same rabbi and receive different directives about the appropriate fertility treatment, either due to differences in age between the couples, different mediating circumstances, or other factors. In short, each couple's situation is evaluated on a case-by-case basis.

In addition, rabbis must negotiate a range of practical questions regarding the Halakhic hazards of various forms of reproductive technology. The entire process of handling and manipulating reproductive genetic material is a source of enormous rabbinic concern, and laboratory procedures involving the preparation and combination of sperm and ova are integral to many forms of infertility treatment. During these procedures, sperm and ova must be withdrawn or procured from human bodies by a variety of methods, transferred through pipettes, catheters, and syringes to petri dishes and test tubes, manipulated, treated, or "washed" by trained technicians, placed into new petri dishes and test tubes, and then transferred back into pipettes and catheters for reimplantation in a woman's body. These procedures take place in busy laboratories where several patients' reproductive material may be circulating at any one time. To ensure that there is no untoward mixing of sperm and eggs, all petri dishes and test tubes are clearly marked with patients' names and all instruments are used only once and then discarded. Potential problems arise when lab technicians mistakenly reuse pipettes or other instruments, particularly when transferring or working with sperm. In such instances, sperm from one procedure may become inadvertently mixed with sperm from another procedure, creating the potential for an unintended fertilization and subsequent pregnancy. To avoid such mistakes, which are obviously undesirable for anyone but which would have disastrous kinship consequences for ultraorthodox Jews (as explained below), Halakhic infertility treatment inspectors called *mashgichot* are employed by hospitals in Israel where ultraorthodox patients are treated. These mashgichot are all ultraorthodox women. They receive training from rabbis who educate them as to the Halakhic importance of their duties,[9] and from doctors, who explain the mechanics of laboratory procedures. The mashgichot sit in infertility laboratories and watch to make sure that instruments are used and disposed of properly, that test tubes containing sperm and petri dishes containing eggs are appropriately matched, and that embryos are implanted in the woman for whom they are designated. PUAH is actively involved in coordinating training programs for mashgichot and for recruiting them.

In the infertility laboratory in which I did fieldwork, mashgichot were employed full time and monitored every procedure that involved reproductive genetic material. The mashgichot and the lab technicians worked side by side, with the mashgichot literally peering over the technicians' shoulders all day long as they did their jobs. Amazingly, there seemed to be little animosity bred from what would seem to be an annoyance; on the contrary, one lab technician said she felt there was a need for supervision. "Four eyes are always better than two," she said, "and we also don't want to make any mistakes."

One *mashgicha* (singular of *mashgichot*) told me that all of this technology would work only if God Almighty wanted it to work; she explained that what she does is "holy work" and is more important than what the doctors and scientists do to achieve pregnancy.

INFERTILITY TREATMENT: THEORETICAL CONCERNS FOR ULTRAORTHODOX JEWS

It is clear that there are a plethora of practical concerns that must be negotiated in order for ultraorthodox Jews to receive infertility treatment. Let us now examine some of the theoretical questions that have fueled the intense and ongoing rabbinic debates about these issues. First, it must be understood that there is nothing unusual about debate and disagreement in the ultraorthodox Jewish world. Since rabbinic decision making is, by its very nature, decentralized and variable yet binding, there exists a great diversity of rabbinic opinion on many issues, from the number of hours one waits to drink milk after eating meat to the appropriate way to procure sperm for medical analysis.

Rabbinic debates about reproductive technology began substantively in the 1940s with debates about artificial insemination and continue today. By the 1990s many of the questions fundamental to the appropriate use of reproductive technology have been effectively resolved, although there are large and vocal minorities in the rabbinic world who vehemently reject the majority opinions. The dissenting opinions of these rabbinic decisors directly limit the choices available to their followers.

Artificial Insemination

Artificial insemination using Jewish sperm, either from the husband or from a Jewish donor, raises numerous Halakhic questions that have been central to rabbinic debate. These questions range from practical concerns regarding sperm procurement to more complex concerns regarding the act of artificial insemination and its conceptual repercussions.

For example, one of the central issues of rabbinic concern is, does artificial insemination with Jewish donor sperm from a third party constitute adultery?[10] If so, it must be prohibited, as the children born of adulterous unions, *mamzerim*, carry a range of severe and intractable social stigmas. The traditional Halakhic definition of adultery is sexual intercourse that occurs between a married Jewish woman and a Jewish man who is not her husband. According to certain rabbinic interpretations, the sin in adultery is not confined to the physical act of intercourse but inheres in the resulting conception as well. Therefore, the resulting stigma is indelibly stamped on the children who are born from such unions. In other words, the physical act of illicit sexual intercourse between a man and a woman has a direct relationship to the subsequent biological act of the sperm and egg joining in conception.

If this definition of adultery is applied to fertility treatments using Jewish donor sperm from a third party, then certainly a married Jewish woman's egg should be prohibited from achieving conception with sperm that has been procured from a Jewish man who is not her husband, because the child so conceived would be effectively the product of an adulterous union. As a result of these rabbinic concerns about the status of children conceived with Jewish donor sperm from a third party, its use is entirely prohibited for ultraorthodox Jews facing severe male-factor infertility.

The rabbinic definition of adultery refers only to illicit sexual unions between Jews; it does not refer to sexual unions between Jews and non-Jews. An interesting possibility is thus presented; if a Jewish woman is married to an infertile Jewish man and is inseminated with non-Jewish donor sperm instead of Jewish donor sperm from a third party, the resulting conception will not have adulterous overtones. The child so conceived will therefore not be a *mamzer* and yet he or she *will* be a full-fledged Jew, as Jewishness is conferred through the matriline. And so it is in the rulings of the majority of contemporary rabbinic decisors who allow for artificial insemination by third-party donor, provided that the donor sperm that is used in these cases is donated by a non-Jew.[11]

Artificial insemination with non-Jewish donor sperm is not the only innovative solution for male-factor infertility. Some rabbis have advocated IVF and embryo transfer (ET) as another possible avenue for treating male-factor infertility with donor sperm while circumventing the adulterous combination of sperm and eggs. For there is a clear Halakhic distinction between the act of sperm being introduced into the vagina of a woman and the act of an embryo being placed in a woman's uterus (or fallopian tube) as the prohibition against adultery is derived from the biblical verse, "Thou shalt not implant thy seed into thy neighbor's wife" (Lev. 18:20). The prohibition, then, is against putting "seed" in thy neighbor's wife; it is not against putting an embryo in her, and it is clear that an embryo is a fundamentally different entity than sperm. Thus IVF and ET are preferred by many rabbis as a form of infertility treatment that does not violate the literal Halakhic precepts against adultery (Waldenburg, 1982).

Certainly, the advent of intracytoplasmic sperm injection (ICSI) in the mid-1990s has decreased the practical need to use donor sperm from a third party altogether. With ICSI, individual sperm cells are retrieved and injected into oocytes in the laboratory, allowing men with extremely low sperm counts to contribute their own genetic material to conception instead of using third-party donor sperm. Many of the Halakhic problems intrinsic to sperm donation from a third party have been thus eliminated. ICSI has quickly become common practice in IVF clinics in Israel.

The confluence of rabbinic innovation and technological possibility has a range of remarkable applications. Take, for example, the following ethnographic anecdote about a couple who was treated by one of the infertility specialists I interviewed in Jerusalem.

After being diagnosed with severe male-factor infertility and receiving medical advice that the only treatment was artificial insemination by donor, the couple in question consulted their rabbi, who advised them to receive treatment using non-Jewish donor sperm. This was not unusual for the reasons outlined above. What was unusual was the way they dealt with the problem of the husband's status as a Kohen, a patrilineal status that designates membership in the priestly class, a status which passes from father to son. The woman was given hormonal treatment to stimulate her ovaries so that they would produce an abundance of eggs. These eggs were then surgically removed and fertilized with the donated non-Jewish sperm, and the resulting embryos were implanted in her uterus. As often happens in these cases, an overabundance of fertilized embryos began to grow in the uterus and the woman had to undergo an "embryo reduction" to prevent the spontaneous abortion of all the embryos. In this case, the couple had access to advanced technology that allowed the doctor to determine the sex of the developing embryos. The couple had the embryos sexed and then asked to have the male embryos aborted so that only daughters would be born. Since Kohen status is passed through the patriline from father to son, sons born to a man who is a Kohen would be expected to perform the many public duties of a Kohen. These duties include the recitation of the "priestly benediction" in synagogue and the observance of restrictions imposed on a Kohen, including not visiting cemeteries and not marrying divorced women. But sons born from non-Jewish donor sperm do not inherit identity from their Jewish social fathers, so a son conceived with non-Jewish donor sperm whose social father is a Kohen is not a Kohen himself (even though some rabbis have innovatively ruled that in such a case the son could inherit Kohen status from his mother if her father was a Kohen) (Auerbach, 1958). This couple decided, then, that because daughters born to a Kohen do not have the public obligations of a Kohen, a daughter born from non-Jewish donor sperm would avoid the social expectations that would be demanded of her brother. By choosing to have daughters, this couple succeeded in having legitimate Jewish children while avoiding Halakhic and social complications related to the patrilineal inheritance of Kohen status. This story offers a remarkable contrast to popular accounts of how sex-determining technologies have been used to ensure the birth of boys in other cultural contexts.

Ovum Donation

The Halakhic questions regarding ovum donation are extremely complex and are made more difficult by the fact that Jewishness is conferred through the matriline, so any concerns about determining the origins of maternity become concerns about determining the origins of Jewishness. Contemporary rabbis seeking to legislate for the appropriate uses of NRTs have to isolate and reify the essential elements of maternity, which makes for some dizzying and as yet unresolved debates about where Jewishness comes from. Are Jews born from Jewish ova? From Jewish wombs? From some combination of the two? Persuasive rabbinic arguments have been made that, in light of these new technologies, maternity should be understood to have both a genetic and a gestational source and that both variables should be considered in the determination of a child's identity.[12] Other traditional precedents strongly suggest, however, that maternity is solely established at birth—precedents that have persuaded the majority of contemporary orthodox rabbis that gestation and parturition should continue to be the sole determinants of maternity and, ergo, the fundamental source of Jewish identity. [13]

This Halakhic crisis, whereby the determination of maternity has been so profoundly destabilized by the advent of ovum-related technologies, has not prevented the practice of ovum donation, however. The drive to reproduce and the technological potential presented by ovum donation seem to have superseded any desire to await conclusive rabbinic rulings on the subject, even among the ultraorthodox population. To be sure, as with artificial insemination, ultraorthodox Jews follow the opinions of different rabbis, and some rabbis are much more lenient than others when it comes to ovum donation.

The Halakhic questions inherent in ovum donation echo rabbinic concerns about artificial insemination, particularly with regard to whether it is preferable for an ultraorthodox Jewish woman to receive a donated ovum from a Jewish or a non-Jewish woman. The practical questions regarding ovum donation are fundamentally different, however, for unlike sperm, which can be readily obtained and frozen, ova must be surgically extracted from a woman's hormonally hyperstimulated ovaries and then fertilized within hours or else they expire.

I asked the office manager of PUAH about the use of donated non-Jewish eggs to conceive Jewish children. He explained that for those rabbis who believe that maternal identity is determined at parturition, a Jewish woman can give birth to a Jewish baby even if the baby is conceived with a non-Jewish egg. Other rabbis who believe in the genetic basis for maternal identity suggest that a child born of a non-Jewish egg to a Jewish mother needs to be converted to "sanctify the people of Israel" (Bleich, 1991, pp. 88–

89).[14] In practice, potential egg recipients are informed of the ethnic and religious identity of the egg donor and may refuse to accept an egg donation from a woman on those bases, depending on her rabbi's rulings regarding ovum donation.

ETHNOGRAPHIC SILENCES

Unfortunately, no in-depth ethnographic research has been done on how ultraorthodox Jews experience fertility treatments. Because this population is extremely resistant to efforts of social scientists to survey and question them about any issue, let alone an issue like infertility, which is both intensely personal and highly stigmatized, it is difficult to draw all but the sketchiest conclusions about individual attitudes toward and experiences of these treatments. In interviews with infertility specialists and in informal conversations with infertile ultraorthodox patients who were receiving treatments in the infertility clinics in which I did fieldwork, I learned that most ultraorthodox couples who are undergoing infertility treatment do so quietly, and, in fact, many try to keep it a secret. They are concerned that if their problems with fertility become known, the stigma may devolve onto their children, making it difficult for them to find spouses when they are adults, since they, too, may be assumed to have difficulty with conception. Although there is no Halakhic injunction to overcome infertility, the social pressure to pursue these treatments remains intense. One ultraorthodox woman I encountered in an infertility clinic in Jerusalem was receiving extensive IVF treatments, including hormonal injections and the surgical extraction of her ova, because she had been diagnosed with secondary infertility after the birth of her fifth child. Everyone else in her neighborhood had at least eight children, and she was desperate to do what she could to keep up.

What was particularly troubling about the methodological difficulties in gaining access to the lived experience of infertility treatment among ultraorthodox Jews was the silence of ultraorthodox women. Rabbinic debates and directives about these technologies are articulated by ultraorthodox rabbis, all of whom are male and all of whom are primarily concerned about the Halakhic implications of conceiving Jews through assisted reproduction. Ultraorthodox women's opinions about these treatments, let alone their experiences of invasive, ongoing, and often futile treatments, are of secondary concern at best, and they certainly have no formal outlet beyond the individual's complaint to her doctor or rabbi. Such silencing is particularly deafening when women are under intense pressure to bear children, when this pressure is reinforced by rabbinic directives that explicitly prescribe fertility treatment, and when fertility treatment is provided by the state virtually free of charge. Under these circumstances, there is little room and few excuses for noncompliance with the technological pursuit of motherhood.

The convergence of pronatalist social pressure, rabbinic permission, and economic accessibility makes fertility treatment all but inevitable for infertile ultraorthodox women in Israel. How ironic it is, then, that so many of the hormonal therapies and surgical procedures integral to these high-tech treatments are performed on their bodies regardless of whether the fertility problem is theirs or their husbands'.

Recent accounts of assisted conception describe the ways in which women experience infertility treatment in less coercive cultural contexts, where these treatments are more costly and the imperative to reproduce is not reinforced by the mandates of religious authorities. These studies suggest that women seek out such treatments on a more explicitly voluntary basis as consumers living in consumer-oriented societies (Franklin, 1997; Sandelowski, 1993).

Ultraorthodox women who undergo infertility treatment in Israel do not do so as atomized consumers in a free-market context; they do so as participants in a pronatalist religious system and as citizens of a pronatalist state. Though it is unlikely that they would articulate criticism of these treatments, for the imperative to reproduce is one they presumably share as ultraorthodox Jews, the contours of their compliance remain to be charted and the narratives of their fertility treatments remain to be told. Until we hear their stories, we are left with their silence.

NOTES

1. This study emerges out of a larger project in which I examined the social uses of new reproductive technologies in Israel more broadly (Kahn, 2000).

2. The National Health Insurance Law (1994) provides universal coverage for all resident Israelis, both Jewish and Arab. However, while Jewish residents of the Occupied Territories are covered by this law, Palestinian residents are not. The law guarantees that every Israeli citizen has the right to receive health care and obligates health funds to accept all applicants as members and to provide them with a basic basket of services.

3. In the 1950s David Ben Gurion gave 100-lira awards to "Heroine Mothers" who had ten or more children (a policy that was discontinued after it became apparent that more Israeli Arab women were receiving these awards than Israeli Jewish women). In 1967 the Israeli demographic center was established "to act systematically to realize a demographic policy directed at creating an atmosphere and the conditions for encouraging a birth rate, which is so vital to the future of the Jewish people." In 1968 the Fund for Encouraging Birth was established to offer subsidized housing loans and increased child allowances for Jewish families with three or more children. In 1983 the Law on Families Blessed with Children was passed, which

made provisions for a host of subsidies for families with three or more children (Yuval-Davis, 1987). Today the Israeli government grants small allowances to families for the birth of each child.

4. Ultraorthodox Jews are known as *haredim* in Hebrew, a Hebrew word that comes from the biblical phrase in Isaiah, "Hear the word of the Lord, you who tremble *[haredim]* at His word" (66:5). "Ultraorthodox" is not considered a pejorative term.

5. The ultraorthodox community is not geographically isolated in Israel. Ultraorthodox Jews live in the United States, Canada, South America, and indeed all over the world. Despite their geographic dispersion and the fact that they are divided into more than forty sects, each of which has distinct customs, the laws they follow and their dependence on rabbinic guidance to resolve conflicts and answer questions about their lives remain remarkably uniform.

6. One reason for this increase in birthrates among ultraorthodox Jews is suggested by Israeli (1997). Israeli argues that the high fertility rate among the ultraorthodox is attributable to evolving social norms that encourage childbirth, such as low marital ages (20–24 for men, 18–21 for women). She suggests that the rising fertility rate among the ultraorthodox "serves the present goals of ultraorthodox society by contributing to its growth, preserving the family structure and role distribution, and enhancing its patriarchal forces" (Israeli, 1997, p.16). She points out that after the Holocaust, average ultraorthodox families had 4 to 5 children and that since then birthrates have steadily climbed to present-day levels where 12 children are considered "a respectable family."

7. It is important to point out that infertile Jews are under no strict obligation to take extraordinary measures to overcome their infertility and that there are Halakhic precedents that suggest that if a couple is unable to have children, the commandment to be fruitful and multiply no longer applies, for one can only be commanded to do what one is capable of (Dorff, 1998, p. 41).

8. "Sephardi" literally denotes "Spanish" heritage but is commonly used in Israel to include Jews of Mizrachi, that is, North African or Asian, heritage as well.

9. It was explained to me that all of the maschigchot are women, because women patients in the clinics are often partially naked in the course of their treatments, an immodest work environment for a male ultraorthodox Jew.

10. Additional rabbinic questions regarding artificial insemination include the following: Has a married Jewish woman who consents to artificial insemination by donor consented to a form of adulterous relationship, and must she therefore be punished as an adulteress? Is the sperm donor considered to be the father of a child conceived with his sperm? If so, is he obligated to support the child financially? Has a man fulfilled his obligation to be fruitful and multiply when his sperm, which was not emitted during the intentional act of sexual intercourse, conceives a child? Does a child conceived without sexual intercourse have parents? If a Jewish man who is married but childless donates sperm and then subsequently dies, is he considered to be childless even though his sperm has successfully conceived children, albeit not with his wife? And if so, is his brother still obligated to marry his wife in order to carry on his name, commensurate with the obligation of levirate marriage (*yibbum*)?

11. For a more thorough discussion of this issue, see Kahn (1998a). There are two primary sources for frozen, non-Jewish sperm in Israel. It can be ordered from the "non-Jewish" sperm bank in Afula, Israel, which accepts sperm donations from resident non-Jews as well as non-Jewish tourists in Israel, such as kibbutz volunteers. It is also sometimes imported from the United States.

12. See Kahn (1998b, pp. 30–31).

13. It is important to understand that the traditional precedents that privilege birth as the determining factor of maternity were codified during historical periods in which ova were not known to exist.

14. See Bleich (1991, supra n. 38). Bleich also provides an interesting discussion of rabbinic attitudes toward conversion of a child in utero in response to the question, could a Jewish woman carrying an embryo conceived with a non-Jewish egg immerse in a ritual bath and thereby convert the child in utero?

REFERENCES

Auerbach, S. (1958). *Noam, 1,* 165. [In Hebrew]

Berman, E. (2000). Sect, subsidy and sacrifice: An economist's view of ultraorthodox Jews. *Quarterly Journal of Economics, 115(3),* 905–953.

Bleich, D. J. (1991). In-vitro fertilization: Questions of maternal identity and conversion. *Tradition, 25(4),* 82–102.

Dorff, E. (1998). *Matters of life and death: A Jewish approach to modern medical ethics.* Philadelphia: Jewish Publication Society.

Franklin, S. (1997). *Embodied progress: A cultural account of assisted conception.* London: Routledge.

Heilman, S. (1992). *Defenders of the faith: Inside ultraorthodox Jewry.* New York: Schocken Books.

Howards, S. (1995). Treatment of male infertility. *New England Journal of Medicine, 2(February).*

Inhorn, M. C. (1994). *Quest for conception: Gender, infertility and Egyptian medical traditions.* Philadelphia: University of Pennsylvania Press.

Israeli, H. (1997). Religiosity and fertility: The influence of social structure on fertility in religious communities in Israel. M.A. thesis, Ben Gurion University of the Negev.

Kahn, S. M. (1998a). Gentile sperm and the rabbinic uses of non-Jewish bodies for Jewish reproduction. Paper presented at the annual meeting of the American Anthropological Association.

Kahn, S. M. (1998b). Putting Jewish wombs to work: Israelis confront the new reproductive technologies. *Lilith, 23(2),* 30–31.

Kahn, S. M. (2000). *Reproducing Jews: A cultural account of assisted conception in Israel.* Durham, NC: Duke University Press.

Reminnick, L. I. (1996). *Fertility regulation problem: The Israeli scene in the international context.* Jerusalem: Israel Women's Network.

Sandelowski, M. (1993). *With child in mind: Studies in the personal encounter with infertility.* Philadelphia: University of Pennsylvania Press.

Shalev, C. (1998). Halakha and patriarchal motherhood: An anatomy of the new Israeli surrogacy law. *Israel Law Review, 32(1)*, 51–81.

Waldenburg, R. E. (1982). In-vitro fertilization: A medical Halakhic discussion. *Assia, 33*. [In Hebrew]

Yuval-Davis, N. (1987). The Jewish collectivity. In S. Magida (Ed.), *Women in the Middle East*. London: Zed Books.

SIXTEEN

The Politics of Making Modern Babies in China

Reproductive Technologies and the "New" Eugenics

Lisa Handwerker

Since the late 1980s, there has been increased interest in and use of new reproductive technologies (NRTs), resulting in a "new" eugenics in the People's Republic of China. In March 1988 in Beijing, a thirty-nine-year-old woman from rural China gave birth to China's first test-tube baby. By December 1993, one of China's major teaching hospitals had produced more than fifty test-tube babies through the combined efforts of in vitro fertilization (IVF) and gamete intrafallopian transfer (GIFT). In other cases, babies have been conceived with the help of donated eggs, donated embryos, artificial insemination (Chao, 1988), sperm intrafallopian transfer (SIFT), and gamete intrauterine transfer (GIUT). Today in China, major urban hospitals and research institutes are pushing the limits of reproductive technologies to include eugenic-oriented practices of sex selection and human reproductive cloning.

In China, a country with an explicit and restrictive birth planning campaign, there is no official policy to foster IVF programs, and high-tech baby making is viewed ambivalently by both professionals and the public. Nonetheless, in this chapter, I argue that the growth of a reproductive technology industry has been unwittingly encouraged through the combined influences of (1) a long-standing cultural imperative for women to become mothers and, ideally, to produce sons; (2) Maoist social ideology and practices; (3) the one-child birth policy; and (4) post-1980 global market influences.

In the context of the birth planning policy, NRT-assisted pregnancies and births have also resulted in a new obligation on the part of educated parents to have a mentally and physically superior baby. A new reproductive standard has been established through NRTs, creating a scenario for a eugenics based on medical ideology and practices and a corresponding elitism in China for an improved single child.

To illustrate these points, this chapter is divided into three main sections. Following a discussion of research methodology, I first explore Chinese birth control policy. I argue that the intent of the birth policy is quite different from its actual impact on women, especially infertile women. Next I analyze the growth of the reproductive technology industry despite this restrictive birth policy and despite ambivalence about NRTs among professionals and the public. In the last section I show how NRTs and the one-child policy are on a collision course in China, in the form of a "new" eugenics made possible by doctors using these technologies to purportedly produce the "perfect" child.

METHODOLOGY

This chapter, based on the first comprehensive ethnographic study of infertility and reproductive technologies in modern China, draws on a wide range of anthropological methods and sources (Handwerker, 1990, 1993). For twelve months, in 1990–1991, I observed patient-doctor interactions at three well-established, infertility clinics in Beijing, two based in biomedical hospitals and one based in a traditional Chinese medicine hospital. I also took two brief side trips, including a two-week trip to Hunan Province where I met with both the founder of China's first sperm bank and the founder of China's eugenics movement.

Using a formal, thirty-eight-page written questionnaire, I, along with a research assistant, interviewed one hundred women, mostly Han Chinese. In Mandarin, we asked open- and closed-ended questions about a variety of subjects, including demographic information, women's roles, marriage, fertility beliefs (including pregnancy, menstruation, prenatal education, and childbirth), sexuality, gynecological disorders, infertility, and medical treatments for infertility, including NRTs.

In addition, I interviewed approximately fifty other women and five men, asking open-ended questions about family relations, marriage, the birth policy, children, sex preference, sexuality, and infertility and its treatment, including NRTs, adoption, and eugenics. I also interviewed physicians, including seven family planning experts, two representatives from international family planning agencies, seven infertility specialists, the team of doctors who produced China's first test-tube baby, and the founder of China's first sperm bank, as noted above. At the request of one IVF director, I also designed a brief structured questionnaire on attitudes toward egg and sperm donation, which I administered to twenty-three women in her clinic.

Since I had arrived in China six months after the Tiananmen Square massacre and was not sure whether I would face fieldwork restrictions, I complemented interviews and observations with folklore and popular materials. As it turned out, I was not restricted, but these materials added richly to my other data. I collected and analyzed newspaper and magazine articles, to illuminate ideas about gender, reproduction, and medicine. Finally, I had translated and analyzed more than fifty letters written by patients to an infertility specialist at one hospital.

All of these methods were important in that each revealed a particular aspect of Chinese culture. Together, they provided important insights into how the broader cultural, economic, and social milieu—especially medical knowledge and practice—frames the politics of gender and reproduction for infertile women.

Although a single-locality study does not permit me to draw conclusions about all of China, this study, conducted mainly in Beijing from 1990 to 1991 and during a brief follow-up visit in 1997, provides insights into other regions as well. I selected Beijing as my primary research site because it is a city with numerous infertility clinics of both *xiyi* (Western medicine) and *zhongyi* (traditional Chinese medicine) and the birthplace of China's first test-tube baby. As a result, I interviewed women who came to Beijing from all parts of China to seek treatment in well-known hospitals. Moreover, because Beijing is the administrative capital from which family planning decisions disseminate, it is an important place to observe the tensions between policies that discourage and those that unwittingly encourage births.

THE IMPACT OF CHINA'S BIRTH PLANNING POLICY ON WOMEN

Until the 1950s, with little demographic information available, Chinese leaders supported large families and the growing population. The idea of *renkou* (population) as a negative force to be managed is a modern concept linked to the emergence of Chinese socialist development policies. In 1954, with the first national survey results reported, Mao Zedong and other leaders relaxed their opposition to birth control in response to mounting public pressures and economic concerns (Wang, 1988, p. 54). Nevertheless, in part because of the political atmosphere of the Cultural Revolution, mandatory population control measures were not pursued for another twenty years.

Only in the mid-1970s did China, under the influence of international health agency agendas, make population control a top national priority. Low birthrates became a symbol of modernity for developing countries in general and China in particular. In the 1970s, when surveys revealed 10 million women of childbearing age amid a rapidly growing population (Davin, 1987, p. 1), Chinese Communist Party (CCP) leaders became alarmed. Leaders such as Mao shifted from an earlier reluctance to implement birth control measures because of a long-standing cultural imperative for women to reproduce (ideally, sons) to a Chinese socialist perspective viewing population growth as a problem that required a compulsory one-child policy (Banister, 1987; Croll, Davin, & Kane, 1985; Greenhalgh, 1986, 1990a, 1990b, 1993).

With the introduction of the one-child policy in 1979 and subsequent changes in birth policies, such as allowing some families two children[1] (Croll, 1985; Greenhalgh, 1990a, 1990b), the most intimate realms of family life have been made objects of control within the panoptic gaze of the state (Anagnost, 1988, 1989; Foucault, 1979, 1980). Enforcement of the birth planning policy has led to unprecedented surveillance and regulation of the Chinese social body (population) in general and the female body in particular.

Whereas census statistics on men of childbearing age are rare, statistics on women's fertility and sexual and reproductive practices are gathered and widely circulated. Information is collected on the number of women of childbearing age, live births, abortions, miscarriages, pregnancies, and contraceptive use and knowledge. Furthermore, since the 1990s, semiannual gynecological examinations have been required for some married women of reproductive age (Greenhalgh, 1993, p. 32) to enforce contraceptive use or to detect hidden pregnancies. Unmarried women are required to undergo premarital examinations to detect any visible structural problems in their reproductive organs and family history of genetic abnormalities that would interfere with the birth of a "normal" child.

In urban areas, where the government has been able to enforce the one-child policy, mechanisms of female fertility surveillance have also been achieved through charting menstrual cycles, granting permission for and documenting births, and distributing free contraceptives, especially intrauterine devices (IUDs) that require implantation and removal by a medical professional. When combined, all of this information becomes the means through which the state-party mobilizes social pressure to influence the reproductive and sexual practices of households and families (Anagnost, 1988, 1989). This birth campaign and its results exemplify what Foucault (1980) has referred to as a "technology of normalization," which systematically scrutinizes, classifies, and controls anomalies of the body, especially the female body.

Although the CCP's attempt to regulate female reproduction through birth planning has been, in many ways, an effective means of control and normalization, it paradoxically defines and reinforces childless women as Other, or different from other women. During an in-depth interview, one woman told me:

I am sure the pressure to have children in China is greater than in any other country. I especially feel a lot of pressure from my work unit. I think if I didn't work the pressure might be less. . . . I feel so much pressure because of the mandatory birth certificate which provides me with permission to have a child. I have had to turn in my certificate the last three years because I couldn't have a child. I felt terrible. Here they give you permission and then you can't even give birth. I feel so humiliated to have to get a new certificate each year. This year I didn't even go to the planning authorities; they automatically gave me a new one in April. (July 4, 1990)

Another woman from my sample of one hundred interviews, summarizing the sentiment of many, said, "The one-child policy is really the 'you *must* have one child policy.' " While the pressure on women to produce a child and ideally a son is a "cultural imperative" dating back long before recent birth planning programs, the assumption that all women of reproductive age should be fertile appears even stronger under the one-child policy. In other words, the intent and the impact of the birth policy are different for infertile women.

THE GROWTH OF A HIGH-TECH BABY-MAKING INDUSTRY

Responses from the Medical Profession

The obligatory call for women to control family size in response to modernization pressures appears in stark contrast to an obligatory call to reproduce. However, *fuke* (women's health specialty) doctors—who promote birth control and abortion, on the one hand, yet aggressively assist infertile women, on the other hand—perceive no conflict. During my interviews with fuke doctors, they argued that their efforts, including the use of NRTs, to help infertile women are justified for humanitarian and scientific reasons.

With respect to the humanitarian dimensions, fuke doctors perceive that they are fulfilling a social need. Historically, the purpose of marriage in China has been to produce heirs to carry on the family line. In Confucian society, failure to have children, especially sons, was a disgrace to one's ancestors and a shameful act. The classical Confucian writer Mencius stated, "There are three things that are unfilial, and to have no posterity is the greatest of these" (Waltner, 1990, p. 13). Without a son, there was no one to continue the family line and to make ancestral sacrifices, and family property would fall into the hands of strangers (Waltner, 1990, p. 13). While ancient Chinese classical medical texts acknowledge male as well as female infertility, in cultural terms, infertility was a condition for which women were held culpable. Thus, historically, fuke doctors had the important role of ensuring the continuity of the patrilineal family by guaranteeing women's reproductive health (Furth, 1999).

Today, with public perceptions that infertility is on the rise,[2] the role of fuke doctors in addressing infertility continues. One fuke doctor stated:

> Too many births cause havoc, but no births at all produces greater anxiety. The treatment of infertility remains a worthy topic as long as the Chinese family remains. . . . In China, a country in its initial stages of development, infertile patients are more overwhelmed with anxieties and stronger in their appeals for the test-tube baby.

An infertility specialist showed me numerous letters that she had received from women all over China, begging for the chance to bear a child and detailing their suffering. One letter reads:

> Have pity on my family, please, my dear doctor. My family has just had one successor for three generations. When I was six months old my father died a violent death. When I was only one and a half, my brother breathed his last breath, leaving me the only child to take care of my aging grandparents. Later my grandmother died. My grandfather, now almost 90 years old, has been waiting for me to bear a child for twenty years but still I am barren. I am almost 40 years old, my husband is a peasant. Without a child, my family is at a loss about our future.

After listening to an interview with a woman who had lost her only child in a tragic accident, I was told by her physician that the effective implementation of the state family planning policy required that fuke specialists be adept not only in contraception and birth control but also in reverse sterilization in case of an accidental death of an only child.

To defend the "aggressive" treatment and use of NRTs given the restrictive birth policy, one doctor responded to a local reporter who asked, "Why should we [China] have test-tube babies when Chinese hospitals are busy with abortions in the context of a population explosion?" The doctor, founder of China's first IVF clinic, replied:

> China has a huge population. Surely, there should be family planning, which includes both contraception and abortion for control of birthrates and infertility treatment in some men and women. One may ask, There are too many pregnant women, why treat infertility? In this logic, since China is overpopulated, why bother to treat diseases? Why help the disabled? Why cure the wounded and save the dying? Why set up hospitals? Why are we doctors needed?

Medical practitioners are motivated to assist infertile couples for a number of reasons. Many practitioners are driven by the need to help infertile couples, especially women, whom they feel suffer enormously in Chinese society. Some are motivated by their interest in medical innovations and in nation-state building. Still others are motivated by the potential for economic profits. Today, in a competitive health care economy that promotes medical privatization and the marketing of medicine and technological products, infertility has become a potentially lucrative business for hospitals, doctors, and pharmaceutical factories. An international population officer explained:

> We provide money annually toward the development of contraceptive research and technology in China. We presently fund five major factories for contraceptive production in various parts of China. During a recent site visit, we discovered that officials have been using our money to secretly manufacture medicines to treat the infertile and sexually impotent because of the potential for large private profits.

Overall, increased dependency on international funding and technological transfers in science and medicine have contributed to a post-1980 consumer market for infertility treatment, research, and products. Despite these forces, some government officials, doctors, and citizens are ambivalent at best and even largely unsympathetic to infertility research and clinical medicine. State doctors addressing infertility issues often have to justify their work and need for resources. One doctor, who worked at a state-sponsored hospital, angrily told me how much initial resistance to conducting IVF research she faced. Refusing to give her or her colleagues funds, the state acknowledged the importance of their work only after their first successful IVF birth. Even her own son reproached her, saying, "What are you doing? Everyone is going to hate you. China has enough people." Other doctors asked her, "Why treat infertile couples when they can help our population problem?" Some health care professionals voiced their concerns to me about my project and expressed hope that I would not find a "solution to infertility" in the context of China's population problem. A well-known endocrinologist specializing in infertility treatment refused to open an IVF clinic. Instead, she argued that in China, a country with limited goods, there needs to be more emphasis on the prevention of diseases leading to infertility, including chlamydia and other sexually transmitted diseases. Yet, at the time of my initial research, chlamydia testing was still routinely unavailable even at the largest urban hospitals.

Post-1980 Consumer Demand for High-Tech Baby Making

Although there are contradictory responses to the introduction of NRTs among medical professionals, this has not slowed down the development or use of NRTs in China. In a society that values reproduction and stigmatizes childlessness and in which adoption is either difficult or viewed as a last resort, high-tech baby making is also driven by consumers, infertile women who desire a child. While women speak of distinct pressures depending on their geographic locations, social class, educational background, and work and family circumstances, all women feel pressured by the condition of childlessness—regardless of whether or not it is "her" problem. In my interviews, infertile women presented six major reasons for their desire to have a child: "everyone wants a child," "lineage continuity," "to provide care in old age," "to relieve loneliness and add interest to life," "societal pressure," and "spouse's or mother-in-law's insistence." One woman cried, "If I don't have the ability to give birth, I am not a woman." In such a state of vulnerability, there is ample opportunity for exploitation of infertile women.

In the post-1980 global market, there is also a belief among infertile Chinese women that the best medicine is often the most technical and expensive. The recent equation of "Western" medicine with modernity and prestige has led to the incorporation of more and more Western biomedical techniques into an increasingly competitive market. Medical competence is now redefined by the quantity and variety of technology brought to bear on infertility. While women from diverse backgrounds seek out and use both traditional Chinese medicine and biomedicine, they place their final hopes in the "miracles" brought by Chinese medical specialists who have trained in the West with the latest technologies. Yet, these miracles, widely reported on by Chinese newspapers and television, sharply contrast with the realities of women's lives. One woman, who suffered from infertility for ten years, recounts her story as follows:

> I have been a primary school teacher all my life. I work with children daily and I love kids, so I couldn't understand how this could have happened to me. You have no idea what a terrible disease this is, this infertility. It is the worst disease possible in China. I suffered so much in my life. My parents died when I was young, so I was raised by my grandparents. After my grandmother died, my grandfather continued to take care of me and now he is in his eighties and my only surviving relative. I must care for him. When my husband and I married his family agreed to my unusual family circumstances. First, rather than I move in with his family, he would move in with me and my grandfather. Second, our first child would be named after my grandfather and any subsequent children after his name. Who would have predicted I would be infertile? For ten years we tried every treatment in our area. We were poor and couldn't seek medical help in the larger cities. Then, in 1988, after we had already given up hope, my relative heard an interview with Professor Zhang on television and told me about the test-tube baby. At first I didn't understand it—I thought you go and pick out a baby from a tube and bring it home. We saved our money, as it costs almost 2,000 to 3,000 yuan to do the operation. Because of the economic reforms, my family is much wealthier now, so it wasn't like before when we had no money. When I became pregnant, I was so happy. After the baby was born I named her after Professor Zhang and my grandfather. When my husband found out he was furious. Before this birth, even though I was infertile, he was always good to me, but

now he has started beating me. It is terrible and I don't know what to do. I came here to ask the doctor for a chance for a second baby, and this time, I'll name the baby after him.

Rather than offer a magical solution, IVF exacerbated the old social tension of reproducing the patrilineal line and created new social problems for this woman. She returned to the clinic hoping for a second baby—maybe even a boy—born through IVF.

Society cannot always keep pace with the introduction of new technologies. In my interviews with twenty-three women about their willingness to use and their attitudes toward egg and sperm donation, they were confused about what should count as "natural" and how this might influence kinship relations. On the one hand, the women I interviewed told me they would use an egg donor, as long as the egg was combined with their husband's sperm. The use of their husband's sperm was the most important factor in considering the child their own. On the other hand, women expressed great ambivalence about accepting sperm from an anonymous male donor out of fear that their husbands or in-laws might reject the child.[3]

Despite these and other reservations, infertile women who desire a biological baby are seduced by the promise of NRTs. Clinics are overflowing with patients seeking out these services, and doctors are trying to keep up with the demand. It appears that current expectations and reactions to NRTs are linked to earlier long-standing norms about reproduction, including an imperative for women in China to be mothers—ideally, mothers of sons. Thus, while high-tech baby making is still viewed ambivalently by some professionals and the public, I would argue that China has unwittingly encouraged the growth of infertility treatment and research, including high-tech baby making. Furthermore, China has backed into a "new" eugenics based on clinical practices involving NRTs and other technologies, a subject to which I now turn.

EUGENIC PRACTICES IN CHINA: THEN AND NOW

China's birth planning policy is a call not only for fewer births but also for improved-quality births, or what might best be called a "new" eugenics. The push to improve offspring is both a consequence of the one-child policy and, more recently, an additional policy in and of itself. "Eugenics," a term referring to the improvement of the human race by controlling breeding, has serious negative connotations in the West, where it evokes the Nazi campaign for racial purification through forced sterilization and extermination of the ostensibly unfit (Rosenthal, 2000). Yet the founder of China's eugenic movement, a ninety-year-old man, told me in an interview that the term "eugenics" in China has a more positive association, where it retains much of the original sense of "excellent birth."

Eugenic practices in China are not new but rather date to late Imperial China (1550–1911) (Dikötter, 1998; Furth, 1999). During this period, ideas about the importance of both environmental and hereditary factors to good breeding thrived in the patrilineal society. Since reproductive behavior was key in continuing the male lineage—the indispensable link connecting past ancestors and future descendants—individuals had to be closely regulated (Dikötter, 1998; Furth, 1999). Medical texts at this time were consumed with concern about eliminating birth defects through reproductive regulation (Furth, 1999).

The Chinese Medical Profession and the "New" Eugenics

Currently in China, a "new" eugenics, drawing on old cultural principles, has emerged under the guise of modern scientific knowledge in clinical practice (Dikötter, 1998). Since the 1980s NRTs are one of the ways in which eugenic practices have become legitimated. NRTs are cited not only as a cure for infertility, but as medical services arguably needed to reproduce healthy offspring. In 1984 in Beijing, as part of China's Seventh Five Year Plan, IVF and embryo transfer research began under the title, "Eugenics Research on the Protection, Preservation, and Development of Early Embryos." In an interview, the doctor who gained fame for producing China's first test-tube baby stated,

> Programs such as IVF, ET [embryo transfer], and gamete intrafallopian transfer [GIFT] open up a new avenue to promote basic medical research in genetics, immunology, and early embryology. . . . I am sure a day will come when a man can design his own body according to [society's] need, just as in engineering. By that time, humans will have been able to select chromosomes with the best genetic material for artificial fertilization so as to raise the qualities of the human body in all its aspects. Scientific research is endless and scientific thinking is beautiful. . . . Some scientists even dream of asexual human propagation. . . . All this is but a fantasy. But fantasies prove a thoroughfare to ideals. Isn't the birth of the test-tube baby proof of this? (Tu, 1988, p. 303)

The founder of China's first sperm bank, also the daughter of one of the founders of China's eugenics movement, emphasized the need for superior babies produced through the insemination of "quality" sperm. Moreover, she emphasized how research on sperm would lead to cloning and new techniques in assisted reproduction.

Chinese Consumers and the "New" Eugenics

In addition to medical professionals' perceptions of enhancing birth quality through NRTs, couples using NRTs believe that test-tube babies are smarter than those born through "natural" reproduction. One male patient asked me, "If I pay more money can I get a better-quality baby?" Another man whose wife had undergone IVF to compensate for his low sperm count insisted that his child, from the moment of birth, was smarter than all the other babies born that day. Beliefs about the superiority of babies born through reproductive technologies are both reflected in and reinforced by the media. A newspaper account describing one of China's first IVF babies, who was four and a half years old at the time, reads:

> Meng Zhu has never been sick. She was trained to brush her teeth and put on her clothes at the age of three. She is taller than children her age by half a head. Her intelligence is also higher than children of her age. At present, Meng Zhu has mastered 500 Chinese words, can recite 20 poems, sing 30 songs and perform 10 different dances. She can also do simple arithmetic skillfully. (*China Industrial and Commercial News*, 1993)

The cultivation of the superior or "perfect" IVF child is clearly related to the one-child policy, which has from its inception been accompanied by a series of informational materials promoting the healthy development of a single child (Nathanson Milwertz, 1997, p. 128). For example, in 1992, the first national exhibition, "Eugenics, Improved Childbearing and Child-rearing," was held in Beijing (Guofang, 1992; Nathanson Milwertz, 1997, p.130). The exhibition linked the one-child policy with the need for an improved single child. At one booth, doctors from the National Defense Scientific Working Committee Hospital, No. 514, offered visitors the opportunity to test a computer program that calculates the optimal conception date to achieve a healthy and intelligent child. Calculations are based on information about the intelligence, emotions, and physical cycles of future parents. Older cultural beliefs such as *feng shui* (Chinese geomancy) were thus creatively blended with new scientific language through computers.

In clinical settings, pregnant women, who are considered primarily responsible for giving birth and raising a superior single child, are exposed to educational materials promoting a morally and physically superior baby. With public anxiety high about the healthy development of a single child, health materials encouraging women to take action to achieve the production of such a child are proliferating (Dikötter, 1998, p.124). Materials range from practical discussions of prenatal care, including nutrition, to more complex concerns about genetics and heredity. During my interviews, many women expressed strong beliefs about what constituted good prenatal care and education, including a couple's abstinence from sex for at least the first three months of pregnancy to prevent fetal harm. One woman described how she used a specially designed earphone placed on her belly for her fetus to listen to music to encourage intellectual growth. Interestingly, it was Western classical music that was believed to be more advantageous to fetal development and intelligence. And, regardless of the techniques used, the responsibility for superior fetal development was clearly believed to rest with the mother.

Chinese Leaders and the "New" Eugenics

In a recent effort to improve China's overall population quality, leaders, including public health officials, proposed national legislation in 1993 called the Eugenics Law. Later renamed the Maternal and Infant Health Care Law after international criticism, it was established to guarantee prenatal and pediatric health care to poor women and children. But it contained a highly controversial stipulation that couples, especially women, undergo premarital physical examinations to learn of any genetic prob lems. And doctors who discover a problem are charged with taking steps to stop "abnormal" pregnancies through long-term contraceptives and sterilizations (Tyler, 1993). This proposed legislation, furthermore, requires even tighter surveillance of women who are already pregnant, for any woman diagnosed with an abnormal fetus would be advised to abort. This was not the first time such legislation had been proposed and enforced. Five years earlier, in northwestern Gansu Province, legislation was passed to prevent mentally disabled women from having children (Tyler, 1993).

One troublesome aspect of the new eugenic legislation is that the right to reproduce and even the right to exist are determined by ill-defined and partial ideas about genetic fitness. For example, mental retardation is not always genetic but can be caused by malnutrition and inadequate prenatal care. Eugenics is not so much a clear set of scientific principles as a modern way of talking about social problems in biologizing terms (Dikötter, 1998).

In addition, the "new" eugenics colludes with Chinese patriarchal culture. In China, where the cultural preference in rural areas is for a son, the female embryo may be considered a defect in and of itself (Dikötter, 1998). Worldwide, birthrates are estimated at 106 males to every 100 females (Kristof & Wudunn, 1994, pp. 228–231). In China, until the 1980s, census data showed no shortfall of baby girls. But since the 1980s and as a consequence of a strict population policy, census data indicate that baby girls are "missing." In 1992 the gender ratio in China had widened to 118.5 boys to every 100 girls. A possible explanation for these skewed statistics is female infanticide, formerly practiced in rural China, or the recent trend of concealing the births of baby girls from authorities in rural areas so that a couple can try for a baby boy in a second or third pregnancy. Another explanation is the now widespread use of ultrasound testing in China. As early as 1979 China began manufacturing ultrasound scanners. By the late 1980s China was importing more than 2,000 ultrasound scanners and making 10,000 of its own. By 1990 one Chinese demographer estimated 100,000 scanners in use (Kristof & Wudunn, 1994, pp. 228–231). Ultrasound technology is used to confirm women's use of IUD contraception and to check for healthy fetal development, but it is also a sex-selection technique.

As ultrasound use has become routine in China, the sex favor ratio has been skewed even further (Coale & Banister, 1994; Dikötter, 1998, p. 181). In 1987 the government issued a ban on ultrasound technology for purposes of sex identification and prohibited technicians from telling the parents the fetal sex. Ironically, this prohibition seems only to have raised the cost of bribes to ultrasound technicians or encouraged private doctors to purchase the equipment for profit. For example, a private pharmacist who purchased an ultrasound machine for $1,000 said he can see up to one hundred pregnant women daily, at a charge of $50 for a brief consultation (Kristof & Wudunn, 1994, p. 230). In other words, despite the ban, ultrasound technology for the purposes of sex selection is more, not less, accessible.

Thus today the determination in China to control virtually every facet of childbirth includes the use of sex-selection methods originally developed in the United States and then imported to China. Supporters of the technique argue that it will allow couples the reproductive freedom to chose their babies' sex. However, in China, especially in rural areas, where boys are still the precious gem, the search for the "perfect" baby may translate into the search for the "perfect" boy. Thus the most recent developments in NRTs, which include choosing the sex of one's embryo, may create devastating consequences for female embryos in China.

CONCLUSION

This chapter addresses an important and timely issue in feminist studies—namely, the use of NRTs in the promotion of "new" eugenics in modern China. Several key issues are highlighted. First, Chinese birth policy aimed at reducing births has ironically led to the further stigmatization of infertile women as Other. Second, although no official policy promotes infertility treatment and research and although medical professionals and the public remain highly ambivalent about the NRTs, China has unwittingly encouraged the growth of a high-tech baby-making industry. The combined influences of a long-standing cultural imperative to reproduce (ideally, sons), Maoist social ideology and practices, the one-child policy, post-1980 global market forces, and the importation of Western reproductive technologies have played out in China in unique ways. Perhaps most ironically, high-tech baby making in this cultural setting has become a potent signifier of

Chinese "modernity," even though modernity is also signaled by the country's low birthrate. Third, permission to have a child has become an obligation to have a mentally and physically superior single child. This has created a "new" eugenics and a corresponding elitism that plays out in clinical settings. New technologies such as IVF, ultrasound, and sex-selection techniques allow for even greater intervention in reproduction. Unfortunately, this superior single child may be visualized by many parents as male, creating a further imbalance in the unequal gender ratio documented in China.

Clearly, this study shows that the implementation of new reproductive practices and their consequences are not always coercive but rather operate in a subtler way to create new standards of reproductive normality among both professionals and the public. In short, the example of China allows us to understand the complex ways in which technology is more than just a tool; it is also an organizing principle of human life, with specific implications for women's lives in particular locations.

NOTES

The research for this chapter was generously supported by a joint grant from the Fulbright-Hays Doctoral Dissertation Award Committee and the Committee on Scholarly Communication with the PRC. Assistance was also provided by the Wenner-Gren Anthropological Association Dissertation Fund, a National Science Foundation Doctoral Dissertation Improvement Grant (No. BNS89–13347), and the Association for Women in Science. In addition, the Soroptomist International Award and the University of California, San Francisco, Humanities Award provided dissertation writing support. The Institute for the Study of Social Change, Women and Gender at the University of California, Berkeley, provided me with important writing time. I appreciate the editorial insights of Marcia Inhorn, Frank van Balen, and Cindy Fulton as well as anonymous reviewers for *Women's Studies International Forum*. My work has benefited from the support of many people, including J. Ablon, G. Becker, A. Clarke, T. Gold, the Handwerkers, A. Ong, and Y. Verdoner. Thanks to Drs. Zhang Li Zhu, Zuo Wen Li, Chai, Gao, and Lu. I am warmly indebted to Dr. Yuan Hong and the women with whom I worked, for without them this project could not have been as comprehensive or as exciting. I also thank Meera Jaffrey, a dear friend, for my initiation to China. The above persons bear no responsibility for my data results or interpretations.

1. In April 2000 Elizabeth Rosenthal reported in the *New York Times,* "[I]n a country best known for its excruciatingly tough one-child policy, large young families today are scattered throughout the countryside. Although, technically, rural families can have only up to two children—and then only if the first child is a girl—families with three, four, five or more children are now the norm in many areas, including Lufeng, a southern coastal region of Guangdong."

2. Although existing statistical information suggests no increase in the incidence of infertility over the past decade, there is nonetheless a public perception that infertility is on the rise in China. There is also the belief that female infertility is greater than male infertility, despite recent statistics suggesting an equal proportion of male and female infertility problems. A recent article in *Women in China* (Yuan, 1991, pp. 8–10) suggests a 10 percent infertility rate in large cities in China, with 40 percent male infertility, 40 percent female infertility, and 10 percent couple or "unidentified" infertility.

3. In fact, these women have reason to be concerned. In one widely publicized case from Shanghai, a couple secretly underwent artificial insemination by donor (AID). After the child was born, the paternal grandparents became suspicious on the grounds that the child did not look like their son. They accused the wife of having an extramarital affair. Under pressure, the man admitted that as a result of his sterility his wife had undergone AID. His parents refused to believe their son was sterile and rejected the child. The husband, forced to choose between his parents and his wife, decided to divorce.

REFERENCES

Anagnost, A. (1988). Family violence and magical violence: Woman as victim in China's one-child family policy. *Women and Language, 11,* 16–22.

Anagnost, A. (1989). Transformations of gender in modern China. In S. Morgen (Ed.), *Gender and anthropology* (pp. 313–342). Washington, DC: American Anthropological Association.

Banister, J. (1987). *China's changing population.* Stanford, CA: Stanford University Press.

Beijing Review. (1988). First test-tube baby on Mainland. *31, March 21–27,* 11. (Chinese announcement appeared in *Renmin Ribao,* March 1988.)

Chao, J. (1988). More than three hundred women in Tianjin have received artificial insemination. *Renmin Ribao* (overseas edition), *October 24.*

China Industrial and Commercial News. (1993). China's first test-tube baby goes to school. *September 27.*

Coale, J., & Banister, J. (1994). Five decades of missing females in China. *Demography, 31(3),* 459–479.

Croll, E., Davin, D., & Kane, P. (Eds.). (1985). *China's one-child family policy.* London: Macmillan.

Davin, D. (1987). Gender and population in the People's Republic of China. In H. Afshar (Ed.), *Women, state and ideology: Studies from Africa and Asia* (pp. 111–130). Albany: State University of New York Press.

Dikötter, F. (1998). *Imperfect conceptions: Medical knowledge, birth defects and eugenics in China.* New York: Columbia University Press.

Foucault, M. (1979). *Discipline and punish.* New York: Vintage.

Foucault, M. (1980). *The history of sexuality, volume 1: An introduction.* New York: Vintage.

Furth, C. (1999). *A flourishing yin: Gender in China's medical history, 960–1665.* Berkeley: University of California Press.

Greenhalgh, S. (1986). Shifts in China's population policy, 1984–86: Views from the central, provincial, and local levels. *Population and Development Review, 12(3)*, 491–515.

Greenhalgh, S. (1990a). The evolution of the one-child policy in Shanxi, 1979–1988. *China Quarterly 122*, 191–229.

Greenhalgh, S. (1990b). *The peasantization of population policy in Shanxi: Cadre mediation of the state-society conflict.* Working Paper No. 21. New York: Population Council.

Greenhalgh, S. (1993). The peasantization of the one-child policy in Shanxi: Negotiating birth control in China. In D. Davis & S. Harrell (Eds.), *Chinese Families in the post-Mao era* (pp. 29–250). Berkeley: University of California Press.

Greenhalgh, S., & Bongaarts, J. (1985). An alternative to the one-child policy in China. *Population and Development Review, 11(4)*, 585–617.

Guofang kegongwei wuyisi yiyuan yiwusuo (National Defense Scientific Working Committee No. 514 Clinic) (1992). *Guogang kegongwei can zhan xiangmu jianjie* (A brief introduction to the National Defense Scientific Working Committee projects included in the exhibition). Beijing: Guofang kegongwei jihua shengyu ligdao xiazu bangongshu banli. June.

Handwerker, L. (1990). The hen that can't lay an egg: Preliminary thoughts on infertility research in China. Paper presented at the Center for Chinese Studies, Fall Regional Seminar, University of California, Berkeley.

Handwerker, L. (1993). The hen that can't lay an egg *(Bu xia dan de mu ji):* The stigmatization of female infertility in late-twentieth-century People's Republic of China. Ph.D. dissertation,University of California, San Francisco/Berkeley.

Handwerker, L. (1995). The hen that can't lay an egg *(Bu xia dan de mu ji):* Conceptions of female infertility in modern China. In J. Terry & J. Urla (Eds.), *Deviant bodies: Critical perspectives on difference in science and popular culture* (pp. 358–379). Bloomington: Indiana University Press.

Handwerker, L. (1998). The consequences of modernity for childless women in China: Medicalization and resistance. In M. Lock & P. A. Kaufert (Eds.), *Pragmatic women and body politics* (pp. 178–206). New York: Cambridge University Press.

Henderson, G. E., & Cohen, M. S. (1984). *The Chinese socialist work unit.* New Haven, CT: Yale University Press.

Kane, P. (1987). *The second billion: Population and family planning in China.* London: Penguin Books.

Kristof, N. D., & Wudunn, S. (1994). *China wakes: The struggle for the soul of a rising power.* New York: Vintage.

Lampton, D. M. (1987). *Policy implementation in post-Mao China.* Berkeley: University of California Press.

Landler, M. (2000). Clinic caters to couples seeking "precious gem." *New York Times, July 1*, p. A4.

Nathansen Milwertz, C. (1997). *Accepting population control: Urban Chinese women and the one-child family policy.* Nordic Institute of Asian Studies Series. Surrey: Curzon.

Ng, V. W. (1990). *Madness in late imperial China: From illness to deviance.* Norman: University of Oklahoma Press.

Parker, A., Russo, M., Sommer, D., & Yaeger, P. (Eds.). (1992). *Nationalisms and sexualities.* New York: Routledge.

Potter, S. H., & Potter, J. (1990). *China's peasants: The anthropology of a revolution.* Cambridge: Cambridge University Press.

Rosenthal, E. (1998). Scientists debate China's law on sterilizing the carriers of genetic defects. *New York Times, August 16,* A14.

Rosenthal, E. (2000). Rural flouting of one-child policy undercuts China's census. *New York Times, August 14,* p. A6.

Sawicki, J. (1991). *Disciplining Foucault: Feminism, power and the body.* London: Routledge.

Simon, D. F., & Goldman, M. (Eds.). (1989). *Science and technology in post-Mao China.* Harvard Contemporary China Series, 5. Cambridge, MA: Harvard University Press.

Smith, C. (1991). *China: People and places in the land of one billion.* Boulder, CO: Westview Press.

Smith, C. (1993). (Over)eating success: The health consequences of capitalism in rural China. *Social Science & Medicine, 37,* 761–770.

Suttmeier, R. (1982). Science and technology in China's socialist development. Paper presented at the World Bank Science and Technology Unit, Project Advisory Staff. January.

Tu, N. (1988). Revealing the secrets of human reproduction—recording the birth of a test-tube baby. (Translated from unidentified magazine article.)

Tyler, P. E. (1993). China weighs using sterilization and abortions to stop "abnormal" births. *New York Times, December 22.*

Waltner, A. (1990). *Getting an heir: Adoption and the construction of kinship in late imperial China.* Honolulu: University of Hawaii Press.

Wang, F. (1988). Historical demography in China. *Review and Perspective, 236,* 53–69.

Wolf, S. M. (Ed.). (1996). *Feminism and bioethics: Beyond reproduction.* New York: Oxford University Press.

Zeng Yi, Tu Ping, Gu Baochang, and Xu Pi et al. (1993). Causes and implications of the recent increase in the reported sex ratio at birth in China. *Population and Development Review, 19(2),* 283–396.

Zhang, X., & Yang, C. (1981). Qianjin zhing de xin wenti (New problems in the forward march). *Guangming Ribao* (Bright Daily), *2(September),* p. 29.

Zhao, Z. (1985). Gaige keji tizhi, tuidong keji he jingsi, shehui xietao (Reform the science and technology system, and promote its coordination with the economy and society). *People's Daily, 12(March),* pp. 1–3.

SEVENTEEN

Conception Politics

Medical Egos, Media Spotlights, and the Contest over Test-Tube Firsts in India

Aditya Bharadwaj

The history of in vitro fertilization (IVF) in India is arguably as old as the history of IVF itself. Its origin has been controversial and its subsequent development no less so. In vitro fertilization laid the foundation for assisted conception in India and created a terrain on which wars for the legitimate ownership of the first "test-tube baby miracle" are being fought.[1] The story of the first IVF baby in India has exposed scientific intolerance to knowledge claims that do not pass under the gaze of peer review. Assisted conception in India today is a contested terrain in part because of the reckless pursuit for credit (reward) and credibility (ability to do science) by its practitioners (Latour & Woolgar, 1986).[2] This pursuit is accentuated by an entrenched multimedia rhetoric on assisted conceptive techniques as a long-awaited solution to the biosocial problem of human infertility.[3]

This chapter represents my attempt to chart the trajectory of assisted conception in India by stringing together various key moments in its growth. The politics of conception are unveiled by focusing on the contested nature of the claims of various medical practitioners to being responsible for producing the first test-tube baby in India. I intend to provide substance to the idea that pursuit of peer-endorsed credibility is not always pivotal in motivating scientists and scientific work and that scientific credibility generation and ascription is inherently multicentered. In so asserting the importance of politics and power relations in the practice of science, I ultimately emphasize the ways in which scientific "facts" are constructed and contested.

The chapter opens with a short description of the data and methodology, then goes on to contextualize the politics behind the development and growth of assisted conception in India. The role played by the state in introducing assisted conception in India is stressed, along with other policies that directly or indirectly launched assisted conception there. The remaining three sections deal with the controversy surrounding the birth of India's first test-tube baby and the way in which the media helped experts compete for legitimacy and recognition.

METHODOLOGY

The chapter is based on a multisited research project looking at the day-to-day working of infertility clinics, as well as the views of patients and infertility experts, in five Indian cities. The main data were collected through a series of in-depth, semistructured and open-ended qualitative interviews with some forty-three treatment-seeking individuals and thirty medical practitioners.

Material for this chapter is also culled from academic texts, extensive media reports (both print and electronic), and excerpts from a few in-depth interviews with scientists engaged in researching human fertility in India. While following the media reports and debates, I made no attempt to conceal identities as the names were already present in the public domain. I also draw extensively on a published article by an eminent assisted conception expert. In this way I endeavor to piece together the controversy over the birth of India's first test-tube baby and the subsequent politicization and playing out of this contentious issue in the mainstream media. To achieve this, I undertake an extensive narrative analysis of both primary (interviews) and secondary data (textual and media reports). Through such an analysis, this chapter attempts to expose the political underbelly of the scientific enterprise.

THE POLITICS OF CONCEPTION: THE CONTEXT

The presence of infertility and its clinical management in India surprises some. In an overpopulated country of nearly one billion people pursuing an aggressive state-sponsored policy of population control—not to mention the poverty and the growth pains typically associated with transitional economies—infertility and its high-tech management does not resonate with Western perceptions. Inhorn (1994, p. 459), however, has quite rightly argued:

> Infertility is inherently political in that it threatens the perpetuation of the body politic. Thus, even when the State attempts to "control" fertility among a reluctant populace, infertility is rarely viewed as a tenable option, as apparent in the recent proliferation of "high-tech" infertility clinics in purportedly "overpopulated," developing countries.

To understand conception politics in contemporary India, it is important to understand India's postcolonial biomedical development. The evident growth of high-tech infertility treatment facilities in the ostensibly overpopulated country is rooted in state policies and social structures that both contain and explain this exponential growth.

Despite its avowed commitment to providing health care and planning, the state in independent India has not curtailed private interest in health provision. On the contrary, under the shelter of a mixed-economy model, the private and public health care sectors have managed to establish a protracted symbiotic coexistence (Baru, 1998). In the closing decades of the twentieth century, however, there was a rapid growth in private sector health care in India. The reason for this can be located in part in the nature of state policy and in part in medical personnel's own strategies of career furtherance. With better pecuniary returns, minimal state interference, control over working conditions, and higher status, the lure of the private sector has managed to attract a significant number of doctors from the public sector. Even when in state employment, doctors are widely known to continue to practice privately (Baru, 1998; Venkatratnam, 1973, 1987). Against this backdrop, a peculiar feature of Indian health services must be confronted. To cite Jeffery (1988, p. 167):

> Health services are not central to class interests in India, either as benefits to be fought over or as important elements in the reproduction of a class-based social structure. The main protagonists are the various kinds of medical practitioners who fight over shares of the cake, rather than the broader ideological issues.

High-tech infertility management in India originated in the public sector. This may appear surprising given the Indian state's long-standing commitment to controlling population. The first scientifically recognized breakthrough in producing an IVF baby resulted from a collaboration between the Institute of Research in Reproduction (IRR), controlled by the Indian Council for Medical Research (ICMR), and a Bombay public hospital. ICMR's annual report of 1986–1987 justified the practice of IVF in a state-controlled research institute by positioning the diagnosis and treatment of infertility as "complementary to an effective Family Welfare Program" (p. 47). The rationale behind this approach was that if the causes of infertility, as well as how fertility could be induced in the infertile, could be known, it would provide new insights into how human fertility could be controlled through clinical and nonclinical interventions. In a 1987 interview, the director of IRR, Dr. T. C. Anand Kumar, stated:

> The IVF-ET technique has now provided a major and justifiable reason to investigate infertile couples thoroughly and thus has offered many opportunities to identify and study factors contributing to infertility. And, an understanding of these factors may provide clues as to how to induce infertility in fertile couples as a means of family planning. There are number of lessons to

be learnt from Nature's Workshop which has created the infertile couple.
(Cited in Lingham, 1990, p. 15)

Interestingly, however, fierce infighting and ego clashes—according to those who were either associated with the project or had a ringside view of its development—led to the demise of the public sector's fleeting but significant tryst with assisted conception.[4] By the end of the 1980s, assisted conception was almost entirely taken over by the private sector. The main protagonists responsible for India's first "official" IVF baby fairly rapidly moved out of state sector employment and set up thriving private practices of their own.

Development of assisted conception in India is therefore contingent on several interrelated factors. First, the "experts" were able to successfully move out of the state sector in order to function with a degree of autonomy and freedom that the public sector did not allow. Second, once out, they were able to use the media to not only carve a niche in the infertility market but also set in motion a contest for respect, status, and credit hitherto unknown to them. Indeed, many media accounts of assisted conception appear no more than attempts to promote the reach and penetration of various practitioners in the infertility market—creating a media/medicine nexus (Bharadwaj, 2000). Third, the state in the past decade offered several incentives in line with its policy of liberalizing the Indian economy, which greatly assisted the growth of technological management of infertility.[5] Fourth, the stigma attached to infertility and an almost oppressive cultural expectation to contribute living children to society (Bharadwaj, 1999) increased the existing demand for treatment in the face of new technological breakthroughs.

Thus, to summarize, the collapse of the state-sponsored IVF program, coupled with the experts leaving the public sector, accompanied by success in the private sector primarily as a result of liberal state policies and lack of regulatory mechanisms, soon fueled a contest for proper credit allocation and recognition, the roots of which go as far back as 1978. It is to this history that I now turn.

REWRITING THE PAST

With the birth of the first scientifically documented test-tube baby, Harsha, on August 6, 1986, India officially entered the brave new world of assisted conception. The use of the term "scientifically documented" is significant as it is repeated ad nauseam in scientific circles to negate the parallel claims of a similar breakthrough made by an Indian doctor in 1978, months after the birth of the world's first test-tube baby, Louise Brown, in Britain.

On October 3, 1978, the birth of the world's second test-tube baby was announced by Dr. Subhas Mukerji in Calcutta. The news was widely reported in the media in India and to some extent abroad. Mukerji's claim, however, was contested because he did not publish the bulk of his research work in the standard peer-reviewed journals. Ironically, nineteen years later the story of Mukerji's test-tube baby was retold by the man most closely associated with India's first "scientifically documented" IVF baby.

It was Dr. Anand Kumar and his collaborators in Bombay who produced the baby girl Harsha. Anand Kumar (1977, p. 526) himself admits, "Harsha was described as India's first 'scientifically documented' test-tube baby because the details of Mukerji's work were not then available."

Delivering the Subhas Mukerji Memorial Oration at the third National Congress on Assisted Reproductive Technology and Advances in Infertility Management held in Calcutta on February 8, 1997, Anand Kumar made an appeal to posthumously credit Mukerji for creating India's first test-tube baby. On April 10, 1997, he followed this appeal with the publication of an article in the journal *Current Science* titled, "Architect of India's First Test Tube Baby: Dr. Subhas Mukerji (January 16, 1931 to July 19, 1981)." The story of Mukerji's long-forgotten past was resurrected with the publication of this article, and Anand Kumar presented a forceful argument to support the claim—which he personally came to believe—that Mukerji did produce a test-tube baby in 1978.

Mukerji had been a medical graduate of Calcutta University, where he also obtained a D.Phil. degree. He was awarded the Colombo Plan scholarship to work in the MRC Clinical Endocrinology Research Unit in Edinburgh under John A. Loraine, a reproductive physiologist. In his *Current Science* article, Anand Kumar offers exhaustive documentation of Mukerji's presentations at various scientific and public forums, along with a detailed description of his research interests and an analysis of the IVF technique that he employed to produce a baby girl who was given a pseudonym, Durga. Anand Kumar undertakes this systematic exercise to demonstrate that even in the absence of published scientific papers in leading journals, Mukerji's work was truly monumental and pathbreaking. According to Anand Kumar (1997, p. 529), Mukerji was "far ahead of his time in successfully using an ovarian stimulation protocol before anyone else in the world had thought of doing so." Similarly, he adds (p. 530),

> It may be noted that Subhas Mukerji reported the successful cryopreservation of an 8-cell embryo, storing it for 53 days, thawing and replacing it into the mother's womb, resulting in a successful and live birth as early as 1978—a full 5 years before anyone else had done so. This small publication of Mukerji in 1978 clearly shows that Mukerji was on the right line of thinking much before anyone else had demonstrated the successful outcome of a pregnancy following the transfer of an 8-cell frozen-thawed embryo into human subjects transferring 8-cell cryopreserved embryos.

Mukerji's happiness, however, was short lived. The government of West Bengal appointed an "expert committee" under the Indian Medical Association and the Bengal Obstetrics and Gynecology Association to investigate the veracity of Mukerji's claims. The inquiry committee met on November 18, 1978, to critically review the report given by Mukerji to the director of health services (DHS), West Bengal Government, and they ultimately rejected Mukerji's claim. Anand Kumar questions this outcome, as the committee was headed by a professor of radiophysics and composed of a gynecologist, a physiologist, and a neurophysiologist. None of these committee members, he argues, "could have had any background or insight into modern Reproductive Technologies, a subject upon which they were to hold an inquiry" (Anand Kumar, 1997, p. 528).

Mukerji had tried to explain his position in a letter to the DHS dated December 1, 1978. He stated that he needed adequate time to prepare the report on his work. Because the report was put together hurriedly in about two weeks' time before the committee's judgment, Mukerji felt he was not able to plead his case in sufficient detail. Anand Kumar (1997, p. 528), however, claims:

> With very sound reasoning, he did not reveal all his data because he wanted to "publish these in recognized scientific journals after the reproducibility of the work is reasonably assured." He went on to state: "The final concentration of DMSO used before freezing as well as the exact indigenous method of cooling were deliberately omitted from the report, like (also) the steps for removal of DMSO before thawing. Certain essential intermediate steps, during the whole procedures also involving the use of undisclosed and enriched media[,] were completely omitted. I had to be careful to guard our unpublished data, because by that time I became aware of the penetrating efficiency of the tentacles of the mass media."

Mukerji had to pay dearly for withholding this crucial information. Not only was his claim rejected by the committee, but the DHS imposed strict restrictions, including preventing him from attending conferences without first obtaining permission. Anand Kumar (1997, pp. 530–531) provides a copious account of events leading up to Mukerji's physical, mental, and emotional deterioration:

> Mukerji was invited by the Primate Research Center of the Kyoto University, Japan, on 25 January 1979 to attend a closed meeting at their expense to discuss details of Mukerji's work. Mukerji applied to the DHS for permission, which was promptly denied via their letter of 16 February 1979. The letter directed Mukerji not to leave the country without prior clearance from the Government. Subhas Mukerji shortly afterwards suffered a heart attack. His request for special leave was declined but his request for transfer was promptly accepted and, at "pleasure of the Governor of West Bengal" he was transferred to the Regional Institute of Ophthalmology as Professor of electrophysiology

on 5 June 1981. The Government, preventing him from presenting his work at scientific meetings, denying him leave to write up his results, and humiliation he was subjected to by his colleagues in Calcutta were some of the things that the sensitive Subhas Mukerji could not bear. His transfer to a department in which he had no expertise was the last straw on the proverbial camel's back for Mukerji. This transfer order was dated 5 June 1981. Mukerji gave up fighting the system and ended his life on 19 July 1981, 44 days after the transfer order was issued. Much of Mukerji's work remained unpublished not because he did not have data but because he was not given a chance to do so by his administrative Ministry in the Government.[6]

The impact of Anand Kumar's appeal extended beyond the medical community. A Calcutta English daily, the *Telegraph,* carried the following report on February 21, 1997:

India's medical establishment is under pressure to recognize the doctor's work 16 years after he committed suicide, following a leading scientist's assertion on this count. Dr. T. C. Anand Kumar, an authority on human infertility management and assisted reproductive technology, has rekindled the debate on India's first test tube baby by crediting Dr. Mukherjee *[sic]* with engineering it.

The same article reported that Mukerji's wife, Namita Mukerji, was living in "a twilight of physical pain and bitter-sweet memories and believed that all the moves to recognize her husband's work posthumously would not 'bring him back.' " She, on the contrary, hoped for an establishment that would create an environment where a scientist would not driven to death if his genius was not evaluated correctly. This sentiment notwithstanding, Anand Kumar's assertions at the Calcutta conference were published in major national dailies, and the regional press included such remarks as "Let me tell you that Subhash Mukerji must be given credit for producing the first test tube baby"and "All other achievements dwarf in comparison to what he achieved."

The focus simultaneously shifted to Mukerji's miracle baby, Durga, whose identity and that of her parents was kept under wraps for eighteen years. Headlines such as "Test Tube Baby's Parents Reveal All, Resurrect Scorned Scientist" ([Calcutta] *Telegraph,* 1997), and "Test Tube Baby, Now 18, Is Ready to Talk" ([New Delhi] *Hindustan Times,* 1997) added to the drama unfolding in Calcutta. Some media accounts unanimously identified Mukerji's biggest shortcoming as his inability to produce the baby as evidence to consolidate his claim; he either did not understand then, as we now do, or resisted the notion that babies legitimate the use of new conceptive technologies in very powerful ways (Stanworth, 1987). Moreover, parents of the Calcutta baby, fearing social ostracism, did not allow Mukerji to go public with the details in 1978. Anand Kumar himself spoke of the Indian psyche that considers barrenness a curse. According to the media,

After hearing the lecture, Durga's parents met him [Anand Kumar] to explain why they did not want Durga's identity revealed at that time when IVF was a novel procedure and how they felt differently now. According to Anand Kumar, Durga[,] who is a "delightful young lady of 18, well educated and articulate," did not have an objection to revealing facts of her birth "if it helped advancement of knowledge." But she did not want the press to intrude on her or her parents' privacy. (*Hindustan Times,* February 19, 1997)

Basically, four things were against Mukerji at the time. First, he did not have a baby to show to the world because of patient confidentiality. Second, he did not have a sufficient number of publications to support his claims. Third, the all-important peer review was absent. Fourth, bureaucratic hostility made it impossible for Mukerji to present his work to the world at large.

Twenty years later, Mukerji is news in India because of the efforts of Anand Kumar. What is particularly interesting is the evangelical zeal with which Anand Kumar took on the campaign to clear Mukerji's name. The situation is complicated by the fact that Anand Kumar stands to lose his claim of being associated with the first scientifically documented test-tube baby, Harsha. Recognizing Mukerji as the scientific father of the very first Indian test-tube baby and the second test-tube baby in the world would require a degree of peer recognition and scientific validation from the Indian scientific community that would mark a fundamental shift in the definition of the first "scientifically documented test-tube baby in India." That is to say, the present claim to the first test-tube baby will have to be abandoned in favor of the earlier claim of Mukerji, and Harsha will have to be replaced by Durga. This construction of the first baby born from a test tube is at the heart of the contested terrain that assisted conception has now become in India. The contests are being fought to salvage and restructure scientific reputations in a thinly disguised rhetoric of scientific and peer documentation. I attempt to problematize these strategies and clashes of ambition in the next section.

BIRTH OF A CONTEST

The genesis of the ascription of "proper credit" for producing the first test-tube baby may be traced back to the birth of Harsha, when the actual credit allocation, following the media aftermath of the breakthrough, completely disrupted the credibility of the scientific team responsible for the feat. What emerged was a fundamental distinction between the multisited nature of both credibility production and credibility allocation. That is, there was a divergence between credit and credibility as they emerged from peers versus their emergence in the media.

Baby Harsha was the product of a collaboration between an institute controlled by the Indian Council for Medical Research and a Bombay public hospital. The scientific team was popularly believed to be headed by the collaborating pair of Anand Kumar, the medical director of the Institute for Research in Reproduction, and Indira Hinduja, a gynecologist from the King Edward Memorial (KEM) Hospital. The rest of the team comprised both senior and junior scientists. With the publication of the IVF project results in 1985–1986, India's first test-tube baby became a peer-reviewed reality. Although the information first appeared in the ICMR annual report and did not offer the exact scientific details, it opened the way for scientific engagement and peer review. The publication (ICMR, 1986, pp. 73–74) cited the contributing team members before more detailed data on the technique and other accomplishments were revealed.

Title of Project	11.8. In vitro Transfer: A collaborative project between the KEM Hospital and the Institute for Research in Reproduction
Project leader	Dr. T. C. Anand Kumar
Project staff	Dr. J. V. Iyer, Dr. G. M. Ranga
Project collaborators	Dr. I. Hinduja, KEM Hospital
	Dr. C. P. Puri, IRR
	Dr. T. D. Nandedkar, IRR
	Dr. K. Gopalkrishnan, IRR
	Dr. R. Asok Kumar, IRR
Start date	August 1985
Approximate duration	Five Years
Provisional date of completion	1990

The article goes on to state, "[The] In Vitro Fertilization and Embryo transfer technique has been perfected and performed as a collaborative project between the KEM Hospital and the IRR. This has resulted in the birth of the country's first ever, scientifically documented, test tube baby" (ICMR, 1986, p. 74).

The project leader and project collaborators were very clearly defined in the article. Dr. Hinduja was but one among five collaborators under the project leader, Dr. Anand Kumar. The inclusion of the KEM Hospital as a collaborating partner recognized Hinduja's links with the hospital. Together, they (IRR and KEM) made India's first scientifically documented test-tube baby.

India learned of this breakthrough on national television's "Doordar-shan" evening news.[7] On the evening of August 6, 1986, the program carried the following report:

> The first test-tube baby in India was born to Mrs. Mani Chawda a twenty-four-year-old housewife at the KEM Hospital, Bombay. Our Bombay correspondent reports: "A pretty and healthy baby girl weighing 2.8 kg has become India's first scientifically documented test-tube baby. She was born to Mani Shanti Chawda at KEM Hospital this afternoon at the hands of Dr. Indira Hinduja. The baby was delivered by cesarean section. This tiny bundle is India's first successful case of conception using the in vitro fertilization technique where the sperm and ovum are fertilized outside the mother's womb and fetus transferred inside her for development. Dr. Hinduja successfully used the technique in close cooperation with Dr. Anand Kumar and his Institute for Research in Reproduction in Bombay. We spoke to Dr. Hinduja and the child's father, Shanti Kumar."

The first media account shifted the balance of credit allocation in favor of Indira Hinduja. Throughout the news report, Hinduja was shown with the baby and the hospital staff, and even as she was interviewed on camera, the project leader, Anand Kumar, was seen standing quietly next to her. In subsequent coverage, the reporter found it more newsworthy to interview the father of the baby and not the project leader, whose name was mentioned in passing as a close collaborator. Thus, in the evening news, Hinduja practically walked away as the project leader who produced India's first scientifically documented test-tube baby. In a matter of hours, she was transformed from one of the five project collaborators into the person who delivered India's first test-tube baby, and Anand Kumar fell from the position of project leader to that of close collaborator.

The media frenzy that followed the announcement of August 6, 1986, further developed the account in the evening bulletin announced on "Doordarshan." All leading dailies were splashed with pictures of and news items on Hinduja, the newborn wonder Harsha, and her parents. Anand Kumar and rest of the scientific team were lost to the public gaze in this media melee. Media interest did not abate with time. With the dawn of the 1990s, the field of assisted conception was fully entrenched in the popular media. Coverage on infertility and on scientific advancements in its management had become louder and more shrill. The uproar over and interest in assisted conception that was generated in the media was accentuated by the entrance of newer players in the field. Hinduja herself, however, had become a cult figure as far as IVF was concerned. No media account could begin without paying tribute to the groundbreaking achievement of the lady doctor "who did it first." Some examples are as follows: "Dr. Indira Hinduja of Bombay is the only doctor in India doing microfertilization.

She has a number of other medical firsts to her credit: the first test tube baby in India, the first GIFT [gamete intrafallopian transfer] baby, the first IVF baby from donor sperm" (*The Week*, December 13, 1992); "[Dr. Indira Hinduja is] the woman who headed the team responsible for the birth of Harsha Chawda, India's first officially recognized test tube baby" (*Sunday Times of India*, February 6, 1994); "Dr. Indira Hinduja . . . was responsible for the birth of Harsha Chawda, India's first test tube baby, in 1986" (*Sunday Times of India Review*, January 7, 1996).

Hinduja's superstardom is not confined to the print media alone. She has continued to make appearances since 1986 on television talk shows and continues to be interviewed by reporters. Even a long-running television series on parenting has featured her in episodes concerning infertility. In one such episode, the Chadwa couple was interviewed:

> Q: The Chawda couple has a special place for Dr. Hinduja in their heart.
>
> Mani Chadwa (Mother): I was never . . . I was not meant to have a child . . . but madam did the test tube and gave me a baby. We consider Indira Hinduja God. She is our God. Madam made it possible, everything she did, I feel she [Harsha] is her daughter.

In another episode Hinduja was extolled as follows: "After all, what is a test tube baby? Let us meet the person responsible for the sensational news; the world's second and India's first test-tube baby's creator, Dr. Indira Hinduja!" With dramatic, high-pitched voice-over, the "goddess" of artificial conception was unveiled to the audience. This small introduction offers insight into the limits crossed by popular representations in their pursuit for glorification. Such coverage is an abject misrepresentation of "documented" facts—as Hinduja's name literally comes to replace Mukerji's. Yet, curiously, there is a certain consonance with Mukerji's claim of producing the world's second test-tube baby and India's first. In the 1980s, in one of her earlier television appearances, Hinduja was asked directly and at the start of an interview about Mukerji's claim:

> Q: Is this India's first test-tube baby, or have there been such cases in the past?
>
> Hinduja: First of all I would like to say that this procedure was a product of collaboration between [the] Institute for Research in Reproduction, which is ICMR's branch, and the other one KEM, Bombay. These two institutes together researched and established this. Your second question was whether this is the first baby. I would like to say that [on] 6th August 1986 the child that was born was scientifically documented, [the] first IVF baby in India.
>
> Q: It was heard that in Calcutta a similar baby was born. That was not documented . . . it was not scientifically documented?
>
> Hinduja: Yes, I would only say this, that this procedure was not repeated and no other child was born because of this procedure.

Hinduja took the line of least resistance in answering these questions. That the 1986 baby was a product of collaboration between two institutes provided the credibility Mukerji lacked in an obvious sense. Besides, viability of any IVF project could only be measured by how successful subsequent applications were. Once again, on that count, Mukerji was silent, and Hinduja was able to produce a number of ongoing pregnancies and live births. What is interesting, however, is that this line of questioning and answering disappeared in subsequent media accounts. The phrase "collaboration between two institutes" is absent from most accounts that emerged in the print and electronic media. Hinduja became virtually synonymous with India's first test-tube baby. Mukerji, on the other hand, was to remain completely invisible until the beginning of 1997, when for the first time since 1978 the media reported the details of his past—details made available to them by Anand Kumar.

CONTESTING CLAIMS

On November 4, 1990, in an English-language magazine, *The Week,* an article appeared titled "An Ill-Conceived Move: Research Rivalry Leads to Winding Up of Test Tube Baby Project." The article blamed the ICMR for closing the project at the IRR in Bombay. It began by asserting dramatically that the IRR is barely a "test tube's throw away" from the King Edward Memorial Hospital of Bombay and yet a "yawning gulf" has suddenly emerged between the two whose joint effort saw the birth of India's first test-tube baby (Rao, 1990, p. 14). The article went on to quote the director of ICMR:

> Dr. A. S. Paintal, director of the Indian Council of Medical Research (ICMR) under whose wings IRR has been hiding cosily all these years, had this belated explanation: "The major reason for winding up the IVF (in vitro fertilization) unit is that Dr. Indira Hinduja's (she was the brain behind India's first test tube baby) project has already proved its success. And we thought she could continue her studies outside whereas the IRR's funds could be utilised for other important projects." (Rao, 1990, p. 14)

There are two very interesting points in the above extract. First, as early as 1990 it was firmly established—even in official (ICMR) circles—that the test-tube baby was Hindujas's project. It is surprising that the director above describes the project, funded by a government council (ICMR) and executed by its own institute (IRR) in collaboration with a public hospital (KEM), as Dr. Hinduja's project. It tells us something interesting about the inroads media and popular representations of India's first scientifically documented test-tube baby had made in the official vocabulary. It can alternatively be referred to as the "synonymous effect"—a product of media elocution that made Hinduja's name synonymous with the first test-tube baby project. Second, the passage exposes the enunciatory function of the media. The all-important parenthetical remark, inserted into the objective quote of the interviewee, is for the less informed reader who might have missed all the crucial details of the central role played by Hinduja. The article goes on to show how the slashing of ICMR's budget of Rs 34 crore by 20 percent is used as the reason for terminating the project and further asserts that the Rs 10 crore "gobbled up by IVF is inflated perhaps to justify its killing" (Rao, 1990, p. 14). Citing modest expenses on the project (from the IRR annual report), the article argues that the test-tube baby research project was never a "white elephant" for the IRR. The problem is attributed to conflict of interest inside IRR:

> Another vital aspect is professional jealousy: the impression that Hinduja, who is on the rolls of the KEM Hospital, has been hogging the limelight and depriving the IRR scientists, who have been handling the lab side of the IVF project, [of] their share of the glory. Ironically, there was perfect harmony within the IVF unit, but the so-called experts within the IRR who have nothing to do with the IVF project have been fomenting trouble. This led to increasing non-cooperation, raising of hurdles, deprival of facilities and at times open antagonism, which steeply brought down the tally of IVF babies. (Rao, 1990, p. 14)

The article makes a strong case for perfect harmony within the IVF team. However, when I contacted some of the team members, they gave very different accounts—on the condition of strict anonymity. One team member, for instance, when first contacted on April 13, 1998, spoke of the "arrogant" and "uncompromising" attitude of the gynecologists that led to the collapse of the project. The informant went on to say that "the publicity-hungry individuals associated with the project created an atmosphere of dejection and frustration" among the real scientific "think tank" behind the project. Those involved were pulling in different directions. Whereas some were more interested in "promoting themselves," others became too "disgruntled" because their "behind-the-scenes hard work was not being appreciated" and they were being "systematically sidetracked," as the bulk of the limelight remained on only a chosen few.

I contacted this respondent again on April 21, 1998, and requested elaboration on the earlier interview. The respondent now talked of moves to "stifle people who wanted to be heard." The example given was of a research officer who was transferred without reason because she wanted to be included; she was replaced by someone who would not question the authority of the top project management. The respondent added that "no data" came "from the top"; all the hard work was being done in the lab, and the data were simply "passed on" to the principals. The informant continued:

Nobody was trained; neither there was any second in line to take up from where the top people involved in the project left off. Repeated pleas were ignored, and people did not even have access to biological material to research with. They decided who got what, and when the whole thing got over the entire IVF lab was dismantled and equipment was distributed within the institute to different departments on a piecemeal basis.

These two interviews were not tape recorded as the respondent was extremely anxious about talking on record. However, the notes taken throughout the course of the interview and afterward revealed a deep sense of disappointment and anger in someone who was associated with the scientific team that was purportedly "in perfect harmony."

I had some success in interviewing another individual who, once again, asked to remain anonymous but gave a brief tape-recorded interview that revealed some interesting grudges and resentments about the way things were handled.

You see, if at that time we had also trained up some people to take over, like when a person goes away that would have been much better . . . that couldn't happen . . . but that was very sad the way she was given publicity, which is wrong, why the council and the government and the . . . was not questioning our director? Why should she get so much publicity? All the facilities, everything at the cost of the other research, all the money was diverted to this IVF program, and then my God! the credit should have been given equally to the institute. That is why our current director more or less goes on emphasizing that—he goes on projecting our institute at the ministry that it was our institute, our funds, our this, our effort and that has brought about this [the IVF baby].

Q: Who was the director when this was happening?

A: Anand Kumar . . . he was there, I don't know, he got carried away by the lady. We have a scientific advisory committee who usually assesses our projects and gives advice, healthy criticism. There it was also questioned that you have okay . . . you've developed a technology, you are enforcing it, you are doing it but the technology is going—it is not going for further research. Who are the next in line or would you conduct a workshop so that other people are trained, so that if one person goes, the technology carries forward. But he just gave some vague reason.

The tendency to eclipse the other emerges as the basis on which the ensuing contest for credibility seems to be constructed. On the one hand, the scientific team claims that it was kept at arm's length from credit (reward) and that because they were marginalized, their credibility (ability to do science) could not attain its potential. On the other hand, the principals, Anand Kumar and Hinduja, appear to pursue an approach of mutual obfuscation. There have been few documented media accounts in which there is an open reference to the other as collaborating partner. The earliest accounts, such as the evening news of August 6, 1986, have passing references to both individuals as collaborators. But the closest one protagonist comes to acknowledging the other in interviews and in other accounts on the issue of the first test-tube baby is to name the collaborating institutes. The two institutes have been bestowed with a metonymic quality as they almost step in to contain the two collaborators. Anand Kumar (1997, p. 526), for instance, made the following assertion in his article on Mukerji:

> The organisers of the recent Calcutta meeting believed that I was preeminently qualified and experienced to delve into whatever material was available regarding Mukerji's past work and throw light on it. The reason for this assumption perhaps lay in my having played a key role in the birth of another test tube baby, Harsha[,] on 6 August 1986. This birth was announced by myself, when I was the director of the ICMR's Institute for Research in Reproduction and Dr. G. B. Parulekar, Dean of our collaborating institution, King Edward Memorial (KEM) Hospital, Bombay. . . . I published our technical report and procedural details in the ICMR Bulletin. The work leading to Harsha's birth was executed by a team of scientists from the IRR and clinicians from the KEM Hospital working under my direct guidance and supervision.

The argument is blunt on three counts. First, Hinduja's name, synomymous in the media with the birth of the first test-tube baby, is completely eliminated. Her "claims" are openly resisted by reminding the readers of the contents of the report published in the ICMR Bulletin (ICMR, 1986). The primacy of peer-reviewed documentation over popular media accounts is openly asserted. It is also noteworthy that Hinduja is conspicuous by her absence while there is a reference to the KEM Hospital and to the dean of the collaborating institute rather than the more popular collaborator. Second, the distinction between IRR and KEM is constructed on a clear-cut scientific hierarchy of scientists over clinicians. A sense of "our" (IRR) scientists and "their" (KEM) clinicians is asserted to reclaim the "reality" that was glossed over by media representations, such as "Dr. Hinduja, the brain behind the project." Third, and most significantly, the emphasis on terms such as "key role" and "my direct guidance and supervision" completely undermines the importance and even the extent of the contribution of the collaborating hospital and its now-famous collaborating partner, Dr. Indira Hinduja.

For her part, Hinduja has pursued a similar but subtler line of asserting the primacy of her contribution to the breakthrough that led to the birth of Harsha. In a television interview ("Doordarshan" documentary, 1986), for instance, she was asked where she had learned the technique, as it is not taught in India. Hinduja responded:

I did not go abroad to learn the technique, I learned from my own experience. First I started with animal experiments, in humans, people who used to come for sterilization—we tried to study their eggs . . . tried to study fertilization, and when it was found that something is happening, then we started enrolling infertile couples.

Clearly, Hinduja is not "a mere clinician," as Anand Kumar has implied, and this is supported by the fact that she has a successful practice of her own. However, there is consistency in these accounts in not acknowledging anyone beyond the self. Hinduja "did it on her own," Anand Kumar "got it done under his direct guidance and supervision," and the disgruntled team of scientists "couldn't do anything" as they felt completely side-tracked. In short, there is a complete breakdown of credibility ascription to the "other."

CONCLUSION

The analysis in this chapter firmly establishes the multisited nature of credibility production. The credibility generated by the media accounts carries with it the potential to obfuscate peer-reviewed and endorsed credibility. The peer-documented credit shared by Hinduja and Anand Kumar is different from the credit generated by the media accounts, which focused on Hinduja alone.

Credibility, or a scientist's ability to do science, it is therefore argued, is only a point of departure. Its continual upkeep and regeneration, through a quest for credible reward and recognition, is the mainstay of scientific enterprise when it acquires a commercial face. This helps us to understand how scientists have responded to demands from outside the scientific terrain. There, the market (infertility patients) judges the credibility of an expert not from what his or her peers have to say—though that is centrally important to the scientists' survival in the field—but in terms of what is said in the media representation of the experts.

By raising Mukerji's claim, Anand Kumar stands to lose his own claim to be associated with the birth of India's first test-tube baby. However, in light of the foregoing analysis, it can be hypothesized that Anand Kumar stands to lose nothing at all, as his credibility—which is well documented as far as peer citations go—is intact. The professional credit of being associated with the first test-tube baby is more or less secure—as long as he does not prove Mukerji's claim. What he lacks, however, is credit of a different kind that no amount of peer citations can generate. This credit or reward is what his partner, Hinduja, walked away with under the media spotlight (and she also is recognized as an able scientist by her peers). Official recognition of Mukerji would deny Hinduja what was denied to the rest of the collaborating team all along. Should that happen, the media's attention might shift to the man (Anand Kumar) who dismantled one claim (Hinduja's) and replaced it with another more substantial claim (Mukerji's).

Whether this hypothesis will stand the test of time cannot be known with certainty. What emerges with clarity, however, is the fact that attempts are being made to deconstruct the credibility painstakingly constructed in the media and to substitute newer claims to credit and credibility. At the end of the day, scientific credibility and peer recognition are available in plenty to the protagonists of this story. What is lacking, however, is credibility of a different kind—one that only the loving eye of the camera and the affectionate outpouring of the journalist's pen can bestow.

NOTES

1. Stanworth (1987) has quite rightly argued that the use of the "curious term test-tube babies" conjures an odd image of a fetus growing independently of the body of a woman—a miracle of science rather than nature. Even though the term denies women agency, it is used in this chapter, first, as it has come to be normalized in both scientific and nonscientific (media) discourses on infertility in India and, second, to allow continuity between the narratives used in this chapter and their subsequent analysis. Another important implication of the term "test-tube baby" is that it makes the ownership of the expert primary and that of women and couples secondary. The political struggle over the ownership of the first test-tube baby amply demonstrates how babies technologically created are viewed as scientific trophies rather than as mere scientific resolution of infertility.

2. The terms "credit" and "credibility" are used here as developed by Latour and Woolgar (1979) in *Laboratory Life*. Latour and Woolgar make a fundamental distinction, at least analytically, between credit as reward and credit as credibility. They reserve credit as reward for those instances in which there is a sharing of rewards and awards that is also symbolic of peer recognition of a previous scientific achievement. Credit as credibility, they argue, should be taken to mean scientists' actual ability to do science. Interestingly, they give primacy to the notion of credibility as encompassing scientists' ability to do science, investment strategies, the scientific reward system and scientific education, and so on. At the same time, they assert that both credit (reward) and credibility originate essentially from peers' comments about other scientists.

3. The term "multimedia/media" is loosely used to stand for both print (mainly English national dailies and popular magazines) and electronic (mainly television). In places, I use the term "media" to suggest print media only, and "multimedia" alludes to the "total" presence of the media network in India.

4. More on this in the next sections.

5. With the reduction in import duties on high-tech medical equipment, several gynecologists could upgrade their practice and move into "super specialty" areas such as assisted conception. More important, by recognizing medical care as an industry (Baru, 1998), the state made it possible for doctors and private nursing

332   GLOBALIZING TECHNOLOGIES

homes to take loans from banks and other financial institutions. Not surprisingly, therefore, many doctors running IVF clinics in India are backed by bank loans to help pay for their expansion plans.

6. Anand Kumar is not the first to report the events leading up to Mukerji's suicide. Corea (1985) has described in great detail how Steptoe and Edwards's success led to a scramble among gynecologists and physiologists across the world. Drawing on Mukerji's interview given to the CBS reporter Jay McMullen and on the *Sydney Morning Herald* reporter Rajan Gupta's report on Mukerji's suicide, Corea gives an account of Mukerji's claim and eventual suicide on page 139, note 22.

7. Television news bulletins and other programs used in this chapter for the purpose of elaborating the argument could not be cited as either the exact date of telecast or the channel on which they were broadcast could not be ascertained. The accounts were obtained during fieldwork from one of the informant doctors, who had copies of the various television programs telecast since 1986—on the subject of infertility and test-tube babies in India—on a personal videotape.

REFERENCES

Anand Kumar, T. C. (1997). Architect of India's first test tube baby: Dr Subhas Mukerji (16 January 1931 to 19 July 1981). *Current Science, 72,* 526–531.

Baru, R. V. (1998). *Private health care in India: Social characteristics and trends.* New Delhi: Sage.

Bharadwaj, A. (1999). Barren wives and sterile husbands: Infertility and assisted conception in India. Paper read at the conference, Gender, health and healing: Reflections on the public and private divide, April 23–24, Warwick, U.K.

Bharadwaj, A. (2000). How some Indian baby makers are made: Media narratives and assisted conception in India. *Anthropology and Medicine, 7,* 63–78.

Corea, G. (1985). *The mother machine: Reproductive technologies from artificial insemination to artificial wombs.* London: Women's Press.

Hindustan Times. (1997). Test-tube baby, now 18, is ready to talk. February 19, New Delhi.

ICMR (Indian Council for Medical Research) (1986). *In vitro fertilization & embryo transfer: A collaborative project between the KEM Hospital and the Institute for Research in Reproduction.* Annual report.

Inhorn, M. C. (1994). Interpreting infertility: Medical anthropological perspectives. *Social Science & Medicine, 39,* 459–461.

Jeffery, R. (1988). *The politics of health in India.* Berkeley: University of California Press.

Latour, B., & Woolgar, S. (1986). *Laboratory life: The social construction of scientific facts.* 2d ed. Princeton, NJ: Princeton University Press.

Lingam, L. 1990. New reproductive technologies in India: A print media analysis. *Issues in Reproductive and Genetic Engineering, 3,* 13–21.

Mukherjee, M. (1997). Test-tube baby's parents reveal all, resurrect scorned scientist. Amends won't bring him back, rues doctor's widow. *Telegraph,* February 21, Calcutta.

Rao, C. (1990). An ill-conceived move: Research rivalry leads to winding up of test-tube baby project. *The Week*, November 4, pp. 14–15.

Stanworth, M. (1987). Reproductive technologies and the deconstruction of motherhood. In M. Stanworth (Ed.), *Reproductive technologies: Gender, motherhood and medicine* (pp. 10–35). Cambridge: Polity Press.

The Sunday Times of India. (1994). A storm in a test tube. February 6, Bombay.

The Sunday Times of India Review. (1996). The baby-shopping boom. January 7, New Delhi.

The Week. (1992). How some Indian babies are made. December 13, pp. 30–35.

Venkatratnam, R. (1973). *Medical sociology in an Indian setting.* New Delhi: Macmillan.

Venkatratnam, R. (1987). Health system and the polity: A note on Indian scene. In S. K. Lal & A. Chandani (Eds.), *Medical care: Readings in medical sociology* (pp. 16–27). New Delhi: Jainsons Publications.

CONTRIBUTORS

Gay Becker is Professor in Residence, Social and Behavioral Sciences and Medical Anthropology, at the University of California, San Francisco. She has been studying infertility and reproductive technologies for more than twenty years, a project that grew out of her own experience with infertility. Her work includes a general study of people's experiences with infertility, which has resulted in the publication of three University of California Press books: *Healing the Infertile Family: Strengthening Your Relationship in the Search for Parenthood, Disrupted Lives: How People Create Meaning in a Chaotic World,* and *The Elusive Embryo: How Women and Men Approach New Reproductive Technologies.* She is also the author, with Robert Nachtigall, of several articles on donor insemination. For four years, she served as editor of the Society for Medical Anthropology's journal, *Medical Anthropology Quarterly.*

Aditya Bharadwaj is Research Fellow at Cardiff University, Wales, having recently completed his doctorate in the Department of Sociology at the University of Bristol. His dissertation, "Conceptions," examines infertility and the increasing use of new reproductive technologies in India. In the past, he has studied the medical management of childbirth, maternal nutrition, and immunization in India. His research on infertility is an outgrowth of his overall research interests in reproductive health care issues, qualitative research methods, and the anthropological study of India. His current research is in the area of new genetics and population screening for susceptibility to genetic diseases in the United Kingdom.

Sheryl de Lacey is Senior Lecturer in the School of Nursing and Midwifery at Flinders University in South Australia and an affiliate with Reproductive Medicine Services offered by the University of Adelaide. She has contributed to the development of practice and policy in the field of infertility and assisted reproduction through membership in several national ethics committees and policy-making councils over the past fifteen years. Her work includes reviews of how information for children should be regulated, surrogacy, counseling and issues of access in assisted reproduction, and the long-term health effects of assisted reproduction. Her research includes study of the experience of egg donors and a discourse analysis of infertility and in vitro fertilization failure.

Pamela Feldman-Savelsberg is Associate Professor in the Department of Sociology and Anthropology, Carleton College. She has conducted research on women's reproductive health care in Cameroon since the early 1980s. Her work focuses on the social conditions that give rise to fear of infertility. Extensive field research in a rural Bamiléké chiefdom as well as research in European archives has resulted in numerous publications, including *Plundered Kitchens, Empty Wombs: Threatened Reproduction and Identity in the Cameroon Grassfields* (University of Michigan Press, 1999). Current research on urban Bamiléké women's ethnic associations, social networks, and reproductive strategies is supported by an Andrew W. Mellon Fellowship in Anthropological Demography and by the National Science Foundation.

Trudie Gerrits is a medical anthropologist and health educator, working as a researcher and lecturer in the Medical Anthropology Unit of the University of Amsterdam. She is project assistant for the Gender, Reproductive Health and Population Policies Project, an international action research project that aims at generating innovative knowledge about women's and men's needs regarding reproductive health services. From 1985 to 1990 she worked at the Ministry of Health in Mozambique, and in 1993 she conducted a study on social and cultural aspects of infertility in Mozambique, about which she has published a number of articles. She was an initiator and organizer (with Frank van Balen) of an international conference, Interpreting Infertility: Social Science Research on Childlessness in a Global Perspective, held in Amsterdam in November 1999. She has six-year-old IVF twins, Carmen and Jaap.

Arthur L. Greil is Professor of Sociology and Health Policy at Alfred University, Alfred, New York, where he has taught since 1977. His main research interests are in the areas of reproductive health, adult socialization and identity change, and the sociology of religion. His book, *Not Yet Pregnant: Infertile Couples in Contemporary America* (Rutgers University Press, 1991), deals with themes of gender and the experience of infertility and is based on the qualitative analysis of interviews with both partners of infertile American couples. He has also published a number of other articles on infertility, including a major review of the literature on infertility and psychological distress. He became interested in infertility as a result of his own experiences, and he and his wife have two adopted children, Robby, seventeen, and Maddie, ten.

Lisa Handwerker, a medical anthropologist, is Visiting Scholar in the Institute for the Study of Social Change at the University of California, Berkeley, and an adjunct professor in the Department of Anthropology at California State University, Hayward, and the Community Studies Department at the University of California, Santa Cruz. She has published numerous articles on female infertility and reproductive technologies in China and on feminist biomedical ethics. An activist, she sits on the Board of the National Women's Health Network and is a member of the Berkeley Health Commission. In addition, she is a consultant in health, organizational development, and fund-raising.

Marcia C. Inhorn is Associate Professor in the Department of Health Behavior and Health Education, School of Public Health, International Institute, and the Department of Anthropology at the University of Michigan. A medical anthropologist, her primary research interests are in the areas of gender and health, particularly women's reproductive health. Her major research project examines the plight of infertile women and men in urban Egypt. She has written two books on this subject, *Quest for Conception: Gender, Infertility, and Egyptian Medical Traditions* (1994) and *Infertility and Patriarchy: The Cultural Politics of Gender and Family Life in Egypt* (1996), both published by the University of Pennsylvania Press. *Quest for Conception* won the Society for Medical Anthropology's Eileen Basker Prize for outstanding research in the area of gender and health. Currently, she is completing a book titled *Egyptian Mothers of Test-Tube Babies: Gender, Islam, and the Globalization of New Reproductive Technologies,* which examines the global spread of new reproductive technologies to the developing world. Following the stillbirth of identical twin daughters, she went on to bear two living children, Carl, six, and Justine, three.

Gwynne L. Jenkins is Assistant Professor of Anthropology and Women's Studies at the University of Kansas. Her primary research interests are the politics of international health programs, nationalism and health, lay perceptions of health and health care, and the production of reproductive decision making in the clinical encounter and social life. Her dissertation, "The Bureaucratization of Birth: Midwifery Programs, National Health Care, and Local Birth Conventions in Rural Costa Rica," won a Presidential Distinguished Doctoral Dissertation Award from the University at Albany–State University of New York in 1999. She recently received a grant to study the experience of infertility and decision making in selective reduction among new reproductive technologies in the United States. Her next research project concerns the history of female sterilization policy in Costa Rica and its political use in discourses of modernization and nationalism.

Susan Martha Kahn is Senior Research Director of the Hadassah International Research Institute on Jewish Women at Brandeis University, where she is also Adjunct Assistant Professor in the Departments of Anthropology and Near Eastern and Judaic Studies. She received her M.A. in Middle Eastern studies and her Ph.D. in social anthropology from Harvard University. Her book, *Reproducing Jews: A Cultural Account of Assisted Conception in Israel* (Duke University Press, 2000), won a National Jewish Book Award (2000), and her dissertation, on which the book is based, won the Foundation for Jewish Culture's 1998 Musher Prize, awarded biennially for an outstanding dissertation on Jewish life in Israel or America.

Lori Leonard is Assistant Professor of International Health at the Johns Hopkins School of Public Health. She received M.S. and Sc.D. degrees in health and social behavior and population and international health from Harvard University. She has worked in sub-Saharan Africa for nearly fifteen years, first as a Peace Corps volunteer in Zaire (now the Democratic Republic of the Congo) and Chad and later on public health research and intervention projects in Chad, Mali, and Senegal. Much of her research has been on the Sara of southern Chad; her dissertation was on the meaning and management of infertility among the Sara, and she has written a series of articles on female circumcision among the Sara, including a chapter in the edited volume, *Female "Circumcision" in Africa: Culture, Controversy, and Change* (2000). Her interests include women's and reproductive health, STD and HIV prevention, community health, and qualitative research methods.

Melissa J. Pashigian is currently completing her Ph.D. in anthropology at the University of California, Los Angeles. Her dissertation, "Conceiving the 'Happy Family': Infertility, Gender and Reproductive Experience in Northern Vietnam," analyzes the social construction of infertility and its relationship to the politics of reproduction in Hanoi and its surrounding provinces. Her research interests include gender in socialist and postsocialist societies, the politics of reproduction, and the global proliferation of new reproductive technologies.

Catherine Kohler Riessman is Research Professor in the Department of Sociology, Boston College. She is Professor Emerita at Boston University School of Social Work. Her research and publications in medical sociology focus on women's health, gender and divorce, qualitative methods, and the narrative study of lives. She conducted fieldwork in South India in 1993–1994, supported by the Indo-American Fellowship Program (Fulbright), and has written a series of publications on women, power, and infertility in the South Indian context. Her methodological specialty is narrative. She is the author of *Narrative Analysis* (Sage, 1993) and *Divorce Talk* (Rutgers University Press, 1990) and editor of a collection on qualitative methods in social work. She has applied narrative methods in studies of disruptive life events, including divorce, chronic illness, and infertility. She has three grown children and two grandchildren.

Margarete Sandelowski is Professor in the School of Nursing at the University of North Carolina at Chapel Hill and a Fellow of the American Academy of Nursing. Her research is in the area of technology and gender, especially reproductive technology and technology in nursing. She has published widely in nursing and social science anthologies and journals. One of her books, *With Child in Mind: Studies of the Personal Encounter with Infertility* (University of Pennsylvania Press, 1993), was awarded the 1994 Eileen Basker Memorial Prize for exemplary work in the field of gender and health from the Society for Medical Anthropology of the American Anthropological Association. Her latest book, a social history of technology in nursing, is titled *Devices and Desires: Gender, Technology, and American Nursing* (University of North Carolina Press, 2000).

Johanne Sundby is Associate Professor, Section for Medical Anthropology, Institute of General Practice and Community Medicine, University of Oslo. She is a physician specializing in gynecology and obstetrics, with research training in both epidemiology and medical anthropology. She teaches international health in postgraduate programs and supervises students majoring in reproductive health from Norway and several African countries. Her Ph.D. dissertation in community medicine is titled "Infertility: Causes, Care and Consequences," and she has since written several books on infertility and women's health. She was the leader of the Norwegian government's Commission for Women's Health for two years. She has conducted studies on infertility in both Norway and Africa and is currently involved in a project in Tanzania in collaboration with Ulla Larsen of the Harvard School of Public Health. She is infertile herself and adopted a son born in 1974. To substitute for the lack of more children, she enjoys being a competitive dogsled musher with ten lovely Siberian huskies.

Charis M. Thompson is Assistant Professor in the Department of the History of Science at Harvard University. She works on selective pronatalism in the area of human reproductive technologies and population policy, as well as in ex situ (zoo) and in situ biodiversity conservation.

Frank van Balen is Associate Professor in the Department of Education, Social and Behavioral Sciences Faculty, University of Amsterdam. After working as a student counselor and planner in the Dutch university organization, he received a grant in 1988 to begin research on involuntary childlessness in the Netherlands. Following the 1991 publication of his dissertation, "A Life without Children: Involuntary Childlessness, Experience, Stress, and Adaptation," he conducted several quantitative and qualitative studies on various aspects of involuntary childlessness, including the epidemiology of infertility, treatment-seeking behavior, the development of IVF children, the prospects of new reproductive technologies, and infertility counseling. He was an initiator and organizer (with Trudie Gerrits) of an international conference, Interpreting Infertility: Social Science Research on Childlessness in a Global Perspective, held in Amsterdam in November 1999. He has one IVF daughter, Roosmarijn, seventeen, and another daughter, Veerle, fifteen, who was conceived just a month after a failed IVF attempt.

INDEX

Compositor:	Binghamton Valley Composition, LLC
Text:	10/12 Baskerville
Display:	Baskerville
Printer and binder:	Maple-Vail Manufacturing Group